K·I·S·S

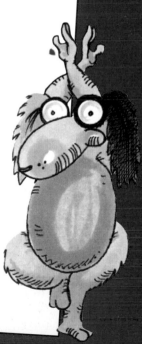

The Only Guides You'll Ever Need!

THIS SERIES IS YOUR TRUSTED GUIDE through all of life's stages and situations. Want to learn how to surf the Internet or care for your new dog? Or maybe you'd like to become a wine connoisseur or an expert gardener? The solution is simple: Just pick up a K.I.S.S. Guide and turn to the first page.

Expert authors will walk you through the subject from start to finish, using simple blocks of knowledge to build your skills one step at a time. Build upon these learning blocks and by the end of the book, you'll be an expert yourself! Or, if you are familiar with the topic but want to learn more, it's easy to dive in and pick up where you left off.

The K.I.S.S. Guides deliver what they promise: Simple access to all the information you'll need on one subject. Other titles you might want to check out include: Weight Loss, Selling, the Internet, Gardening, Pregnancy, Astrology, and many more.

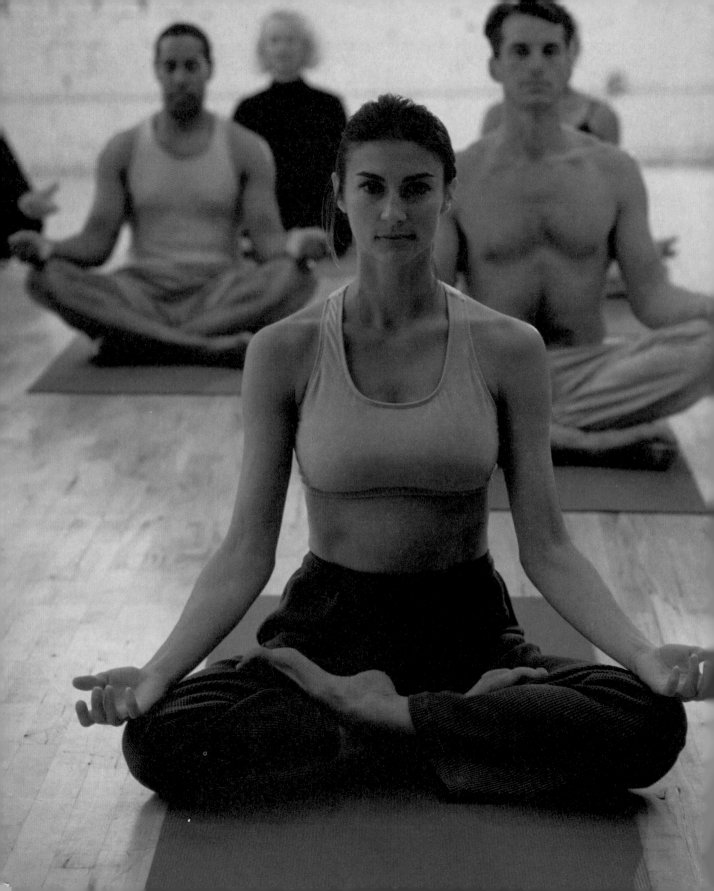

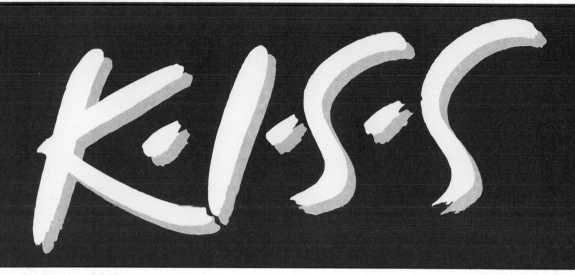

GUIDE TO

Yoga

SHAKTA KAUR KHALSA

Foreword by **Deborah Willoughby**

Editor, *Yoga International* magazine

A Dorling Kindersley Book

LONDON, NEW YORK, SYDNEY, DELHI, PARIS,
MUNICH, AND JOHANNESBURG

DK Publishing, Inc.

Senior Editor Jennifer Williams
Editor Lisa Lenard
Copy Editor Gretchen Fruchey
Category Publisher LaVonne Carlson

Dorling Kindersley Limited

Project Editor Caroline Hunt
Project Art Editor Justin Clow

Managing Editor Maxine Lewis
Managing Art Editor Heather McCarry
Category Publisher Mary Thompson
Production Heather Hughes

Produced for Dorling Kindersley by **Cooling Brown**
9–11 High Street, Hampton, Middlesex TW12 2SA

Creative Director Arthur Brown
Senior Editor Amanda Lebentz
Art Editors Pauline Clarke, Elly King, Hilary Krag, Tish Mills
Editor Helen Ridge

First American Edition, 2001

00 01 02 03 04 05 10 9 8 7 6 5 4 3 2 1

Published in the United States by DK Publishing, Inc.,
95 Madison Avenue, New York, New York 10016

Khalsa, Shakta Kaur, 1950-
    KISS guide to yoga / by Shakta Kaur Khalsa.-- 1st American ed.
        p. cm. -- (Keep it simple series)
    "A Dorling Kindersley Book."
    Includes index.
        ISBN 0-7894-8034-4
        1. Yoga, Hatha.   I. Title. II. Series.
RA781.7 .K484 2001
613.7'046--dc21
                                            2001001483

Color reproduction by ColourScan, Singapore
Printed and bound by Printer Industria Grafica, S.A., Barcelona, Spain

See our complete catalog at
www.dk.com

Contents at a Glance

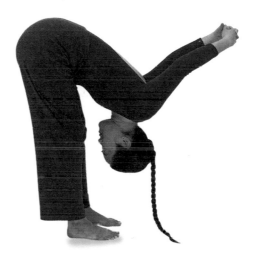

CONTENTS

PART ONE Simplifying Yoga

CHAPTER 1   A Simple Understanding   22

CHAPTER 2   Why Yoga Feels So Good   36

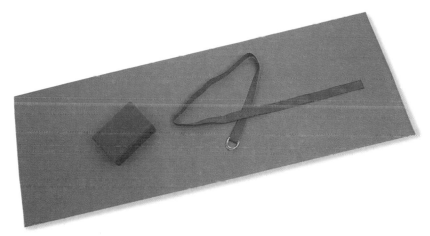

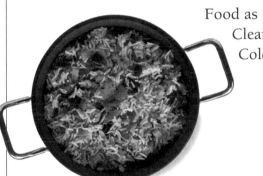

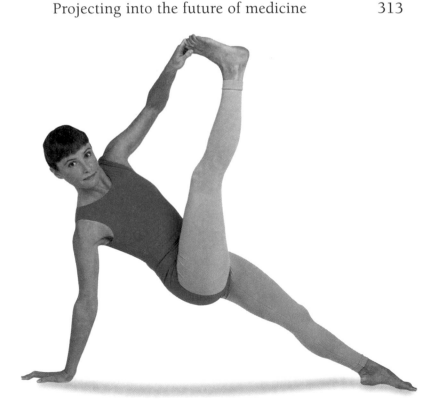

Foreword

THE WORLD IS MOVING TOO FAST *for comfort these days,
leaving most of us feeling harried and a bit stressed. And whether
we admit it or not, there's an undercurrent of disquiet running
through our lives. The practice of yoga offers an antidote. I am
fortunate in that my job as editor of Yoga International magazine
presents me an on-going opportunity to explore yoga's infinite
capacity to calm and center. And that is why I take special
pleasure in introducing this book, which provides you with the
same opportunity.*

*Yoga is an elegant, time-honored system for engendering a
sense of vitality, well-being, and peace. Whatever your age, state
of health, state of mind, or lifestyle, you will find insights and
techniques in these pages that will help you lead a healthier,
more fulfilling, and more joyful life. As its name implies, the
Keep It Simple Series Guide to Yoga is indeed a do-it-yourself
guide to learning about yoga and finding your way, step-by-step,
into a style of practice that works for you. But it is much more
than that, largely because its author, Shakta Kaur Khalsa, is not
only a longtime yoga teacher but also someone who lives her life
by yoga's guiding principles, integrating the body, mind, and spirit
into a unified, peaceful whole.*

*Shakta's gentle, fun-loving spirit permeates this book. Whether
she is guiding the reader one step at a time through a yoga pose,
explaining how to use the breath to get out of a tight spot at the
office, or offering tips on how to trade in unhealthy habits for
healthy ones, Shakta makes the reader feel comfortable and,
more to the point, cared for, every step of the way. The fruitful
pursuit of yoga requires just such a guide, one whose own
immersion in the practice serves as a model. Shakta fills this
challenging role with skill and humor.*

The K.I.S.S. Guide to Yoga is easy to understand and a pleasure to read. Yet it is so comprehensive that it is the only book on yoga you will need for a long time. It not only offers an overview of yoga's seven traditional paths, it also acts as a guide to the major schools of yoga in the West today. You will refer to it again and again, for everything you need is here: How to find the class that's right for you; how to get the most out of your home practice; why and how to include your family in your yoga life; why the yogis believe that the way we eat matters as much as what we eat; how to refresh yourself with relaxation and cleansing practices; why yoga is good for business; and how to meditate and why it is so important.

Paging through this book, I was amazed at both its breadth and depth – I can't think of an aspect of this fascinating topic that isn't covered here. If you have picked it up thinking that yoga is simply a popular system of exercise, you will put it down with the understanding that yoga offers much more than instruction on how to increase your physical strength, grace, and flexibility. What yoga really offers is the opportunity for each of us to rediscover ourselves, to experience who we are at the very core of our beings. All we have to do is find a way to incorporate its wisdom into our daily lives. The K.I.S.S. Guide to Yoga will help you to do just that.

DEBORAH WILLOUGHBY
EDITOR, *YOGA INTERNATIONAL*

Introduction

WELCOME! AND CONGRATULATIONS on *taking an important step to improve the quality of your life, because that's just what you've done by choosing the K.I.S.S. Guide to Yoga. As modern as it is ancient, yoga is one of the most widely practiced forms of exercise in the world. Yoga promises – and delivers – relaxation in place of stress, insight in place of negativity, and courage in the face of conflict.*

If I could name one thing that has made the biggest difference in my life, without a moment's hesitation I would say "yoga." Over the past 30 years, I have taught yoga to hundreds of thousands of men, women, and children, and it is always delightful and super-gratifying to see how effectively yoga benefits each one's life. Yoga changes your life where it counts – from the inside out!

I wrote this book as a simple way for you to touch the essence of yoga – its basic teachings – and to give you ample opportunity to experience a wide array of yoga styles. Knowing that experience is the best teacher, I've included a totally unique feature that you won't find in any other yoga book: An authentic presentation of each of the major styles of yoga that are taught today.

With this K.I.S.S. Guide to Yoga, *there's no need to run around trying different styles of yoga. Just sit down in your own home, open the book, and you can enjoy a fascinating array of yoga experiences. One thing is for certain, no matter what you hope to gain from yoga, by reading this book and practicing the yoga postures you find within its colorful pages, your life will change for the better.*

I am grateful for this opportunity to share the wisdom I've gained by making yoga my partner for life. Enjoy your yoga experience with my best wishes!

Shakta Kaur Khalsa

SHAKTA KAUR KHALSA

Always consult your physician before beginning any exercise program. Nothing in this book is to be construed as medical advice. The benefits attributed to the practice of yoga come from the centuries-old yogic traditions. Results will vary with individuals.

Wherever possible, the information presented in this book has been verified for authenticity through the official organizations and yogic traditions that are represented within these pages.

What's Inside?

THE INFORMATION IN THE K.I.S.S. Guide to Yoga *is arranged from the simple to the more advanced, making it most effective if you start from the beginning and slowly work your way to the more involved chapters.*

PART ONE

In Part One I'll give you information about the ancient beginnings of yoga, and how it has come to arrive at our modern doorsteps. You'll learn about yoga's many health benefits, and how easily yoga can be done by anyone, including you, no matter what your needs and abilities are.

PART TWO

This part's theme is *experience*. In Part Two, I will take you by the hand and lead you through a variety of yoga experiences. Here you get to try every major form of yoga that is available today, from traditional to contemporary forms. Have fun celebrating the wonderful diversity of yoga styles!

PART THREE

Where there's yoga, there's usually meditation. In Part Three you'll learn about the many forms of meditation, and you'll get to experience the essence underlying all forms of meditation. We'll also take a look at different kinds of prayer and chanting and explore their relationship with yoga.

PART FOUR

In Part Four you'll learn to make the most of the many ordinary moments of life into which you can slip a little yoga to increase energy, center yourself, and keep relaxed. You'll also get to try some delicious recipes for healing foods from the great yogi chefs of old!

PART FIVE

Part Five focuses on how yoga is changing our world – in the workplace, in our families, in the way we view medicine, just to name a few. I will present a panoramic view of how yoga can help make a better life for us all, regardless of gender, age, occupation, or physical capabilities.

The Extras

THROUGHOUT THE BOOK, you will notice a number of boxes and symbols. They are there to emphasize certain points I want you to pay special attention to, because they are important to your understanding of yoga. You'll find:

Very Important Point

This symbol points out a topic that deserves careful attention. You really need to know this information before continuing.

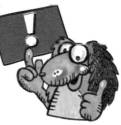

Complete No-No

This is a warning, something I want to advise you not to do or to be aware of.

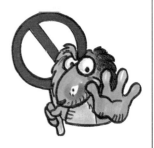

Getting Technical

When the information is about to get a bit technical, I'll let you know so that you can read carefully.

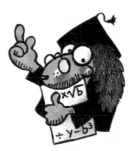

Inside Scoop

These are special suggestions that come from my own personal experience as either a veteran yoga teacher or a practitioner.

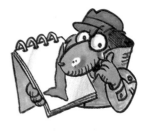

You'll also find some little boxes that include information I think is important, useful, or just plain fun.

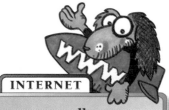

Trivia...

These are simply fun facts that will give you an extra appreciation of yoga in general.

DEFINITION

Here I'll define words and terms for you in an easy-to-understand style. You'll also find a glossary at the back of the book with all the yoga-related lingo, including phonetic pronunciation.

INTERNET

www.dk.com

I think the Internet is a great resource for yoga lovers, so I've scouted out some web sites that will add to your enjoyment and understanding of your yoga experience.

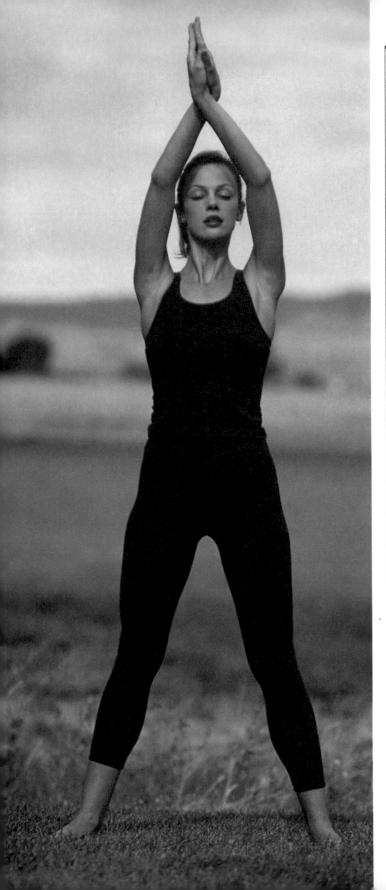

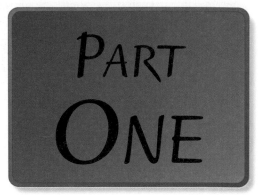

PART ONE

YOGA CREATES A UNION OF BODY, MIND, AND SPIRIT

SIMPLIFYING YOGA

YOGA IS THE NAME given to an ancient practice that helps to create a sense of union in all aspects of ourselves; in body, mind, and spirit. People have been

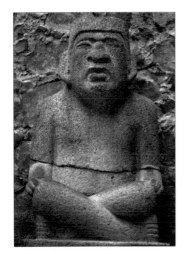

practicing yoga for thousands of years in order to feel at peace with themselves.

Moving your body into poses and exercises is the most commonly known form of yoga. In yoga you will become more aware of your breath and the inner workings of your body and mind. Yoga also helps you become *healthier* and *happier* by circulating vital life energy through all your body systems. The best news about yoga is that it meets you as you are, so rest assured that *you can do yoga*.

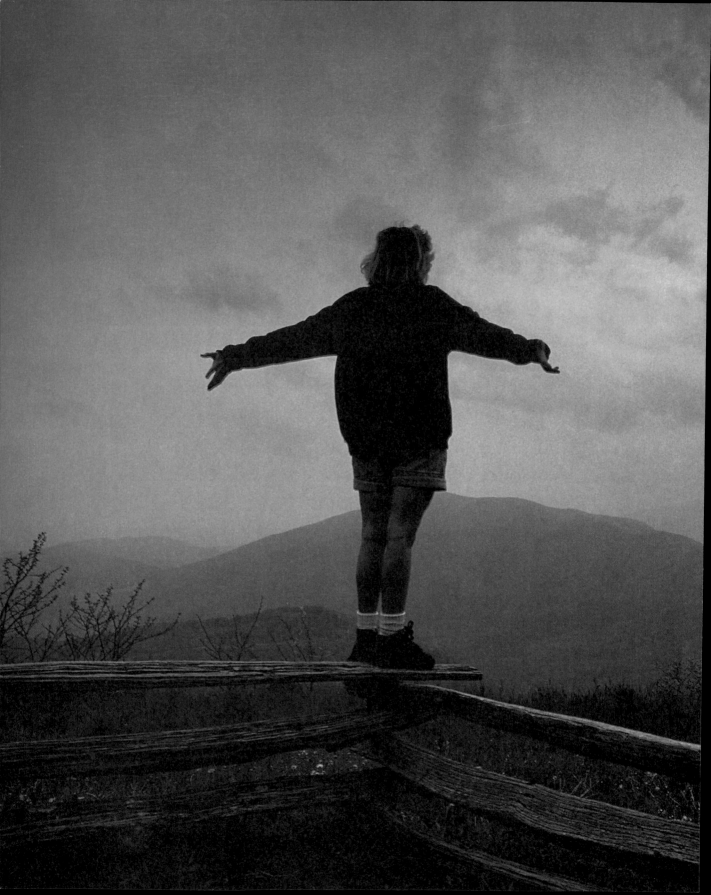

Chapter 1

A Simple Understanding

I T USED TO BE that when I told people I taught yoga, they would often respond with a blank stare or call it "yogurt." That never happens now. Yoga has fast become not only a household word, but a household practice. In fact, it has become the most widely practiced exercise system in the world. Once a totally foreign concept from somewhere "over there," it is now offered as a lunchtime class in forward-thinking corporations. But what is yoga exactly? Let's take a look at its origins.

In this chapter...

✓ Yoga is a yoke

✓ The vast yoga tree

✓ The seven branches of yoga

✓ Go west, young yogi, go west!

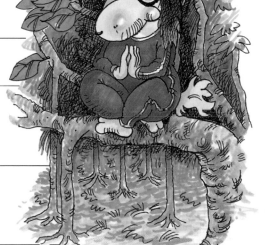

YOGA MEANS "UNION," AND IT PROMOTES A FEELING OF BEING AT ONE WITH LIFE

Yoga is a yoke

EVERY PHILOSOPHY, EVERY RELIGION, *and every therapy addresses the human need to feel whole. That's because when you feel whole, you feel happy, with everything finding its place – and its peace. This is where* yoga *comes in, harmonizing body, mind, and spirit.*

DEFINITION

Yoga *means literally to yoke, to unite, to be whole. It comes from the ancient Indian language of Sanskrit. The Sanskrit word "yug" is the great-grandfather, so to speak, of the English word "yoke." Yoga's aim is to unite the body, mind, and spirit.*

A life that incorporates a practice of yoga is a healthy, happy, whole life, as modern as it is ancient. Even better, you don't have to believe anything in particular, or even give up your own beliefs to practice it, because yoga is just between you and yourself. Yoga "yokes" all the separate parts of you into an integrated whole. This is why many people say that yoga makes them feel peaceful: You feel at peace when you are not conflicted, when your mind is not tugged in ten different directions, and when your body is relaxed.

You may experience what dedicated yoga practitioners confirm: That a peaceful calm seems to emanate from them and transform their relationships with others. When you practice yoga people will say, "You seem different somehow. I can't quite put my finger on it, but it's there." What they are sensing is your inner peace.

Yoga by any other name

"A rose by any other name smells as sweet," and yoga by any other name creates health and inner peace. Taking a few deep breaths before you do something rash is yoga. So is stretching your body toward the sky while taking a deep breath, then letting it hang forward as you exhale, after a long stretch of driving. You can call these practices whatever you like, but the tool, the technology, and the process of getting to a place of peace within yourself began in a land that, in its original language of Sanskrit, called it yoga.

Trivia...
Yoga Journal magazine recently commissioned the Roper Poll in the US to do a nationwide survey exploring people's views on yoga. It found that 6 million Americans practice yoga regularly. An additional 16 million expressed an interest in taking classes.

Forget those images of acrobatic backbends and pretzel-like postures! You are not required to be in perfect physical shape to do yoga. Yoga is vastly adaptable. It works for you simply if you are alive and breathing.

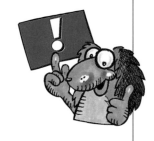

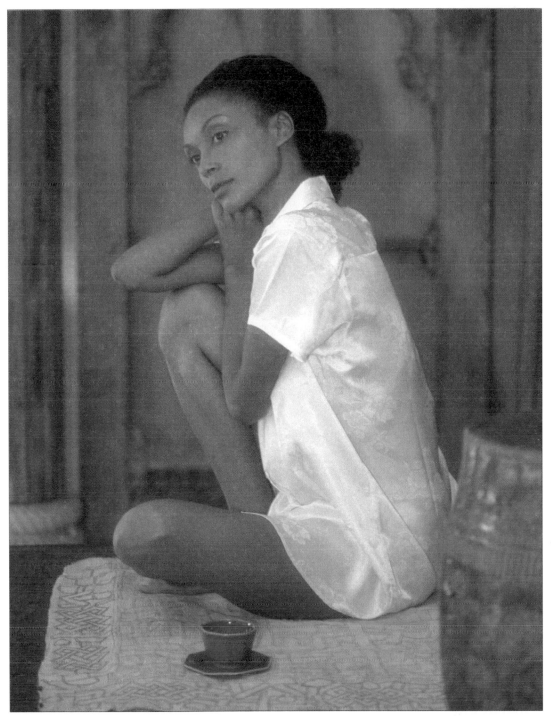

■ **Feeling at peace with yourself** *is one of the many benefits to be gained from regular yoga practice, and that sense of inner calm is often palpable to others.*

The vast yoga tree

A TREE IS OFTEN USED AS AN ANALOGY for explaining the structure of yoga. I like to think of yoga as a large banyan tree. There is nothing common about this common tree of India with its exposed gnarled roots, its trunk so thick that five people holding hands will just about span it, and its snake-like branches that reach down low enough to invite climbers to reach awe-inspiring heights. And, come to think of it, yoga is like that, too. It reaches you exactly where you are, and takes you to your heights, supporting you with its trunk – a solid foundation.

Yoga's roots

The ancient science of yoga developed in more than one wise old civilization, but under different names, of course. Archaeological discoveries have confirmed forms of yoga in ancient Chinese and Mayan cultures, as well as in India and Tibet.

Thousands of years ago, highly evolved humans in each of these civilizations created the system of yoga. Through their own personal experience of yoga, this ancient science developed and eventually was passed on from master to student, from generation to generation.

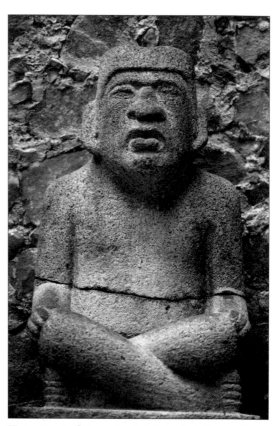

■ **In Central America,** *statues depicting early forms of yoga can be traced back to the ancient Mayan civilization.*

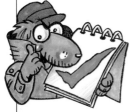

I may say that yoga developed thousands of years ago, but it could be as much as tens of thousands of years ago. No one really knows the absolute beginning of yoga, but ancient scrolls found in Tibet dating as far back as 40,000 BC describe recognizable forms of yoga.

Although forms of yoga have been discovered in various cultures, it was along the ancient Indus River that this body/mind/spirit science was first fully developed and preserved. Imagine an advanced culture flourishing along the banks of the Indus and Saraswati rivers: Multistory baked brick buildings abound; there is a huge public bath waterproofed with bitumen; the brick roads are laid out in geometric patterns; and the sewage system is so advanced it rivals that of the Roman Empire. All of this, dating from somewhere between 3,000–1,900 BC!

Yoga's birth date of somewhere around 3,000–1,900 BC has been confirmed by references in the Rig-Veda, which is the oldest known text in any Indo-European language. Parts of it were composed in the third or even fourth millennium BC.

Within the Rig-Veda, there are references to the Saraswati River, which is believed to have dried up around or before 1,900 BC. This means that this ancient text must have been contemporary with the Indus–Saraswati culture, where yoga first developed.

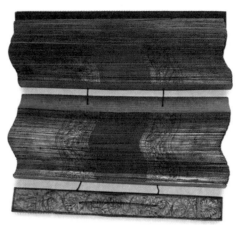

■ **Books made of** *palm leaves were used for the writings of Jnana yoga, one of a number of different yoga paths.*

Yoga's trunk

The trunk, or foundation, of yoga is that we are spiritual beings in human form who are here to find out that we are spiritual beings in human form! I am oversimplifying, of course, but according to the basic science of yoga, there is the soul, or transcendental self, called the atman, and there is the mind–body. Our true identity is found in merging these parts into a unified whole. This, then, is the trunk of yoga from which the spreading limbs, or guiding principles, of yoga emerge and derive their strength. The science of yoga was known and practiced but not clearly documented until AD 200, when a physician-sage named Patanjali systematized and codified the science of yoga into eight limbs. The name given to this text is the *Yoga sutras.*

There is a lucid and very readable book on Patanjali's Yoga sutras called How to Know God, by Christopher Isherwood and Swami Prabhavananda. This work is a "must have" classic for serious students of life!

Yoga's limbs

Patanjali's system of yoga is a map of the process of awakening the possible human in each of us. Although the eight limbs, or basic beliefs, of yoga are intertwined, rather than linear, for clarity's sake I will divide them into two groups. The first four are associated with how a person conducts his life. I think of them as the "goods" of yoga. They are:

- *Yama*. **Do good**. This boils down to the Golden Rule: "Do unto others as you would have them do unto you." The yamas encourage moderation and discourage violence, stealing, lying, and possessiveness.

- *Niyama*. **Be good.** The niyamas give the ground rules for self-discipline and inner awareness. They encourage purity, contentment, chastity, self-study, and awareness of the spirit.

> **DEFINITION**
>
> **Asanas,** *literally "steady poses," are yoga postures and exercises that enhance physical, mental, and spiritual well-being.*

- *Asana*. **Feel good.** The physical body is a temple for the spirit. Yoga postures, or *asanas*, keep the body healthy and the mind calm, creating an atmosphere in which the spirit can more easily flow.

- *Pranayama*. **Live good**. Pranayama focuses on understanding the link between the breath, mind, and body. The practice of conscious breath control allows for a vital and long life.

The importance of these first four limbs is reflected in yoga as it is practiced today. Sometimes yoga is further reduced to a simple emphasis on the physical body through asanas (yoga poses). But, as you will see, the second four teachings are just as important in developing the body/mind/spirit connection. They focus on meditation, which is the process of quieting or controlling the constant waves of thought. They are:

- *Pratyahara*. **Inner focus.** This is the process of becoming aware of, and learning to control, thought patterns. One's attention is drawn away from the five senses of sight, hearing, taste, touch, and smell. Instead, the meditator is focused inwardly in order to quiet the mind.

- *Dharana*. **One-pointedness.** The mind, once withdrawn into itself, is fixed in one-pointed inner concentration.

- *Dhyana*. **Deep meditation**. This is meditation without focus on an object, and is rooted in a deep, inner space of awareness.

- *Samadhi*. **Absorption**. This is the ecstatic state of being in which the meditator becomes one with the object of meditation. Here, one is spiritually awake and absorbed in the Infinite.

The seven branches of yoga

TO EXTEND THE IMAGE OF THE YOGA TREE, with its core trunk
and limbs, let's explore the branches. Remember climbing trees as a kid? Just as
there were many branches to choose from as you climbed, there are many types
of yoga from which to choose as well. You can choose all of them if you like!

① **Hatha yoga.** This is what most people think of as yoga. Here
you find the physical postures, poses, and exercises that work
directly on the body and, in turn, on the mind. People are
attracted to *Hatha* yoga because its benefits are felt
immediately. It relaxes the body, calms the mind, and brings
greater awareness to your life. Much of this book will be
devoted to this important branch of yoga.

② **Raja yoga.** Raja literally means "royal," and it is commonly
known as classic yoga. The eight limbs I discussed earlier fall
under Raja yoga. The focus here is on training the mind to
serve the spirit through meditation. The practice of Raja yoga
typically starts with Hatha yoga in order to prepare the body
and mind for meditation. I've included a whole section on
meditation later in the book, just to get you
started off right.

③ **Karma yoga.** Karma means "right" action.
People who love to serve others and help
out whenever they can, without any
thought of reward, are practicing
Karma yoga. It's amazing, but
you can feel just as great slaving
away for something you really
believe in as you would if you
practiced a lot of Hatha yoga
and meditation.

■ **Raja yoga** *emphasizes
training the mind through
meditation and is
generally preceded by
Hatha yoga, which aids
mental preparation.*

DEFINITION

*The most popular form of
yoga today, **Hatha** can be
defined in two ways. First,
the word divides into "ha,"
which in Sanskrit means sun,
and "tha," which is the moon.
Therefore, Hatha is often
interpreted to mean the
"balance" of opposites (male
and female) within a person.
Another meaning of Hatha is
"forceful" or "effort," which
signifies transformation
through the effort or force
of the physical body.*

TWO GREAT PRACTITIONERS

Two great examples of practitioners of Karma–Bhakti yoga are Mother Teresa and Ma Jaya Sati Bhagavati.

Mother Teresa attended to the needs of India's untouchable caste, people who had leprosy and were dying with no one to care for them. Her love and devotion inspired the world so much that she won the Nobel Peace Prize in 1979.

Ma Jaya Sati Bhagavati, who is known simply as "Ma," carries out her labor of love for people who are dying of cancer and AIDS, helping them make the transition into death. Children of AIDS victims find a loving and spiritual home at her center in Florida. To learn more about Ma's work, see her web site: www.kashi.org.

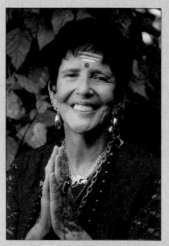

MA JAYA SATI BHAGAVATI

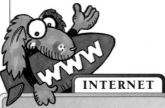

INTERNET

www.yrec.org

Check this site for an in-depth understanding of the who, the what, and the where of yoga. Its founder, Georg Feuerstein, is one of the top yoga scholars and he has written numerous books on yoga, including Living Yoga, *authored with Stephan Bodian, and* The Shambhala Encyclopedia of Yoga.

4 **Bhakti yoga.** Bhakti means devotion and *selfless* love. Have you ever heard someone say, "My heart just went out to her, and I offered to help"? That's Bhakti yoga, and it is Karma yoga, too. Bhakti yoga and Karma yoga often are thought of as two sides of the same coin. When you feel love, you want to serve, and when you serve in a selfless way, you also feel the love and devotion of that action.

5 **Jnana yoga.** This is the path of *wisdom* and of discerning that which is real from that which is unreal. Through this path of wisdom comes the inspiration to view life from the perspective of humans as spiritual beings. The writings of the great sage Jiddu Krishnamurti are a good example of Jnana yoga.

6 **Tantra yoga.** Tantra means the place *where opposites meet* and become one. For this reason, it is often associated with sexual union. But the big picture of Tantra teaches that there is no difference between the *big* opposites – the finite and the infinite, or the Divine with a capital D and the divinity that is ordinary life. Because of the powerful nature of Tantra, it should always be taught by a master teacher.

KRISHNAMURTI

J. Krishnamurti (1895–1986) was undoubtedly one of the greatest philosophical minds of the 20th century. A speaker, author, and educator from India, he conveyed a profound sense of truth to audiences around the world for more than half a century. The following quote is from his book, *Life Ahead*:

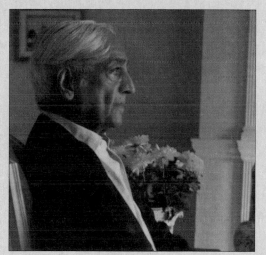

J. KRISHNAMURTI

To experience what is solitude and what is meditation, one must be in a state of inquiry; only a mind that is in a state of inquiry is capable of learning. But when inquiry is suppressed by previous knowledge, or by the authority and experience of another, then learning becomes mere imitation, and imitation causes a human being to repeat what is learnt without experiencing it.

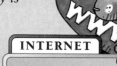

INTERNET

www.kfa.org

www.kinfonet.org

Both these sites are dedicated to the teachings of J. Krishnamurti: One is the site of the Krishnamurti Foundation of America, founded by J. Krishnamurti in 1969, and the other features volumes of books and articles by Krishnamurti.

7 **Mantra yoga.** Sometimes considered an aspect of Tantra yoga, Mantra yoga is the yoga of potent *sound*. The word mantra translates literally as "mind projection." It is a technique for using patterns of sound (through chanting or reciting) to help focus the mind.

At some point in your practice of yoga, you may have a real-life experience of the teachings of the Yoga sutras. "Ah yes!" you might say to yourself. "This is exactly what Patanjali was talking about when he said to draw the attention away from the senses and still the mind."

Go west, young yogi, go west!

WHEN SOMETHING WORKS *as well as yoga does, you can't keep it a secret forever. Considering how long it's been around, it is pretty remarkable that yoga didn't make its debut in the Western world (specifically the United States) until the mid-1800s. At that time groups of intellectual writers discovered yoga through their interest in the esoteric teachings of Ralph Waldo Emerson, Henry David Thoreau, and Amos Bronson Alcott. Some time later, a Victorian-era biography of Guatama Buddha called* The Light of Asia, *by Edwin Arnold, sold half a million copies. So, at least within intellectual circles in the West, Eastern philosophy had arrived.*

A real live *yogi* came on the scene at the Parliament of Religions held in Chicago in 1893. It was at this event that the young *Swami* Vivekananda, who came to the United States at the request of his teacher, even though he didn't know a soul, made a big and lasting impression on the American people. In the years that followed, he traveled and taught widely, attracting many to yoga in the process.

> **DEFINITION**
>
> *A yogi is an accomplished male student of yoga. A female is called a yogini.* Swami *is a title for a spiritual master.*

Early explorations into yoga

Swami Vivekananda taught Raja yoga, which concentrates on meditation and control of the mind. Hatha yoga was introduced to America by Yogendra Mastamani, who came to New York in 1919. Then, in 1920, the International Congress of Religious Liberals hosted the Indian spiritual leader Paramahansa Yogananda at its conference in Boston, and 5 years later he founded the Self Realization Fellowship in Los Angeles. In 1946, Paramahansa Yogananda wrote the classic *Autobiography of a Yogi*, a miraculous story of his spiritual life, which has done more to introduce the Western world to yoga and meditation than any other publication.

> **Trivia...**
> *The British colonization of India helped introduce yoga to the West by translating sacred texts containing yoga themes, like* The Bhagavad Gita, *into English.*

Hatha yoga, the yoga of physical postures, entered mainstream America when the Russian-born Indra Devi opened a studio in Hollywood in 1947 and began to teach movie stars like Jennifer Jones, Gloria Swanson, and Robert Ryan. "The First Lady of Yoga," now in her 90s, is still an influential voice in yoga.

AUTOBIOGRAPHY OF A YOGINI-TO-BE

In 1971, I ran across my best friend and college roommate avidly reading Paramahansa Yogananda's *Autobiography of a Yogi* in our favorite diner. She was so engrossed that at first it bugged me because she wasn't talking to me at all. Then I became curious. What could be so captivating about a paperback book that had a picture of a man in a woman's hairdo on the cover? "Read a little to me," I urged her.

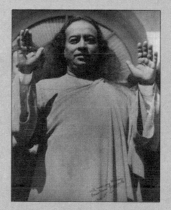

PARAMAHANSA YOGANANDA

She began:
One night, when a cloud of mosquitoes surrounded us, Master failed to issue his usual instructions [to use a mosquito curtain]. I listened nervously to the anticipatory hum of the insects. Getting into bed, I threw a propitiatory prayer in their general direction. A half hour later, I coughed pretentiously to attract my guru's attention. I thought I would go mad with the bites and especially the singing drone as the mosquitoes celebrated bloodthirsty rites.

No responsive stir from Master; I approached him cautiously. He was not breathing. This was my first close observation of him in the yogic trance; it filled me with fright.

His heart must have failed! I placed a mirror under his nose; no breath vapor appeared. To make doubly certain, for minutes I closed his mouth and nostrils with my fingers. His body was cold and motionless. In a daze, I turned toward the door to summon help.

"So! A budding experimentalist! My poor nose!" Master's voice was shaky with laughter. "Why don't you go to bed? Is the whole world going to change for you? Change yourself; be rid of the mosquito consciousness."

Meekly I returned to my bed. Not one insect ventured near. I realized that my guru had previously agreed to the curtains only to please me; he had no fear of mosquitoes. By yogic power he could prevent them from biting him, or, if he chose, he could escape to an inner invulnerability.

I listened to this anecdote with fascination. I was hooked. I bought my own copy of the book, and thus began a life-long journey into Eastern teachings and yoga.

Taking root in new soil

With the advent of television came Richard Hittleman's yoga program, in 1961. Hittleman offered the public a simple exercise plan that matched the standards of the West – minimum effort with maximum results. Ten years later came Lilias Folan's series on public television, which boasts over 500 shows, many of which are still shown today to a large viewership.

The Woodstock generation had a huge influence on bringing yoga to the forefront of American popular culture.

Ram Dass, formerly Dr. Richard Alpert, carried a whole generation on a spiritual journey to India, and to the transcendental self within, when his touchstone book *Be Here Now* was published in 1971. At about the same time, the Beatles' attraction to

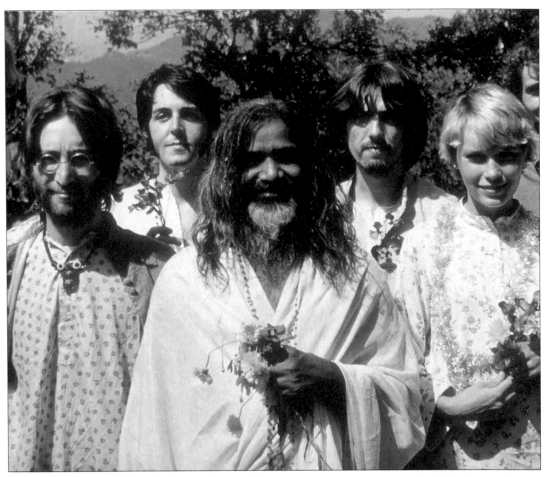

■ **Maharishi Mahesh Yogi** *welcomes famous followers, including John Lennon, Paul McCartney, George Harrison, and Mia Farrow, to his transcendental meditation academy in India in 1968.*

DEFINITION

Guru literally means "one who takes you from the darkness to the light," and is often casually used to denote a teacher or master.

Indian *gurus* and masters not only influenced other young seekers, but exemplified a generation that was looking for something more from life, and was willing to go out and get it.

Eastern teachers and masters of yoga heard the call, and by the late 1970s the West was won. Yoga was making inroads into universities and community centers, and ashrams (spiritual communities) were springing up all over America. The yoga movement, tailored to fit the Western psyche, was here to stay.

INTERNET

www.yogamovement. com

Created for both beginners and experienced yoga practitioners, this site is a great source for everything yoga-related.

A simple summary

✔ Yoga's aim is to unite the body, mind, and spirit. Practicing yoga helps you feel healthy, happy, and whole.

✔ You are not required to be in perfect physical shape to do yoga. Yoga is vastly adaptable to every person's particular needs.

✔ Yoga came into existence thousands of years ago, and was passed on from master to student, from generation to generation.

✔ Yoga provides a system for achieving the union of body, mind, and spirit. Its seven branches represent the paths you can take toward that end.

✔ Hatha yoga is the most popular form of yoga practiced today.

✔ Yoga came to the West in the late 19th century. Hatha yoga entered the mainstream in the late 1940s, and since the 1970s has become the most widely practiced exercise system in the world.

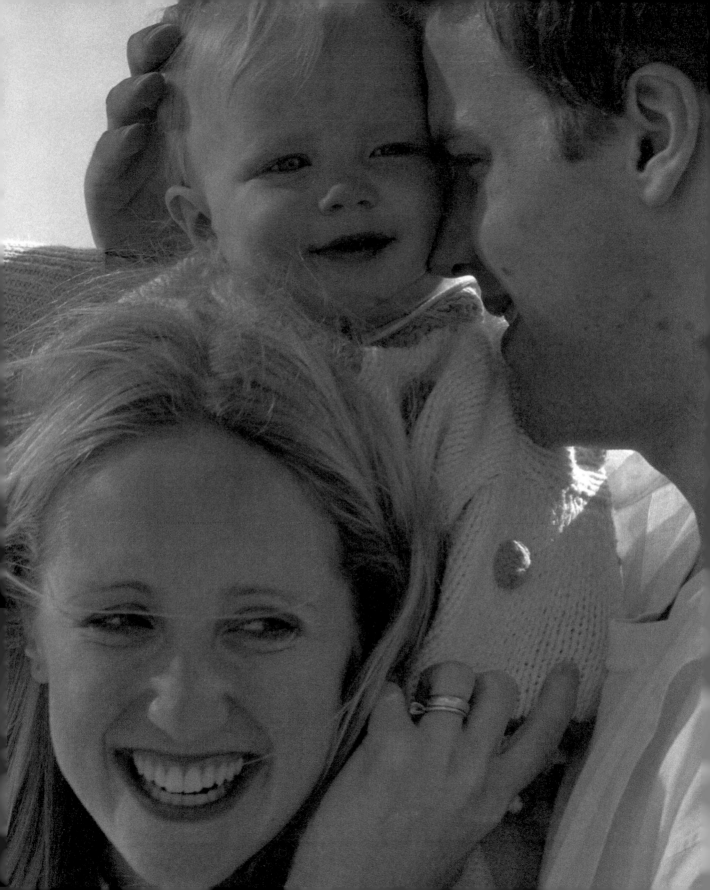

Chapter 2

Why Yoga Feels So Good

YOGA IS THE BEST SELF-HELP TREATMENT you can give yourself. A regular yoga practice revitalizes every single part of you, right down to the cellular level. In this chapter you'll learn how yoga affects your body and mind, and discover that when it comes to effectiveness, nothing quite beats yoga as a great source of natural health care.

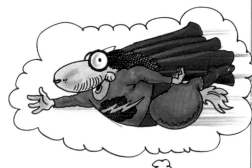

In this chapter...

✓ What yoga can do for you

✓ Conscious breathing

✓ Just want to relax?

✓ The mind–body connection

✓ Acupressure and yoga

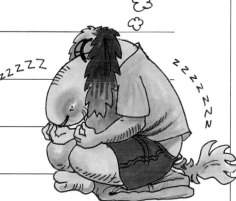

HEALTH, VITALITY, AND MENTAL WELL-BEING ARE AMONG THE MANY POSITIVE EFFECTS OF YOGA PRACTICE

What yoga can do for you

THERE ARE AS MANY REASONS *to practice yoga as there are challenges in our daily lives. Yoga grants physical health and vitality, relief from pain and stress, emotional strength, and clarity during difficult times, and on and on.*

One of my favorite T-shirt sayings is "Whatever the question, the answer is . . . More yoga!" and that seems about right. Of course, not even yoga can be touted as a cure for every ill, but if I find myself needing a mental or physical boost, a little yoga goes a long way. On the next few pages you'll see how simple it is to make yoga work for you.

INTERNET

www.moreyoga.com

You can find inspiring T-shirts and wonderful yoga and relaxation tools at this web site.

Creating a toned, flexible body

How you look has an impact on how you feel, and vice versa. A youthful appearance is one of the many blessings of a consistent yoga practice. Like isometric exercise, yoga postures tone your muscles. When you add inner focus to your yoga stretches, there will be little or no chance of muscle injury. Besides, healthy, toned muscles have less chance of injury, and they hold your posture erect and give you a beautiful physique.

Rather than building muscle, yoga builds muscle tone. Because yoga helps to maintain a balanced metabolism, it also helps to regulate weight. Additionally, yoga stretches muscles lengthwise, causing fat to be eliminated around the cells, thus reducing cellulite.

Yoga can help you look and feel years younger than your age. In India, age is measured by the flexibility of the body and, especially, of the spine. The spine is the "switchboard" of your nervous system and the messenger to your brain. When the spine is flexible, the flow of blood and oxygen to the brain and organs is unrestricted. Many yoga postures and exercises keep the spine flexible by gently twisting or flexing the spine in all directions.

■ **Because yoga tones the muscles,** *improves flexibility and posture, and helps to regulate weight, it keeps you feeling youthful, fit, and full of vitality.*

Less stress, more energy

Stress is an energy zapper. Enjoying life is an energy builder. This explains how a young office worker, who on Friday afternoon says she's exhausted and has no energy left, can go out on the town Friday night and dance until dawn!

What does this have to do with yoga? Yoga gives you the tools to transform stress into energy. If you're wondering how (and since experience is the best teacher), let's try an actual yoga pose right now. Don't worry, it's an easy one – a simple forward stretch.

1. Sit on the floor (use a mat if needed) with your legs stretched out in front of you. Your legs should be about 6 in (15 cm) apart. Lean forward and touch whatever part of you that your hands can reach, whether it's your toes, ankles, or shins. Inhale deeply through your nose and stretch your arms up while lengthening your spine and stretching upward.

2. Now exhale slowly and deeply, and just let yourself fall forward from the hips. Bring your arms down, and hold onto your legs or ankles with your arms relaxed and your elbows bent. Hold this position and take a few more deep breaths. Every time you exhale, let your muscles relax a little more, and allow gravity to draw you even further forward.

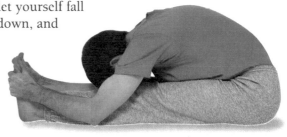

STEP 2

3. Continue stretching and relaxing for five more breaths. Now sit up straight and cross your legs. With your eyes closed, notice how you are feeling from the inside and become aware of your breath moving through your body. Do you feel different? How? As tension is released, can you feel how the subsequent relaxation circulates energy within your body and mind?

If you're wondering what the "stress" is in the previous exercise, it is the tension you feel in your back or legs when you stretch forward, or the tightness in your chest when you attempt to breathe deeply. The "letting go" feeling that you experience on the exhale is the release of that stress.

STEP 3

Off the mat

Let's take yoga off the mat and into the real world for a moment. Imagine you've been practicing the above exercise enough to make it a regular habit and then put yourself in a scenario like this one: Your boss, your child, or your spouse is angry at you about something. At the outset, fear may begin to overtake you. Notice any tightness in your solar plexus (the area above your navel), neck, back, or face, as you prepare your mind for defense and attack. Now, put this scene on "pause" and . . . .

Begin to breathe consciously into the tight spots. Release the need to be defensive. Feel yourself sinking into your body, as you did when you allowed gravity to help you stretch forward. Consciously relax yourself. Feel the ensuing energy. Imagine you have the energy to handle this challenging situation creatively. It takes trust in yourself the first few times you try. But learning this response to stress takes the nasty punches out of life and puts the fun back into it!

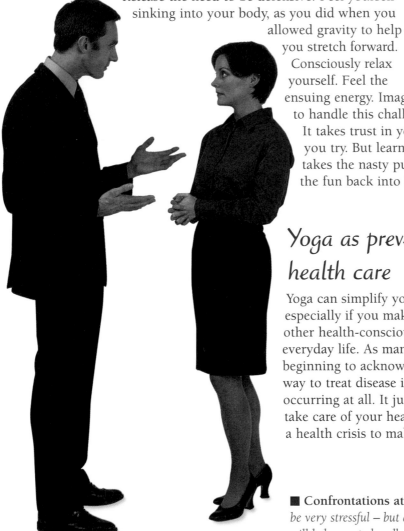

Yoga as preventative health care

Yoga can simplify your healthcare needs, especially if you make good nutrition and other health-conscious choices part of your everyday life. As many healthcare plans are beginning to acknowledge, the most effective way to treat disease is to prevent it from occurring at all. It just makes good sense to take care of your health, instead of waiting for a health crisis to make you pay attention to it.

■ **Confrontations at work** *or in everyday life can be very stressful – but drawing on your yoga practice will help you to handle difficult situations more easily.*

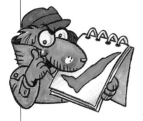

Relief from pain is another reason people turn to yoga.

Pain relief was *my* original motivation for seeking out yoga. In 1972 I didn't know exactly what I was looking for, but I knew my back hurt and my muscles were tense. I was a college student at the time, and it was my good luck that the physical education department at my university offered yoga. I began practicing every day, and loved the way it relaxed not only my back but my entire being.

Peace of mind and higher awareness

Yoga equals freedom: Freedom from the load our minds often carry unconsciously. Once you make a habit of practicing yoga, you'll become more aware of your mental processes. At the same time you may notice how often your mind holds you back. It may be telling you, "I am not good enough to do that," or, "This is not fair, so I'm going to withdraw (or fight)." Becoming aware of the way your mind thinks is the first step toward peace of mind.

After you've practiced yoga for a while, you may have the courage to override any preconceived self-limitations. Once you do, and are successful, you will feel lighter. You may describe this feeling as peace of mind, or an acceptance of your life as it is, with all its challenges. Yoga can help you realize that challenges have their place. Yoga helps you realize your potential, and encourages self-growth toward that potential. With this understanding comes peace of mind.

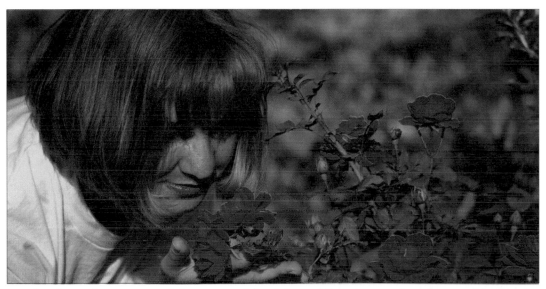

■ **A heightened awareness** *of the senses and the ability to fully appreciate the richness and beauty of your natural surroundings is another bonus of practicing yoga.*

Yoga develops *awareness*. When you first start practicing yoga, you may notice and appreciate the sights, sounds, smells, tastes, and feel of the wondrous variety of life around you, perhaps for the first time. This signals the earliest stage of awareness.

> **DEFINITION**
>
> *Awareness can be described as a state of being that has different levels, including being conscious of your inner and outer surroundings, and your self-identity.*

After some time, you may notice how a thought or a feeling passes through your mind like a bubble – first it is there, then imperceptibly it is gone. Just like that! You begin to realize that there is an observer who is you, who is watching not only your thought processes but everything that happens to you with loving neutrality. This is the beginning of higher awareness.

Higher awareness, as I have come to know it, is directed inward first. Once established within, this consciousness flows outward to help better the world. This is a natural process. You are not limiting your thoughts/insights to yourself; you are creating a foundation from which all good – directed outward – can happen.

Conscious breathing

BREATHING IS THE FIRST THING WE DO *when we come into life, and the last thing we do upon leaving it. In between, most of us are often not aware that we are breathing.*

Have you ever forgotten to breathe? Sometimes it's because whatever is going on is just too exciting, dangerous, or amazing. Think of the many scenarios in which the way you breathe reflects your state of mind: When you are really afraid, your breath becomes rapid and shallow, or you take in sharp breaths; when you finish intense work, you take a deep breath; when you are tired, you yawn and draw in extra oxygen; when you release anxiety, you sigh; when you stand by the ocean with the wind in your face, you take a deep draft of the fresh air to clear your thoughts and emotions.

Taking the unconscious process of breathing and making it conscious is an essential aspect of yoga.

The yogis and sages of old found that when they became aware of the breath as it moved in and out, the mind could be consciously controlled. The yogis then began to use the mind to control the breath, which in turn benefited the mind and body.

Breathing lessons

For beginner yogis and yoginis, here is a very simple way to become aware of the breath. Remember, all yogic breathing is done through the nose, unless otherwise specified. Do not force the breath in any way as you practice this technique.

1 Lie down on your back on a cushioned but firm surface. Bend your knees and tuck your tailbone by tipping your pelvis slightly forward. The arch at the small of your back will be pressed gently toward the floor. This action takes pressure away from the lower spine. A rolled pillow can be placed under your knees for extra comfort. To begin, let your arms rest at your sides.

2 The inhalation will have three parts that flow smoothly from one into the other. When you begin to inhale, your belly will expand as your diaphragm moves downward, drawing air into the lowest part of your lungs. As you continue, your ribcage will expand and air will be pulled into the middle part of your lungs. Lastly, your collarbone will lift and air will fill the upper part of your chest.

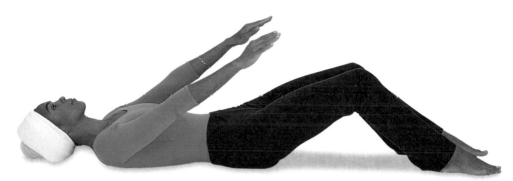

ARMS USED AS "MONITORS" FOR THE INHALATION PROCESS

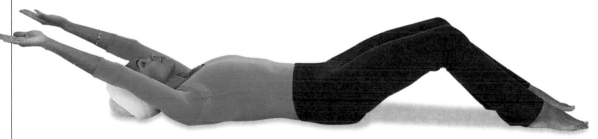

LUNGS FULL AND ARMS FULLY EXTENDED

Try using your arms as "monitors" for the inhalation process. As you begin to fill up the lower part of your lungs with air, raise your arms slowly from your sides. When the air you are breathing in reaches the mid-lungs, your arms should mirror that position. Continue to raise your arms, smoothly mirroring the position of the breath in your lungs until they are full and your arms are fully extended overhead. If you like, pause briefly at the end of the inhalation.

3   With your arms resting overhead, begin to slowly exhale from the top part of the lungs first. Your arm movements will again coordinate with the movement of the lungs. The mid-lungs are emptied next, and your diaphragm moves upward as the last bit of air is emptied from your lungs and your arms come to rest at your sides once more. Pause briefly, then begin a new inhalation.

For a deeper sense of relaxation and calmness, pause a few seconds at the end of each exhalation.

You will notice that the process of exhalation in yogic breathing empties the upper lungs then the lower – the opposite of the inhalation process, which fills the lower lungs then the upper lungs.

4   Practice deep breathing several times a day. When you feel comfortable with this process, change to a sitting posture with a straight spine. Placing a pillow under your buttocks will help to straighten the lower spine and relax the hips downward. Rest your hands on your knees. Take 6–10 seconds for each inhale, and do the same for each exhale. Pause for 1–2 seconds between breaths.

STEP 4

Do not rush the breathing process in this exercise.

May the (life) force be with you!

The ancient yogis were aware of the life energy that all things are made of. They especially took note of the vital energy that enters on the breath, and they called it *prana*. They called the releasing energy of the outbreath *apana*. This interplay of prana and apana keeps us alive by circulating the vital life force and eliminating the used-up energy.

DEFINITION

Prana *is the vital life force in all things, and also refers to the vital energy that is drawn into the body when you inhale.* **Apana** *refers to the release or elimination of waste, and relates to the outbreath when you exhale.*

Just want to relax?

EIGHTY-FIVE PERCENT OF THE PEOPLE who seek out yoga say they are looking for a way to relax: That's because yoga is naturally relaxing. Breathing deeply pours fresh oxygen into the bloodstream and circulates the prana. Yoga postures help muscles unwind and retrain them to relax. In almost all yoga classes, no matter what the style, there is a deep relaxation phase, usually after a series of postures.

DEFINITION

Corpse pose *is a relaxation pose that is done by lying on your back with your hands at the sides of your body, palms up. No energy need be expended to hold the body in this position.*

Relieving muscle tension

A simple technique for systematically relaxing all the muscles of the body is the tense–relax method. You may want someone to read the following instructions, or you can tape record yourself reading them, in order to focus completely on relaxation. To begin, lie down on your back (on a mat, if you like) in what is known as *Corpse pose.* You are going to learn to be dead in life with this pose!

If you like, place a small pillow under your knees to take pressure off the lower spine. Rest your arms at your sides with the palms of your hands facing upward and relaxed.

1 Begin to breathe deeply, as you did in the yogic breathing exercise. While doing this pose, one of my favorite visualizations is to imagine the waves of the ocean rolling up to the shore on the inhale. On the exhale, the waves roll back to the sea.

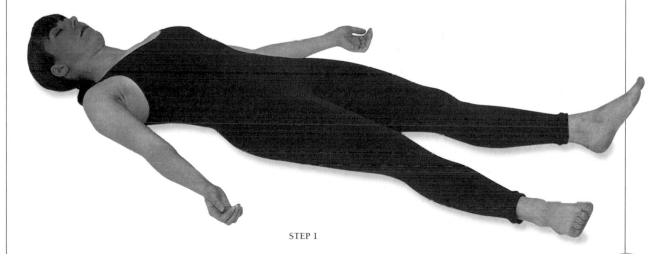

STEP 1

2 To relax all of your muscles, begin with your feet and move upward, isolating and tensing specific parts of your body and then relaxing them. Focus first on your feet, tensing them as you inhale. Hold for a few seconds, then exhale and let all the tension go from your feet.

3 Next, move up to your legs and do the same thing. Then, tense the muscles of your pelvis and lower back on the inhale. Exhale and relax completely. Inhale and tense your solar plexus, chest, and mid-back. Exhale and relax. Move to your shoulders. Tense, then relax. Focus on your arms, tensing on the inhale, relaxing on the exhale. And now tense your hands, and let your breath go. Move up to your neck, head, and face. Inhale and tense your neck, head, and face. Hold the inhale for a few seconds, then exhale completely and relax.

4 For the grand finale, inhale and tense every part of your body at once. Hold your breath for a few seconds, then exhale and relax, releasing all tension on the exhale. Relax for a few more minutes, then stretch your arms overhead with a deep inhale and exhale. Stretch from side to side, and sit up.

Remember, even if your mind wanders while doing yoga, keep away from self-criticism — it will only cause more tension! Just simply remind yourself of what you are doing.

The endorphin connection

Nature provides us with natural feel-good chemicals called *endorphins*. These natural chemicals are the brain's way of responding to the body when it is in an intense phase of physical exertion. Endorphins help to relieve pain caused by intense exertion, and provide a heightened feeling of well-being. If you have ever run a mile at top speed, you may recall that at the end of the run your natural inclination was to flop down in the soft grass. The euphoric feeling you experienced while resting is caused by the release of endorphins. Likewise, at the end of a strong yoga set, the same great feeling can carry you through your day.

■ **Vigorous exercise** *causes endorphins, known as the body's natural opiates, to be released. These produce a pleasurable effect, giving us a mental and physical boost.*

The mind–body connection

YOUR GLANDULAR SYSTEM *is the body's control center. When your glandular system is balanced and healthy, you feel a sense of well-being and a heightened sense of awareness. The hypothalamus, pituitary, and the little-understood pineal glands of the brain are considered the "higher" glands, as they play an important role in the mind–body connection.*

Yoga works directly on the glandular system through breath, postures, and meditation.

During deep breathing, the hypothalamus readjusts the glandular system. Active forms of yoga can awaken the pineal gland. The pituitary gland is

THE BODY'S CONTROL CENTERS

The hypothalamus is the main intermediary between the endocrine and central nervous systems. Anything that has to do with a mind–body connection is controlled by the hypothalamus.

The pituitary is called the master gland because it regulates the secretions of the thyroid, the adrenals, and most of the endocrine glands. The pituitary gets messages from the hypothalamus and is the meeting place between the mind and the body.

The function of the tiny pineal gland has been a mystery for Western science. Scientists know that it produces melatonin, which influences the cyclical levels of sex hormones and regulates sleep. The pineal was originally believed to be active only in children, but recent scientific evidence shows that it may remain active throughout adult life.

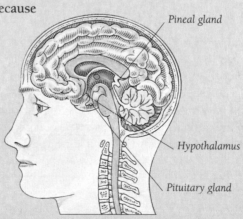

Pineal gland

Hypothalamus

Pituitary gland

■ **The hypothalamus,** *which controls the pituitary, and the pineal gland can be stimulated by deep breathing and active forms of yoga.*

activated by focusing on the pituitary point (between the eyebrows at the forehead level) during meditation.

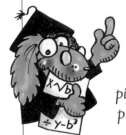

Interestingly, yogic science has understood the importance of the pineal gland for thousands of years. According to yogic teachings, one of the major functions of the pineal is to vibrate and control the nucleus projection of every cell of the body.

Singing the body electric

The body electric is the nervous system. Each of us is equipped with this intricate electrical wiring system. When your nervous system is overstressed, you might say your nerves are "frayed," or that you are like a "live wire." Strong nerves give you endurance and stamina. Yoga postures, especially balancing poses, breathing exercises, and focused meditation, work directly on the nervous system. Deep relaxation techniques directly release pressure on the nervous system.

Trivia...

One of my students, Cheryl, told me that she applies yoga to her trips to the dentist. "Before the dentist starts work, I take some deep breaths, while relaxing any tense areas. Then with my eyes closed, I focus gently at my forehead between the eyebrows. When the dentist hits a nerve, I breathe through the wave of nerve pain, knowing that it will pass very soon. When the momentary nerve pain is gone, I make a point of mentally scanning my body for any tension."

Acupressure and yoga

DEFINITION

*Acupressure, like acupuncture, is an ancient Chinese method of healing. Acupressure directly presses upon and manipulates the body through a system of **acupressure points** and meridians. The pathways through which the life force flows are the **meridians**, and the points are the places where the energy can be tapped.*

WHAT IS THE CONNECTION *between acupressure and yoga?* Acupressure *uses touch to stimulate the* **meridians** *of the body, while yoga uses postures and breath to affect the meridians. Each method has an effect on certain nerves, muscles, and* **acupressure points***. This awakens and balances the flow of energy, which is prana, or chi, as it is known in the terminology of acupressure.*

As you practice yoga, you become much more attuned to your body and mind. Eventually you may cultivate an awareness of the meridians and pressure points in your own body, and intuitively understand which yoga postures or exercises will help you stimulate them.

A tender area is often a sign that a pressure point needs some attention. You can press it firmly and gently, and visualize breathing peace and relaxation into that spot.

If you find the connection between acupressure and yoga fascinating, take a look at the book Acu-Yoga, by Michael Reed Gach. It contains a wealth of practical techniques that combine acupressure and yoga.

■ **Acupressure techniques** *can be practiced at home or at work. To relieve tenderness, use your fingers and thumbs to press directly onto the skin at a pressure point.*

A simple summary

✓ Yoga tones your muscles and keeps your body flexible. It helps with weight control, keeps you young, and is good preventative healthcare.

✓ Practicing yoga gives you tools to transform stress into energy. Peace of mind and higher awareness are developed in yoga.

✓ Taking the unconscious process of breathing and making it conscious has been proven to create beneficial changes in the mind and body.

✓ Yoga strengthens and balances the nervous system and the glandular system, and releases "feel good" chemicals from the brain.

✓ The flow of your internal energy is boosted through yoga, which stimulates pressure points and meridians in much the same way acupressure does.

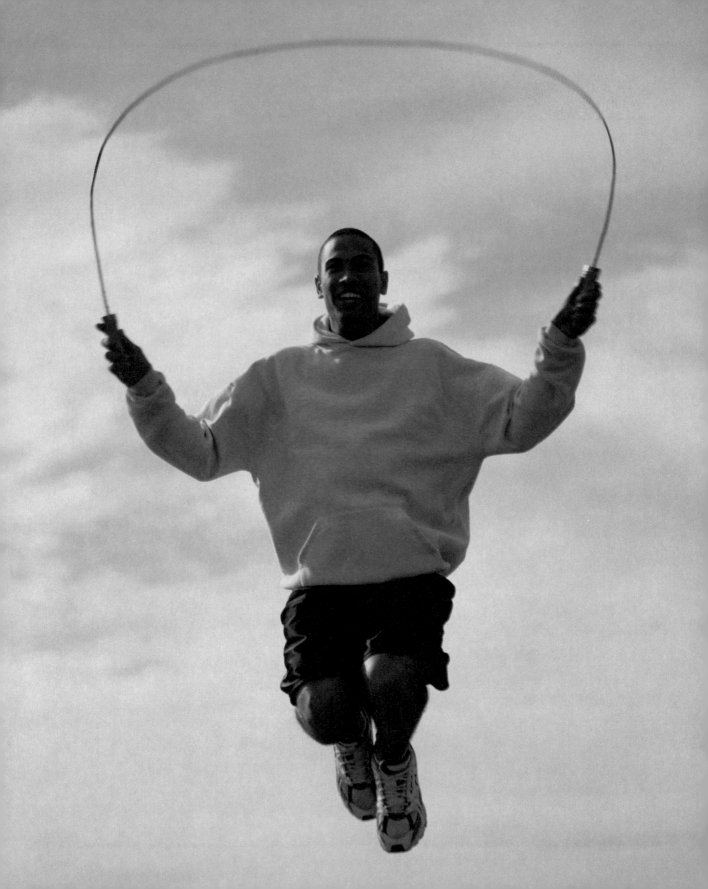

Chapter 3

Your Unseen Energy Centers

THERE'S MORE TO US HUMANS than meets the eye. Within and encircling our bodies are unseen centers of energy that affect everything we do and say. In this chapter you will learn about your energy centers and their relationship with yoga, and you'll have a chance for some first-hand experience with them.

In this chapter...

✓ Getting to know your energy centers

✓ The yoga/chakra connection

✓ Playing in your energy field

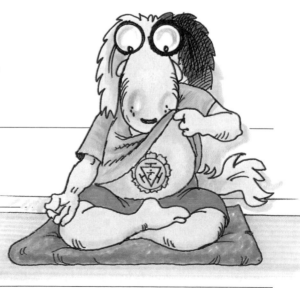

BALANCE YOUR ENERGY CENTERS AND INCREASE YOUR ZEST FOR LIFE

Getting to know your energy centers

ACCORDING TO THE SCIENCE OF YOGA *(and the broader realm of Eastern medicine), the body is made up of centers of energy called chakras that are not visible to most of us. Those who can see chakras say that these fields of energy are like fluid whirlpools of light, each with its own color, that are constantly moving and changing in complex patterns. They say that chakras function as intake organs for energy from the universal life force that is all around us (remember prana and chi from the last chapter?).*

DEFINITION

The energy centers, or vortices, that flow through and around the human body are called chakras, which literally means "circles" or "wheels" in Sanskrit.

Chakras are vital to your health

Eastern medicine recognizes seven major chakras (and many minor ones) that interact with the body, and an eighth chakra that encompasses them all. Though largely unseen, our chakras interact with and influence our thoughts, moods, and health. Chakras are like the air we breathe: invisible yet vital to our lives.

Each chakra is located at a major nerve plexus of the body and is intricately involved in keeping the body organs of that area in proper working order.

Through the intake and assimilation of life energy, each chakra rejuvenates its corresponding body parts. If a chakra stops functioning properly, the intake of energy will be disturbed, and eventually that part of the body will show signs of disease.

The eight chakras

Energy flows through the entire body from the chakras, six of which are located in the body. The seventh chakra is located at the top of the skull, and the eighth chakra is the *aura* that encases and interpenetrates the entire body. All the main chakras are connected by a channel of energy that travels up the center of the spine

DEFINITION

The energy field that surrounds and interpenetrates the body is called the aura. It is considered by yogis and many healers to be the energetic framework upon which the physical body rests.

and around the brain. It is interesting to note that the colors of the chakras follow the same order as the colors of the rainbow, starting with red for the first chakra, and moving through the spectrum of colors as they move upward toward the head.

Each chakra has an important function to perform for you, and you need all of them. The first, second, and third chakras are sometimes referred to as the "lower" chakras, but don't let the word fool you. They are just as important as the "higher" centers (the fourth through eighth chakras). As you learn about the chakras in the section below, you will notice that the first three chakras deal with the physical needs of the body and the basic needs of the mind. The last five chakras work within the psychological and spiritual realms.

1. The **first chakra** is located at the rectum and base of the spine at the conjunction of thousands of nerve endings. This is your root, your basic survival chakra. An imbalance in the first chakra may show up in the form of fear, perversion, and insecurity. When this chakra is working well, you feel grounded and confident.

2. The **second chakra** is located at the third and fourth vertebrae and just above the pubic bone. It governs sex and reproduction, emotions, and creativity. An imbalance in the second chakra brings obsession with sex or unhealthy indulgence of fantasy. A person whose second chakra is in balance is creative, imaginative, adaptable, and has a healthy sex life.

If a chakra is imbalanced, its brilliance and circular movement are weak. When all of the chakras are fairly equal in strength, they are considered to be balanced.

3. The **third chakra** is located at the solar plexus/navel area where the nerve endings meet. It deals with concerns of identity, domain, and judgment. When in a state of imbalance, the third chakra can manifest itself as excessive greed, or an overwhelming drive for personal power. Excessive emotions and susceptibility to illness characterize a weak third chakra. Conversely, a strong third chakra can give good physical health. When in balance, it gives the initiative and courage to persevere and accomplish great deeds.

Trivia...

Just as the umbilical cord connects the unborn child and mother, the third chakra is the connecting cord to our feelings of belonging to and bonding with others.

4. The **fourth chakra,** known as the heart center, is located in the center of the chest, not at the physical heart. A person who has an imbalance in the heart center may seem "cold-hearted," will have trouble expressing love, or will be selfish in matters of the heart. When the heart chakra becomes active, true love can be experienced. It is the center for kindness, compassion, and selfless acts of giving.

Through the heart center, you connect cords to those with whom you have a love relationship. When you say someone is "tugging at your heartstrings," you are expressing this connection absolutely accurately!

5 The **fifth chakra** is located at the throat and is associated with the thyroid gland and lungs. Words that are penetrating, true, and compassionate come from a strong fifth chakra. In an imbalance, blunt or opinionated communication can be the result, or a person may be too fearful to express himself at all. The fifth chakra is also associated with taking responsibility for personal needs – being able to create what you need and receive what is given to you.

6 The **sixth chakra** is located at the center of the forehead, slightly above the eyebrows and 1 in (3 cm) in from the surface. This area is sometimes called the "third eye." It is associated with the pituitary gland, and is considered to be the source of *intuition*. The sixth chakra relates to your capacity to visualize and understand mental concepts, including how you see the world and expect the world to respond to you. When working properly, the sixth chakra can help manifest visions for the benefit of all. When it's imbalanced, a person's basic concepts are not based in reality, and his world may reflect this distortion.

> **DEFINITION**
>
> Intuition *is immediate insight or understanding without conscious reasoning. When you are intuitive, you "know" what is "unknowable" through the senses.*

7 The **seventh chakra** is located at the top of the skull (the crown) and is associated with the pineal gland. It relates to the integration of personality with *spirituality*. If this center is weak, a person may not have an experiential connection to her spirituality or an understanding of what people are talking about when they speak of spiritual experiences. If this center is strong, the person probably will experience her own unique brand of spirituality.

> **DEFINITION**
>
> *The word* **spirituality** *is used to describe a state of being, beyond dogma, that transcends physical existence, and creates a sense of wholeness, peace, and higher purposefulness in a person.*

Trivia...
Kirlian photography is a means of taking pictures of energy patterns and force fields, which are usually unseen by the human eye. Kirlian researchers photographed an image of an entire leaf after half of it was cut away, which revealed that the energy field of the entire leaf was intact.

8 The **eighth chakra**, also called the aura, is the luminous energy field that surrounds and interpenetrates the entire body. The aura is the protective shield that encloses the other chakras. It protects you from incoming negativity and transmittable disease and gives you the power to project your vision into reality.

The aura changes in color, brightness, and size depending upon your general physical health, your thoughts, and your feelings. It normally extends several feet in every direction, and can grow brighter and larger with consistent body/mind/spirit practices, such as yoga and meditation.

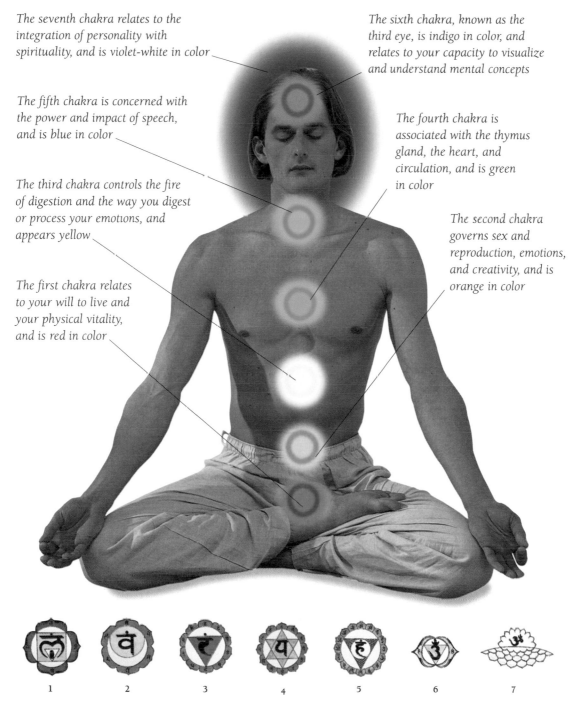

The seventh chakra relates to the integration of personality with spirituality, and is violet-white in color

The sixth chakra, known as the third eye, is indigo in color, and relates to your capacity to visualize and understand mental concepts

The fifth chakra is concerned with the power and impact of speech, and is blue in color

The fourth chakra is associated with the thymus gland, the heart, and circulation, and is green in color

The third chakra controls the fire of digestion and the way you digest or process your emotions, and appears yellow

The second chakra governs sex and reproduction, emotions, and creativity, and is orange in color

The first chakra relates to your will to live and your physical vitality, and is red in color

1   2   3   4   5   6   7

■ **Yogic tradition** often portrays the chakras as lotus flowers, each with a certain number of petals. In the center of each is a letter, or sound, from the Sanskrit alphabet.

CREATING A WATERFALL

To get a sense of just how palpable your aura is, try this yoga relaxation technique, which I introduced as "Waterfall" to my Montessori students.

1. Ask a child or a friend to lie face down, head turned to the side, eyes closed. Begin gently stroking the person from head to foot with short, flowing, feather-light strokes.

2. After a minute, begin to stroke more and more lightly until finally you are stroking a few inches away from the person's physical body.

3. For another minute, imagine you are creating a relaxing waterfall as you brush the aura, stroking downward and off the ends of the feet. Then switch places.

The yoga/chakra connection

NOW THAT YOU ARE AWARE *of your flowing patterns of energy, you may be wondering how the chakras relate to yoga. Or you may have already figured out that yoga helps keep the chakra-wheels spinning and in balance.*

The place where the majority of your energy is centered is your home base, and it influences your basic behavior and outlook on life. Of course, this home base can change, depending on how you grow and change your life, for better or worse.

Each of you has one (or two) particular chakras where most of your energy is focused.

When you practice yoga, you recharge and balance your chakras by bringing circulation and prana to the nerve plexus at each of the chakras.

INTERNET

www.barbarabrennan .com

Barbara Brennan is a remarkable healer and former NASA scientist who works with the human energy field and chakras. This site has information about her books and The Barbara Brennan School of Healing training program.

It may come as no surprise to find out that these centers correspond with the acupressure meridians and pressure points we talked about in Chapter 2.

When you check into the various yoga schools available in your area, you will find a wide range of differences in their emphasis on chakras. Some forms of yoga actively work to balance the chakras and activate the "higher" centers.

Many meditation practices have the intuitive and crown chakras as their focal points. Other schools of yoga do not focus on chakras at all, although a sincere and consistent yoga practice of any tradition will eventually strengthen and balance the chakras and energy field.

It is important to realize that when you practice yoga, you don't need to know or believe anything at all about chakras!

Just as eating wholesome foods will make you healthier, whether you think about it or not, the life energy in your body will circulate more efficiently in the practice of yoga, no matter how you view it.

Playing in your energy field

SO MUCH TALK ABOUT CHAKRAS *has probably put you in your "mental" center, so let's try something to give you a feel for your energy field. Remember, your energy field, or aura, is the surrounding and interpenetrating field of light around and inside you. You have probably felt this field many times before; perhaps you just didn't have a name for the sensation you experienced.*

Have you ever gotten up in the middle of the night to use the bathroom and had a sense of where to go and what to avoid while groping around in the pitch darkness? You may have come within inches of bumping your nose into the wall, but stopped in time.

What made you stop? From the point of view of energy fields, your aura bumped the wall first. You were sensitive to it and automatically stopped moving in that direction.

Trivia...
Those who have studied the human energy field, such as radionics specialist Dr. David Tansley, say that the seven major chakras are formed at the points where the lines of light cross each other 21 times, creating vortices of energy. There are many minor chakras where lines cross each other 14 or 7 times, forming small vortices, which seem to correspond to acupuncture points in the body.

EXPLORING YOUR ENERGY FIELD

It's fun to explore your energy field through your imagination, but even more fun to experience it directly. Here is a little "hands-on" experiment to try:

1. Bring your hands to about the level of your solar plexus. Have your palms facing each other, 2 to 5 in (5 to 13 cm) apart. Slowly move your hands closer together but not touching. Then slowly open them wider until they are about 6 in (15 cm) apart. Keep moving them in and out. Feel the space between your hands as though it were solid matter. Can you feel something building there? What does it feel like?

2. Now slowly move your hands about 8 in (20 cm) apart, and then just as slowly bring them back together to the point at which you feel a pressure pushing against your palms. Notice if you have to use slightly more force to bring them close. You have just touched together the edges of the energy fields of your right and left hands.

3. Keep your left hand still and slowly move your right palm closer to the left until you can actually feel the energy field of your right hand touch the skin on your left palm. How does it feel? Does it have a temperature sensation?

Many people describe the sensation of feeling their energy field as a warmth, a feeling similar to static electricity on the skin, a tickling feeling, or a spongy pressure between the hands.

Don't be discouraged if you didn't feel anything. Remember, this chakra and aura stuff is pretty subtle! If it interests you, try, try again. And keep in mind that your practice of yoga will also help you become aware of these and other subtleties of life.

It is daytime in our next scenario. Imagine you are in an elevator. Another person gets in. He stays 3 ft (1 m) away from you. You are each in your own auric space, so to speak. Then the elevator stops and picks up another person. She naturally positions herself so that the three auras are touching as little as possible.

At the next floor, two more people get in, and since this is a small elevator, everyone is no more than 6 in (15 cm) from each other. A person is standing to your side, 5 or 6 in (13 to 15 cm) away.

Can you feel his energy field overlap with yours? Does it feel warm or cool? Can you sense anything about this person from his aura? How does it feel when he moves away from you after a few people get out of the elevator?

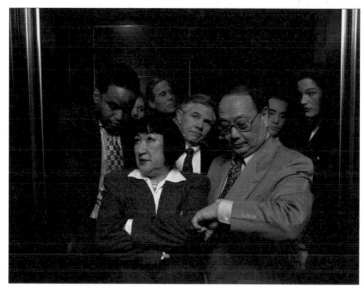

■ **A crowded elevator** *is an ideal place to test your sensitivity to other people's auras. Check out whether you can feel the energy field of the person closest to you, and what you can sense from it.*

A simple summary

✔ Eastern teachings say that the body is made up of eight chakras: Seven major energy centers and a surrounding energy field called the aura.

✔ Our chakras take in universal life energy for use by the physical body. Though mostly unseen, they influence our thoughts, moods, and health.

✔ Yoga helps keep the chakra-wheels spinning and in balance. When you practice yoga, you recharge and balance your chakras with prana (life energy).

✔ You do not need to focus on the chakras, or even believe in their existence, in order to practice yoga. It is totally optional!

✔ You can sensitize yourself to your energy field by becoming aware of the space around you and feeling it.

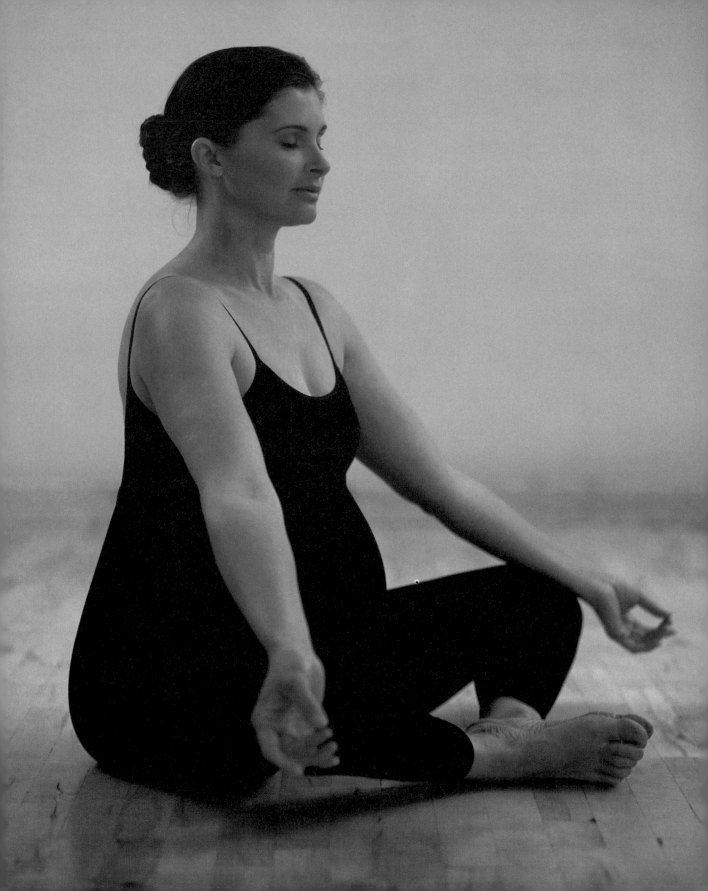

Chapter 4

Who Can Do Yoga?

THE ANSWER TO THIS QUESTION is quite simply you. You can do yoga because it helps you achieve well-being no matter what shape you and your life are in. Many people don't consider themselves candidates for yoga because they feel they would have to make too many dramatic changes in their lifestyle. Some commonly expressed thoughts include, "When I get in shape I can start," or "I have to quit smoking first." In this chapter you'll find encouragement to begin yoga just as you are.

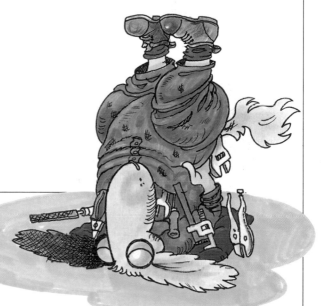

In this chapter...

✓ Something for everyone

✓ Ask yourself what you want

✓ Starting new habits

YOGA'S FOCUS ON BREATHING HELPS MANY WOMEN DURING PREGNANCY AND LABOR

Something for everyone

WHEN SOMETHING HELPS YOU *make positive changes in your life, you want to keep doing it. But when it is totally natural, has no harmful side effects, and goes with you wherever you go as well, you want to tell the world about it! That's how I feel about yoga. And that's why I became a yoga teacher. Twenty-five years and thousands of students later, I cannot say that any two of my yoga students have been in the same shape, have had the same reasons for coming to class, or have gotten the same things out of yoga.*

My students have been office workers, pregnant women, priests, recovering addicts, college students, teens, doctors, mothers, fathers, children, seniors, construction workers, corporate executives, computer whizzes, couch potatoes, heart patients, salespeople, athletes, artists, musicians, school teachers, factory workers, cancer survivors, grandmothers, grandfathers – and babies! I have taught yoga to the overweight, overworked, underpaid, overstressed, undervalued people of this world (which includes most of us!), and the only thing everyone had in common was that each had a unique relationship to yoga.

■ **The beauty of yoga** *is that you're never too old (or too young) to start. And every individual who takes up yoga reaps different benefits from it.*

Unique is the key word. No one can tell you what you will get out of yoga. That journey is yours alone. Think about fingers: Yours – and everyone else's – are made of the same stuff: Skin, bone, muscle. But even though there are millions of us in the world, each of our fingerprints is unique.

Different strokes . . .

Different folks have different reasons for taking up yoga. And different folks bring different abilities to their practice of yoga. Here are a few of their stories:

● Sarah, a young office worker, uses yoga to help her with back and neck pain. Through yoga, she becomes aware of her body's proper alignment, and applies that awareness to her posture while sitting at her desk every day.

- A professional athlete, Stan practices yoga not only to tone muscles but also to strengthen "mental muscles" for better focus and self-control under the pressure of athletic competition.

- Corina is a breast cancer survivor. She feels grateful that she has been given the chance to live, and uses yoga and meditation to help clear out past hurts and fears that she feels were instrumental in causing her cancer.

- Randy is a retail store owner who began coming to yoga classes twice a week after discovering he had heart problems. He says that yoga helps him cope with the pressures of his business without taking a toll on his health.

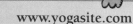

INTERNET

www.yogasite.com

This is an Internet-based resource center for anything related to yoga. It provides lots of great information and links to other yoga sites as well.

- For years Diana has struggled with being overweight. She sees yoga as a way to relax her mind and relieve the desire to overeat. In addition to being a good source of exercise, yoga helps to regulate the glandular system, which controls the metabolism.

- For Mary Ann, a senior citizen, yoga is an opportunity to feel the peace of mind and contentment that is the natural result of a life well lived. Yoga's gentle stretches lessen Mary Ann's arthritis pain by strengthening her muscles and giving protection to her joints.

- Jerry is a corporate executive who uses yoga to lower the stress level and raise the quality of his life. As his blood pressure and heart rate go down, the opportunity to enjoy his life more fully goes up.

- Leslie brings her 9-year-old son, Brian, to yoga classes for help with learning disabilities and hyperactivity. Yoga helps balance the two hemispheres of the brain, and helps Brian develop a calm and focused mind.

■ **As well as being fun,** *yoga can enhance children's physical and mental health, and help develop self-discipline.*

● Janice, who is pregnant, wants to relax and create a calm environment for her unborn baby. She knows yoga will help tremendously when the time comes for the baby to be born. In addition to strengthening and stretching the pelvic muscles, yoga's focus on the breath comes in handy during labor.

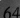

If you have a medical condition, don't practice yoga until you've consulted a medical doctor.

Begin where you are

The body you have is the body you begin with in yoga. All schools and styles of yoga are designed to start you off with poses and exercises that, while they may be challenging, are not impossible.

Always remember that although yoga is highly adaptable, it is designed for people who are in a normal state of health, so be sure that you have your doctor's okay before you begin. Many yoga centers also have props, such as belts, cushions, and blankets, to assist you with more challenging postures.

■ **Yoga is a relaxing** *way to exercise during pregnancy. Combining breathing exercises with muscle-strengthening poses will help you prepare both body and mind for labor.*

Concentrate on your own capabilities

Don't worry about doing yoga wrong. First of all, keep in mind that yoga is non-competitive. Most of the time everyone in the class will close their eyes, and even

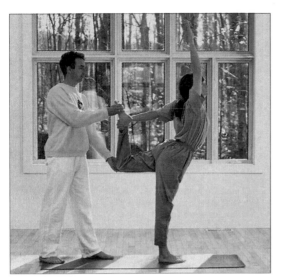

■ **Your yoga instructor** *may help you with gentle adjustments to your posture, so that you can get the most out of yoga.*

when they're open, the focus is inward. Secondly, yoga's motto is, "To the best of your ability." Trained instructors will guide you with clear instruction, kind encouragement, and gentle adjustments to your posture.

If yoga were based on how well you can twist yourself up or perform headstands, then acrobats in the circus would be the best yogis! But that is not true, and why not? Because yoga goes much deeper than this. Yoga accepts your body the way it is, and works with it from there. And because it is *holistic*, yoga affects us positively on every level, from mind, to body, to spirit.

> **DEFINITION**
>
> A holistic *approach to health considers the whole of a person's being (body, mind, and spirit), rather than the separate parts.*

You are not your habits

Many people believe that in order to start practicing yoga, they need to change their lifestyle or even be a different kind of person. Sometimes the feeling is "I'm not good enough, so I shouldn't even start." Perhaps you feel that if you drink alcohol, smoke, or eat meat or "junk food," you will be pressured (either externally or internally) to change your habits overnight. On the contrary, yoga is about moderation, not abstinence! It is for those who want to live in the world, not withdraw from it.

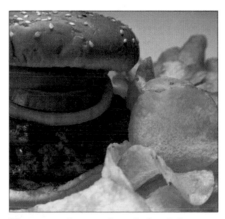

■ **Being a lover of junk food** *doesn't disqualify you from practicing yoga – you can add yoga to your life without having to change your lifestyle in any way.*

The master of your internal house is you, not your habits. When you courageously start yoga with whatever habits you have, soon enough you will find your lifestyle changing. As always, it's up to you to choose how you want your life to change. If you want to keep your life the way it is and add yoga, that is possible, too. The ball is always in your court.

Ask yourself what you want

RIGHT NOW TAKE A COUPLE OF MINUTES
*to jot down as many of your specific goals and desires as
you can think of. They can be on any level you want them
to be – changes in your attitude or the way you respond to
certain situations, changes in your habits, changes in your
physical body, changes in your present life situation –
anything goes! Don't even think about yoga yet. Just focus
on your goals and desires.*

Now look at your list and consider what you know about the
benefits of yoga. You can refer back to Chapter 2, *Why Yoga
Feels So Good*, for help. Visualize how your
needs can be fulfilled by doing yoga.
Whatever the outcome you desire, see if
you can find a match for it through yoga.

Keep this list because you will be able to
use it in the next chapter, where I discuss
how to find a yoga class
that's right for you. You
will find that the different schools of yoga vary as
much as people's individual needs and abilities do.

Trivia...

*Some people find that they
are more interested in
meditation than yoga. If you
are one of them, you are in
luck! Some paths of yoga
focus mainly on meditation.
And although they may start
with yoga postures or
exercises in order to prepare
the body and mind to
meditate, meditation is their
main focus. People who use
a wheelchair, are confined to
bed, or have limited ability
to move often find breath
work and meditation to be a
perfect, powerful match for
their particular needs.*

Opening up to new possibilities

Is your idea of who you are based on your past? If so,
you can let go of those old blocks and swim to a new shore
– or to the wide open sea for that matter! It is your choice to
have a specific goal in mind (the new shore), or to be open to
new possibilities (the wide open sea). Yoga helps you discover
which way you want to go in this process.

Yoga can help you take control of your well-being.
Visualize what you want your life to be like, and have
faith that it can become a reality. Add a practice of
yoga to that vision, and you can change your life.
It may be gradual, or it may be dramatic, but change
happens with yoga.

■ **Writing down** *your goals and desires
will help you focus on the ways in which
yoga can be used to achieve them.*

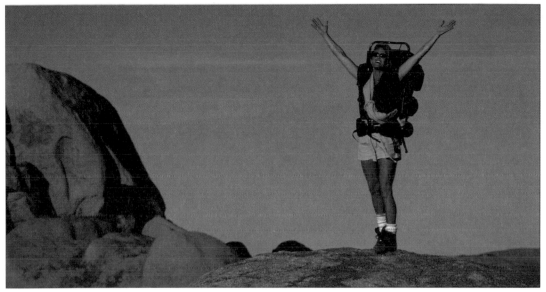

■ **Imagine achieving a long-term goal,** *such as traveling to a place you have always longed to visit. Add a practice of yoga to that vision and you can more easily realize your dream.*

Starting new habits

IN THE SCIENCE OF YOGA, *it is said that it takes 40 days to change a habit, 90 days to confirm the new habit, 120 days for the new habit to become who you are, and in 1,000 days, you will have mastered the habit! Just as the steady dripping of water will eventually wear a hole in stone, little by little and step by step you can change old habits. Remember that the habit you want to change has been functioning as an internal pattern for a long time, so it will take a while for your body and brain to adjust to new patterns.*

Give yourself some room to grow, and most of all be kind to yourself through the process.

Recognizing your anxiety

Looking for the best time to start your new yoga habit can slow you down. Yogi Bhajan, a great yoga master, put it this way. "When the time is on you, start, and the pressure will be off." For most people, the anxiety of anticipation is much worse than actually doing the thing they're so anxious about!

For example, it seems like every time I start writing a new book, I am excited and anxious at the same time. I go through a mountain of mental blocks. Will I be able to communicate what I want to say? How well can I do this? What if this and what if that? Eventually I manage to begin the project. Then, it is just me and the book, and I find a flow with it. I have to laugh when I think of all the mental energy I wasted in anticipating problems!

Substitute a positive thought

Remember the Yoga sutras of Patanjali from Chapter 1? One of the guiding principles is called pratyahara. This is the process of becoming aware of and controlling the thought waves of your mind. In practical terms, it can mean substituting negative thoughts with positive ones.

This concept is not as unusual as it might seem. Many of you learned about pratyahara as children when you read the story *The Little Engine That Could*. Remember the little engine's mantra, "I think I can, I think I can," as she puffed and pulled herself up the hill, and "I knew I could, I knew I could," as she triumphantly came down the hill? You don't tell

Trivia...

According to a study done at the American Public Health Institute, middle-aged people who give up hope are at a greater risk of dying of heart disease. The study followed the subjects' attitudes toward life, and used ultrasound scans on their arteries. Four years and 942 people later, the conclusion was that giving up hope has the same effect on the arteries of a middle-aged person as smoking 20 cigarettes a day.

that story to your children for nothing. You tell it because you believe innately that "as you think so shall you be."

When you catch yourself thinking, "I am a failure," or "This won't work out," substitute these thoughts with, "I can do it," or "Everything's coming my way." A positive mantra goes a long way, especially if you truly believe it.

Pratyahara applies to habits, too. Every time you have the urge to repeat a habit you no longer want, substitute it with a positive habit. People do this all the time without thinking too much about it. Smokers, for example, often quit by substituting chewing gum for cigarettes.

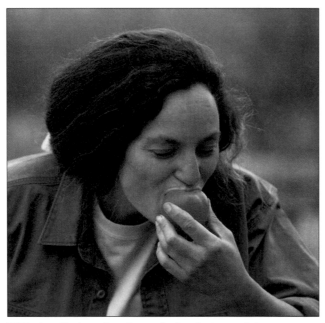

■ **Eating fruit** *rather than a high-calorie snack is one way that dieters substitute a positive habit for a negative one.*

As you practice yoga and your internal state of being begins to change, you may find that some of your old habits no longer serve you. Often they fade away naturally, and are replaced by healthy new habits.

Yoga students often tell me that they no longer feel like eating the foods they used to love but which had harmful effects on their bodies and minds.

Many people feel that the practice of yoga sensitizes them to what they are putting into their bodies. They consistently say that they like the feeling of being healthy more than the momentary enjoyment of eating something tasty but unhealthy. Most of them attribute this change directly to their practice of yoga.

So, now that you know yoga is right for you, can we declare this pep talk a success, and move on to the next chapter in which you will begin the process of finding a yoga class that's right for you?

A simple summary

✔ What you get out of a yoga practice is uniquely yours. No two people come to yoga with the same goals, and yoga is adaptable to everyone's needs.

✔ Yoga is non-competitive. Everyone participates to the best of his or her ability.

✔ Yoga fits with any lifestyle. You don't have to change your habits, but if you have habits you would like to change, they will be affected positively by a continued practice of yoga.

✔ You can use a yogic technique called pratyahara to substitute a new positive thought for an old thought that you feel is holding you back. You can also apply this technique to changing habits.

✔ Give yourself room to grow, and be kind to yourself in the process.

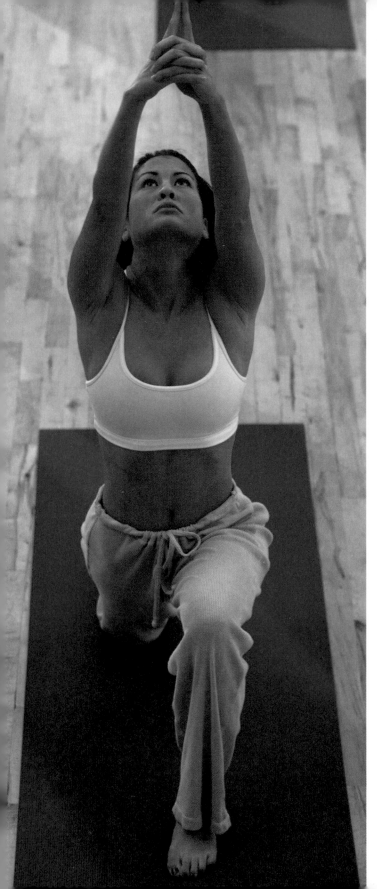

PART TWO

DISCOVER WHAT YOGA CAN DO FOR YOU

EXPLORING STYLES OF YOGA

THE PLACE TO START is simply to know what you want from yoga, and then where to find it. There are as many reasons to do yoga as there are people. And everyone brings different capabilities to yoga. You will find that different styles of yoga will agree with different people's needs and capabilities.

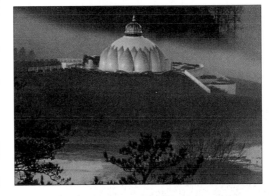

A wide variety of styles and schools of yoga awaits you within these pages. I would suggest you try all of them at some time or another to *experience* and *celebrate* the unity within the *wonderful diversity* of yoga.

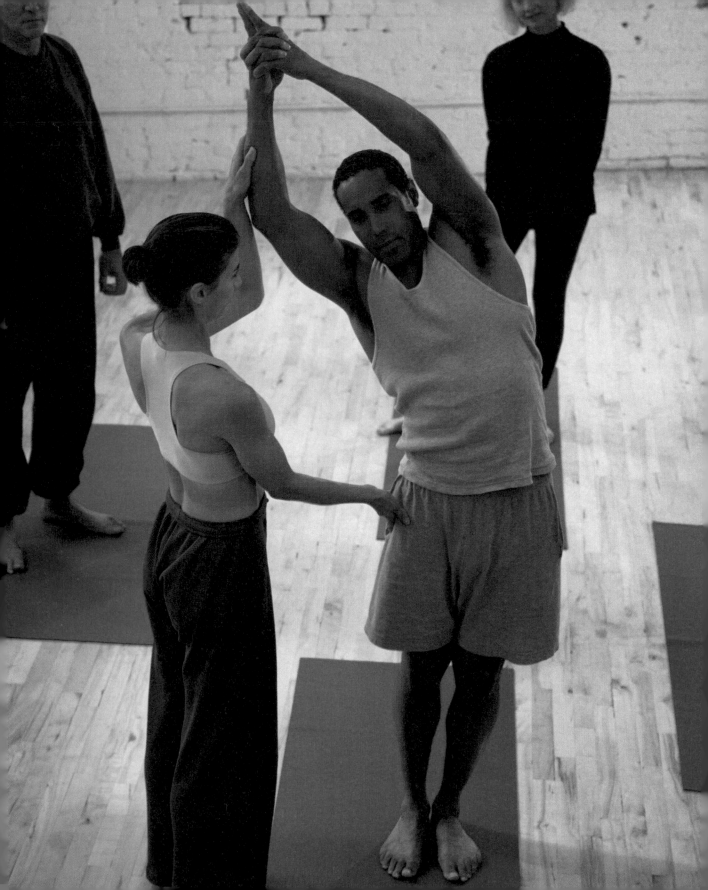

Chapter 5

Getting Started

How do you shop for yoga? Together we'll sort through the practicalities of finding yoga classes that fit with you. You'll find out who to call, where to look, what kind of paraphernalia you might need, how to stay motivated, and how to practice yoga on your own.

In this chapter...

✓ Questions to ask yourself

✓ Where to look

✓ Questions for the teacher

✓ Be prepared

✓ Staying aware

✓ Give it a chance

✓ Your home practice

✓ Warm-up yoga

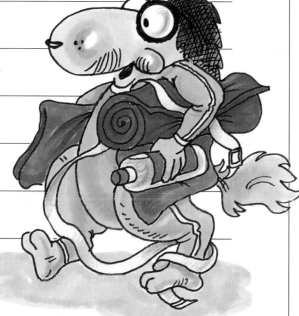

FINDING A GOOD TEACHER IS AN IMPORTANT FIRST STEP

Questions to ask yourself

HOW TO DECIDE WHICH CLASS TO TAKE? *The decision maker for many people is the answer to the very pragmatic question: How far away is it? If you ask ten people why they take yoga in a particular place, at least five of them will say that the location is convenient. Not that the style of the class isn't important but, in some cases, their attachment to a particular style of yoga grew out of their number-one concern: Location, location, location! You would have to really love a class to drive a long distance to get there and back, and some people will do that. It all depends on your priorities and, to some degree, on your time.*

Is the environment important?

Fortunately, in most areas there are yoga classes in numerous locations. Yoga classes are most often taught in either yoga centers and studios, or in sports and fitness clubs. (In the past 15 years, most sports and fitness clubs have added yoga to their standard offering of classes.) It's good to consider whether you'd like to be in a cozy studio, a room in someone's home, or a large gymnasium with mirrors covering the walls. Some people don't care. Others are very sensitive to their environment. This is one factor, among many, to consider in your search.

What do I want from yoga?

It is time to get out your list from Chapter 4, or, if you didn't write one, make one now, even if you don't write it down. Now, contemplate your list for a moment, and then, without too much thinking, just write down, or say aloud, one or two main ideas that sum up your interest in yoga. Keep these main goals and desires in mind when you call around and check for classes.

My goals

- to relax
- to let go of stress
- to remember to be happy and grateful
- to strengthen my muscles, especially arms and abdominals
- to tone my body
- to be more flexible in body (and mind)
- to help me not get angry
- to help me not feel anxious
- to keep me from overeating
- to give me clarity in making decisions
- to deepen my spiritual side

■ **Your list of reasons** *for taking up yoga may be similar to this one, but it will be unique to you.*

In the next few chapters you will get to know all the yoga "brands," both by reading about them and by experiencing each one. You will also see that within all these different styles and schools of yoga, there are many variations and interpretations, depending on the teacher you choose. Often people go with the teacher they resonate with the best, no matter what the style.

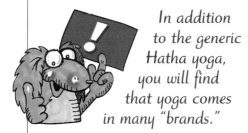

In addition to the generic Hatha yoga, you will find that yoga comes in many "brands."

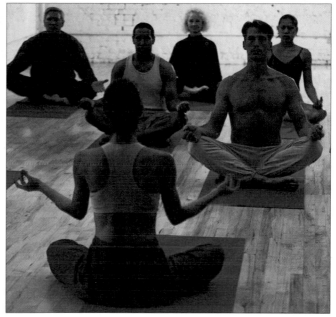

■ **The type of yoga class** *you decide to take may depend on a number of factors, including the teacher, the type of yoga taught, and how convenient the venue is for you.*

What are my limitations?

Your limitations can be physical or psychological. Of course, if you have a serious physical limitation, you should seek the advice of a physician. Let's say you have a situation where your knee cannot bend all the way, or it goes out of place easily. You will want to find out how that fits with the style of yoga you are inquiring about, and mention any physical limitations to the teacher before trying the class.

A psychological limitation might be that you would like yoga classes in which you do postures and exercise your body, but you don't want to sit still and meditate. Decide honestly if what you are expressing is a self-imposed limitation, a simple preference, or a genuine limitation. If it is a genuine limitation, feel fine about not participating. If it is a simple preference, it is your right to decline, and it is your right to push through the limitation. If you are honest enough to assess that it is a self-imposed limitation, you may find great freedom on the other side of those doors. Still, the choice is always yours.

Yoga can be hard work as well as sweet repose. When you push the edge of your comfort zone, you emerge from the experience with a new level of awareness and confidence.

Where to look

THE MOST LOGICAL PLACE to look for yoga classes may well be in the Yellow Pages under the heading Yoga. You can also try looking in local magazines and newspapers that are oriented toward holistic health, including a weekly alternative paper, if your area has one. Flyers and business cards in natural food stores are always a good bet. Plus, be sure to check local community centers and sports clubs. (Some sports club classes are for members only, so make sure to ask.)

INTERNET

www.yogajournal.com

www.yogainternational.com

Both of these online magazines annually print extensive directories of yoga teachers. Both have wonderful articles about yoga, book reviews, yoga retreats, and much more as well.

Finding a teacher through a friend's recommendation is probably the most common way to find a class. If you trust your friend's judgment, you will probably do well to follow her lead. At least it will be a good starting place in your yoga adventure.

Most classes range in price between $8 and $18 per class, depending on the geographic area and the length of the class, and run from 1 to 1½ hours. Often classes are organized into longer sessions, but usually it is possible to try a single class for a fee. Some classes allow you to drop in any time for a slightly higher fee. Others are open classes, meaning anyone can come at any time without committing to a whole session.

INTERNET

www.yogafinder.com

Yoga Finder is a web site specifically to help you find classes and teachers throughout the world.

Many yoga centers have a week or so of "sample" classes before a session starts, so you could try several with different teachers. Generally, centers start classes in the fall, with the next session starting in January, and the spring sessions around April. Classes begin in the summer too, but sometimes there are not as many to choose from because summer vacations take priority, and summer, in general, is a slow time for classes.

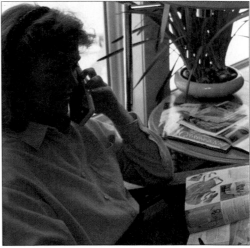

■ **Health and lifestyle magazines** *sometimes feature articles on yoga, with listings of recommended centers. It's a good idea to call and find out more before signing up for a course.*

Questions for the teacher

A TEACHER WILL NOT ONLY INSTRUCT YOU and demonstrate poses, but will observe you, give you personal feedback, and may assist you with hands-on help. Some teachers welcome questions during the class, while others like to keep a meditative atmosphere and will like you to save all but the most urgent questions until the end of class.

Some good questions to ask a teacher before trying the class are:

a What is a typical class like?

b What is the general philosophy of the school of yoga?

c What kind of yoga background does the teacher have?

Trained and experienced?

When you call a yoga teacher or center, you often are asked to leave your name and address for a brochure. In addition to listing a class schedule, most centers will outline their philosophy, training, and experience in a brochure. But I find that

THE YOGA ALLIANCE

Until recently there was no organized way of monitoring the quality and authenticity of yoga teachers. It was especially difficult to have standards, considering the scope and diversity of the many types of yoga that have developed – at least a hundred, probably more!

In 1999 a diverse group of yoga teachers and organizations in the US formed the Yoga Alliance. In addition to working to design a unified minimum standard, Yoga Alliance is a voluntary group dedicated to providing support and upholding the rights of yoga teachers. When teachers are members of Yoga Alliance, they will have the initials R.Y.T. (Registered Yoga Teacher) after their names.

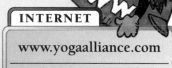

INTERNET

www.yogaalliance.com

Find out more about Yoga Alliance at this web site.

I get a good feel for someone over the phone, and if you're like that too, call and ask to speak with a teacher.

You may want to ask what the teacher's training and experience are, and if they are certified by any particular school of yoga. Teacher training for yoga varies greatly and can be as little as a week and as much as a few years.

You'll want to ask about experience too. There are fantastic teachers who have no certification but who have 20 or 30 years of teaching experience. That ought to count for something!

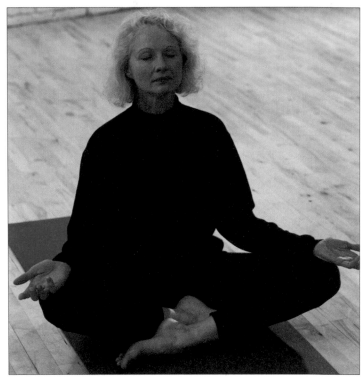

■ **When looking for a yoga instructor,** *remember that certification isn't everything: Many years of teaching experience is a first-rate qualification in itself.*

Use your intuition

Remember your sixth chakra, the center of your intuition? Here's where you get to apply your intuitive sense of what "feels right." You can get a good feel for someone simply by having a conversation with him or her. You may like more than one of the teachers you speak with, so try several classes. What have you got to lose? Yoga shopping may be just what you need. Just don't shop till you drop – that's just not the point of yoga!

A good yoga teacher will:
● know the various effects of yoga and meditation
● have a working understanding of the body's physiology
● give clear instructions and demonstrations
● know how to adapt yoga postures to the individual's capabilities
● distinguish between their personal and/or religious beliefs and yoga
● encourage students with inspiration and kindness

Be prepared

FIND OUT BEFORE CLASS WHAT YOU NEED to bring and wear.
Many yoga centers have mats and equipment that you can use, especially if it
is your first time.

What to wear?

Now that you've found a class that you like, the age-old
question comes up, "What should I wear?" The
answer is simple: Wear something that is
comfortable to move in. Lightweight cotton shirts
and pants with elastic waistbands work well.
Some styles of yoga will prefer no baggy clothes,
as they obscure body alignment. Often leggings
or shorts and T-shirts or tank tops are
recommended. Common sense will tell you to
leave your dangling earrings and pendant at home.
If you are coming from work, bring your yoga
clothes with you.

Mat matters

Most Hatha classes use what is called a sticky mat.
This is a simple piece of thin rubberized material that
fits the length of your body. The advantage of the sticky
mat is that it helps your feet and hands stick when you
need them to – such as when you are balancing on one
foot! It also provides a thin
cushion between you and the
floor (and some yoga centers
have hardwood floors).

A kind of felt-like woolen blanket
is also used in some yoga classes.
You can use it for more
cushioning under your body
when you are lying down, and
it also can be used to sit on.
(More on this in the next few
chapters where we'll talk about
yoga props.)

Trivia...

Yogis of old often wore
nothing more than a
loincloth, a very small body
covering made from a piece of
cotton that wrapped through
the groin and around the
pelvis. Long before TV and
baseball, they were the
original Yogi Bares!

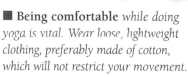
■ **Being comfortable** *while doing*
yoga is vital. Wear loose, lightweight
clothing, preferably made of cotton,
which will not restrict your movement.

If you don't have a mat or blanket, many yoga centers provide them. Most people eventually like to buy their own. That's because in some classes you can really work up a sweat, which finds its way to your mat. And remember, you will be getting quite intimate with your mat every time you lie face down on it.

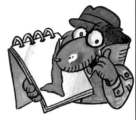

For Hatha yoga, it is important to be able to stick on a thin surface at times. I prefer to have a natural surface underneath me and use a wool blanket, or a sheepskin, which doesn't slip. In the yogic science, it is said animal skins insulate your energy field from that of the Earth, facilitating meditation.

Trivia...

You may want to keep your hair off your face, or at least have a way of tying it back if it is long enough. Hair tied at the nape of the neck may work better than in a ponytail, which can be uncomfortable when you're lying on your back.

Some students like to bring a pillow to sit on and a lightweight shawl for covering during meditation or deep relaxation. During yoga, you can build up an inner (and outer) heat, which then cools off during the relaxation. To avoid feeling a chill, cover yourself. You will probably want to try some classes and see which, if any, of these yoga paraphernalia you will need.

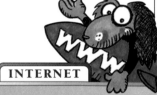

INTERNET

www.gaiam.com

This is one of the finest sources for all kinds of yoga, meditation, and relaxation tools. It is also the producer of the well-known catalog Living Arts. Whether online or browsing the catalog, you'll find yoga mats, pillows, clothing, books, and videos to get you started in yoga.

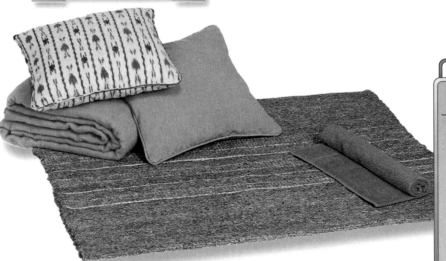

■ **Use a yoga mat** *for extra cushioning, a blanket to keep you warm during relaxation exercises, and a cushion when meditating. Have a towel at hand for wiping off any sweat.*

No to food, yes to water

Try to eat no more than 2 hours prior to your class. If you must eat, make it light, such as fruit or a yogurt at least an hour before class. But do be sure to bring purified water with you. Especially drink if you are sweating, and always drink water after class to rebalance yourself.

DEFINITION

Pure water *is water that has been filtered to remove nitrates, pesticides, and metal traces.* Spring water *is water that is naturally pure, as it comes directly from a mountain spring.*

During yoga, toxins get stirred up and are just waiting to be flushed out. That's where water goes to work. Drink pure water or spring water, not only during yoga, but often during the day — at least 8 cups. When it comes to water, more is better.

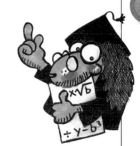

Staying aware

KNOW YOUR BODY *well enough to know what your abilities are. That way you will honestly try your best to perfect the posture or do the exercise, but will not strain muscles or injure yourself in the process.*

To do this you will need to begin to develop a meditative mind in which you become aware of yourself from the inside out. When you feel a tense muscle with a meditative mind, you learn to relax it consciously with the breath. Only then should you allow yourself to stretch more deeply into the posture.

■ **By recognizing your body's limitations** *and not pushing yourself too hard too quickly, you will avoid injury. Increased flexibility will come with time and practice.*

MAXIMIZING YOUR YOGA EXPERIENCE

(a) Give yourself plenty of time to get to class and acclimate. It's best to arrive 10 or 15 minutes early.

(b) Try to join in as best you can, even if something seems strange or odd. Let yourself surrender enough to have an experience.

(c) Be attentive and focused on what the teacher is saying and doing. Put the events of the day aside and create a little yoga oasis for yourself.

(d) Be open to corrections from your teacher, whether verbal or hands-on. Take it in the spirit of friendly guidance.

(e) Don't compare yourself to others. I can't say this enough. So I'll just say, "Know that you are incomparable!"

(f) Let yourself be known. Place yourself where you can see and hear the teacher well. After class ask any questions that arise during the class.

(g) Set reasonable personal goals. Listen to your body, and go at your own pace.

(h) Let your light shine! Be patient with yourself, and grateful to your teacher.

(i) Don't give up hope. The more you practice, the more you grow. The story of the tortoise and the hare applies: Slow and steady wins the race.

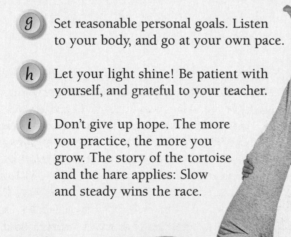

■ **Your yoga teacher** *can help you become more aware of your body's flexibility. If there is any stiffness, it's important not to compensate for it by overstretching your more flexible muscles.*

Give it a chance

EVERYONE HAS A DIFFERENT YOGA STORY. Some students come and go quickly. Others start and stop, and start again. Still others begin, and practice consistently from that day forward.

As your own practice of yoga becomes regular, pay attention to how yoga makes you feel. You will notice subtle and not-so-subtle differences each time you practice. You may feel somewhat tired in a relaxed way, energized and clear, serene and focused, or even agitated and angry.

Wondering why anyone would want to work hard just to feel negative? Yoga cleans all the dark little nooks and crannies of the mind, and brings them to light. Knowing that negative feelings are just passing through as part of yoga's cleansing process makes it easier to just keep going. By continuing to practice yoga, little by little you will feel lighter and lighter.

One of my favorite lines to remember when doing yoga is "Keep up and you'll be kept up!" The universe will keep you going, if you do your part.

Of course, you will have to use your judgment to determine whether the class you've chosen is the right one for you. If not, don't give up on yoga. Try a different teacher, or a different style. But be fair. Give it a chance before you move on. Like life, yoga is a progression. You can experience unlimited progression within one particular school of yoga, or you may find that one school of yoga is perfect for you for a time, but that as you change, so does your yoga path.

■ **Practicing yoga** *regularly will make a difference to how you feel. Whether you start off by experiencing positive or negative emotions, you will eventually feel lighter.*

Your home practice

IT IS SIMPLE TO CONTINUE PRACTICING YOGA at home using videos, audiotapes, and books. Your yoga teacher may have recommendations for your home practice.

Morning is a great time to do yoga, and sets the tone for the day. Evening yoga helps you let go of the busy day, and prepares you for restful sleep. The best time to do yoga is when you need it most.

Teaching children yoga is one of my specialties. I have taught up to 300 children a week. One of my students, a 3½-year-old girl named India, really understood the purpose of yoga. One day when she and her mother were at the playground, things were getting rather chaotic. Children were running and screaming everywhere. With a weary look on her little face, India plopped down beside her mother and said, "Mom I really need some yoga right now!"

Setting a time

Set a time to practice and stick to it as much as possible. Be realistic so you won't be disappointed or pressured. If your home practice consists of 15 minutes on Saturday and Sunday morning, that is fantastic because it is what you can do. You may be able to add another day or two, or increase the time you spend doing yoga. Yoga grows on you if you let it. People often are delighted to discover that instead of trying to force themselves to do more yoga, they naturally feel like increasing their practice simply because it feels so good and so right.

What to include

When you're starting out, the best policy is to keep it simple. Start with a minute or two of deep breathing. Move on to some spine flexing and leg stretching. Then go into some of the postures you've learned in class. End with a few minutes of relaxing on your back. Meditation afterward is almost effortless, so you may want to save a bit of time for that.

Trivia...

Larry is one of my yoga students who has seen substantial changes in his flexibility in the year he has been coming to class. He takes class once a week, which, while commendable, might not be enough to make dramatic changes. But Larry has found a little routine for himself that works. Every morning he does 10 to 15 minutes of warm-up yoga from a class handout. When Larry started class, he could only reach his knees on a forward stretch, and he was not able to relax his upper body forward. Now he can reach his ankles, and has increased his ability to stretch forward, too.

CREATING A YOGA SANCTUARY

a) Choose a quiet, light-filled space in your home that you reserve for yoga and meditation.

b) Add a small bench or altar with simple and meaningful decorations such as flowers, photos, healing stones, and sacred objects.

c) Keep a beautiful sound current of relaxing and spiritual music playing.

d) Have your yoga mat, pillow, and shawl available.

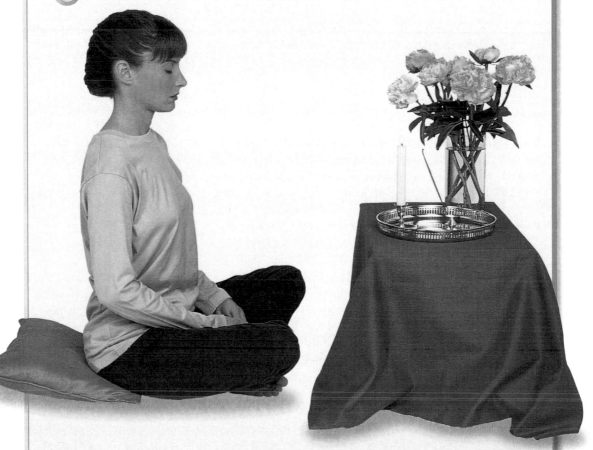

■ **A yoga sanctuary** *should be a place of peace and light. Make the altar your point of focus and face it when practicing yoga or meditating. A cushion will help relieve the pressure on your knees.*

Warm-up yoga

YOU CAN INCREASE YOUR FLEXIBILITY and prepare yourself to do more challenging poses with these yoga exercises. Once you've learned to master them, they'll become a natural addition to your daily routine.

(1) **Tune in.** Sitting on the floor with your legs crossed, straighten your spine by pressing your chest slightly forward and lifting your ribcage. Relax your shoulders and bring your chin level. This is called "Easy" pose. Close your eyes and exhale all your breath out using your abdominal muscles. Then relax and expand your belly as you inhale deeply, using all of your lungs. Repeat two more times.

Pre-yoga centering techniques are done in most yoga traditions, and usually involve the breath. Many yoga paths also include a chanted invocation.

(2) **Spine Flex.** In Easy pose, take hold of the outside of your ankles. Inhale and flex your spine forward, chest out and shoulders back. Then exhale and slump your body. Your shoulders will curve forward, your chest will cave in, and your spine will be rounded. Continue this breathing and movement in a rhythmic, forward-and-backward manner. Focus on rocking the pelvis forward and back, as well as moving the mid- and upper spine. Feel each vertebra of the spine curl and uncurl. As you continue, pick up the pace. Do this for 1 minute, then inhale deeply, holding the breath. Exhale and relax the breath and the pose.

SPINE FLEX

This exercise opens the vertebrae of the spine and increases spinal flexibility.

(3) **Spinal Twists.** Still sitting in Easy pose from number 1, above, bring your hands up to the shoulders with the fingers in the front and the thumbs in the back. Straighten your spine and begin twisting side to side as far as you can in each direction. Keep your upper arms parallel to the ground as you swing freely from side to side.

SPINAL TWIST

Inhale as you twist to the left and exhale as you twist to the right. Breathe rhythmically and powerfully as you continue these motions for 1 minute.

Spinal twisting releases locked places in the spine and massages the internal organs.

(4) **Shoulder Shrugs.** Place your hands on your knees again. Make sure your spine is straight and that your neck is in line with your spine. Inhale and lift your shoulders straight up toward your ears. Imagine that you want to touch your ears with your shoulders. Then exhale and let your shoulders drop down. Use a powerful breath and continue up and down for 1 minute. Then inhale deeply, stretch your shoulders up – hold for a few seconds – and exhale down. Relax and breathe normally for a few seconds. You will feel a warm energy circulating throughout your shoulder and neck area.

SHOULDER SHRUG

Pressurizing the shoulder area squeezes the muscles, then releases tension.

(5) **Neck Rolls.** Gently drop your head forward, and as you inhale begin to rotate your head around to the right. Keep your jaws relaxed and your mouth slack. Your chin will come over your right shoulder as you inhale. The head will drop back in a smooth, continuous motion. As you exhale, your head will move over your left shoulder and back to the front. Move meditatively and slowly, feeling that the weight of your head is taking your neck around in a fluid circle. After two or three slow circles, reverse the direction, inhaling to the left, exhaling as your head comes around to the right. Continue for two or three circles, then inhale and bring your head to the front. Exhale and relax.

Neck rolls relax the head, neck, and face.

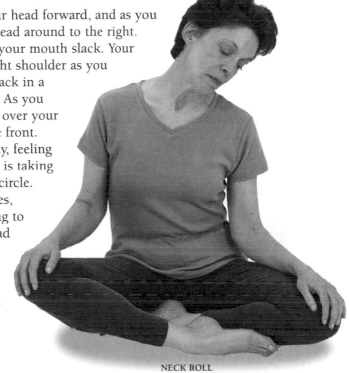

NECK ROLL

6 **Leg Stretches.** Sit with your legs straight out in front, flat on the floor. Reach down as far as you can. If you can, reach your toes. If you cannot, reach what you can – ankles, calves, even your knees are a good start. Exhale and stretch forward, bringing your head toward your knees and your chest toward your thighs. Then inhale and sit up again. On the out-breath, allow yourself to fall more deeply forward each time. On the in-breath, fill the lungs with prana, vital life energy. Continue the up-and-down movement for 1 minute.

This exercise stretches the calves, hamstrings, and sciatic nerve.

LEG STRETCHES

7 **Spread Stretch.** Sitting down, spread your legs as wide apart as is comfortable for you. Inhale and stretch your arms overhead, stretching your spine up tall. Then, exhale and reach to your right foot. If you can, grab hold of your right instep with your hands; otherwise, reach and hold as far down your leg as you comfortably can. Inhale and stretch up to the center again. Exhale and do the same on the left side, stretching toward your left foot. Continue for 1 minute. Then inhale up to the center, and exhale bending forward to the center. Let your hands grasp your feet, ankles, or calves. Hold forward with five more deep breaths. Each time you exhale, relax a little more forward. Then inhale deeply, exhale with maximum stretch, and relax sitting up again.

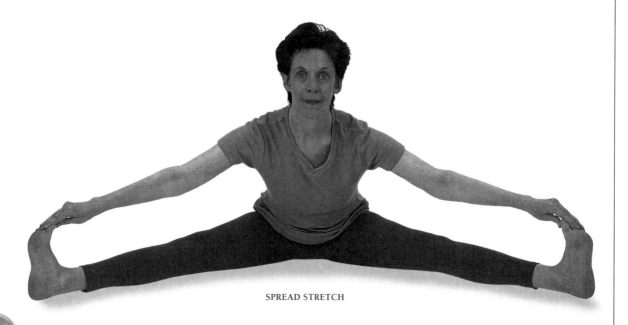

SPREAD STRETCH

Spread stretch tones and stretches the thigh muscles and increases flexibility in the pelvis and hips.

These exercises take 7 to 10 minutes. Do you believe you can find the time for them?

A simple summary

✔ When it comes to choosing a yoga class, ask yourself: What do I want? How far am I willing to drive? What kind of environment and style of class is it? What are my limitations?

✔ Simply look for a class through the Yellow Pages, or ask a friend for a recommendation. When you call a yoga center, ask for their brochure or ask to speak to a teacher.

✔ Find out what a typical class is like, and what kind of training and experience the teacher has. Use intuition along with logic to determine which class feels right for you.

✔ Prepare yourself both in body and mind. Find out what you need to bring and wear to be comfortable. Cultivate a mindset that will allow you to have the most positive yoga experience.

✔ You can deepen your yoga practice by creating a space in your home for yoga. Make a realistic exercise plan that you can stick to.

✔ Begin your home practice by centering with deep breathing or chanting. Then warm up and stretch out your body before doing any yoga postures that require flexibility.

✔ Giving yoga a chance to grow on you will help you grow. Your practice will change as it progresses and may start and stop as well. Just keep going, and it will keep you going.

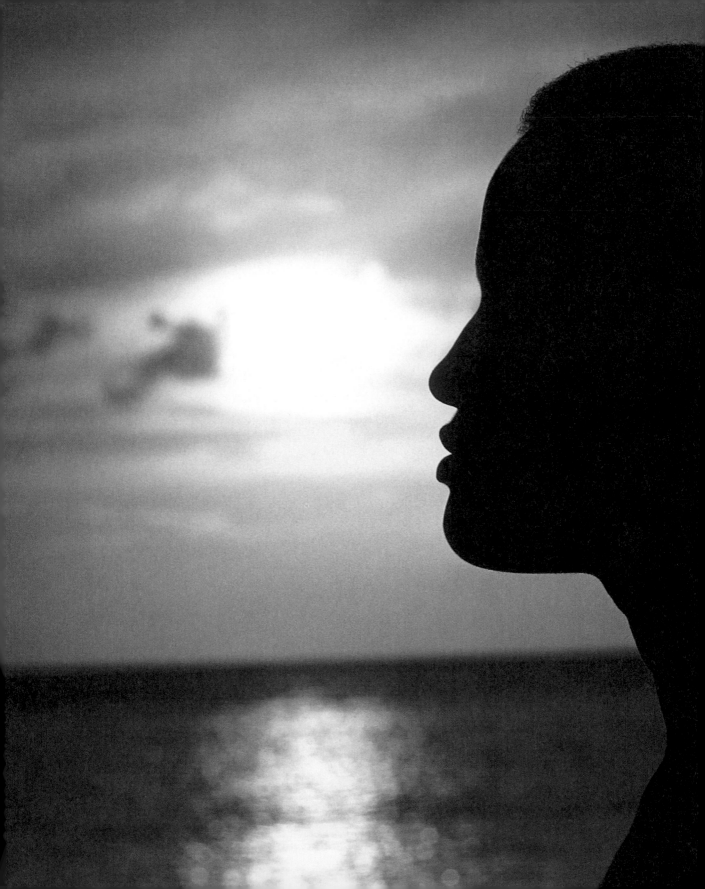

Chapter 6

Simply Hatha

PATANJALI GAVE US THE BLUEPRINT for ways to unite the body, mind, and spirit. One of the most common ways, he tells us, is through asanas, or postures. This is the yoga called Hatha, which involves using the body to change the internal state of mind and consciousness. In this chapter you will learn how to get the best possible experience of Hatha yoga. Then I'd like to invite you to try some basic Hatha yoga postures with me.

In this chapter...

✓ A path for everyone

✓ The yoga of breathing

✓ Ready, "steady"

✓ Centering

✓ Poses – from standing to relaxing

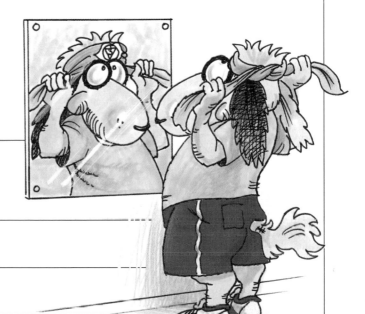

PROPER BREATHING IS AN ESSENTIAL COMPONENT OF HATHA, WHICH IS YOGA IN ITS BASIC FORM

A path for everyone

THE MANY DIFFERENT SCHOOLS *and styles of yoga are like rays of light from one sun. Emanating from the same source, they are all related. It is only natural, though, that distinct differences between the various schools of yoga have developed over time. And thankfully so. There is a path for everyone when it comes to yoga.*

In the next five chapters we will explore each of the major schools of yoga in depth. You will notice that each yoga school has its roots with an individual master teacher who developed a particular style of yoga from ancient teachings or, in some cases, inspired intuition. Those that have stood the test of time have become yoga traditions. Additionally, contemporary styles of yoga have emerged from some of the traditional paths.

The yoga in this chapter is simply Hatha. It is the generic brand, so to speak. And for many people this is the perfect brand.

Most yoga styles incorporate simple Hatha yoga, and each adds its own distinctive character. Hatha yoga is like plain yogurt, while the different schools of yoga are the many varieties of flavored yogurt.

Here you will have the opportunity to experience some of the basic yoga poses for which Hatha is known. First let's take a look at the most essential component of yoga: The breath.

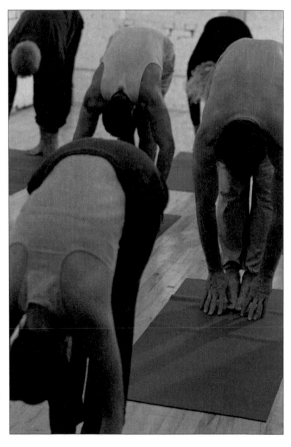

■ **The standing forward bend** *is a basic yoga position, the first of the standing poses. It stretches the body completely, from the scalp to the heels. It also increases the blood supply to the brain.*

The yoga of breathing

ENTIRE BOOKS HAVE *been written on the elements of yogic breathing, or* pranayama. *Actually, yogic breathing in its simplest form is just plain old proper breathing. Some yoga teachers begin their class with pranayama. For some people, this is the best part of a yoga class.*

Many moons ago when I took voice lessons, the teacher had me demonstrate proper breathing to the class. He said I was the only one who really knew how to breathe correctly, and that proper breathing provides maximum lung space for singing. My yogic training really paid off in that class!

Shallow breathing

In general, most of us breathe shallowly. Over time, however, our ineffective ways of breathing lead to fatigue, stress, and worse. That's because we commonly use only the upper portion of our lungs and take in small amounts of oxygen, thus robbing ourselves of vitality. In proper breathing, the diaphragm is fully engaged, and we take in full breaths. Though it may sound funny, we could all use some breathing lessons!

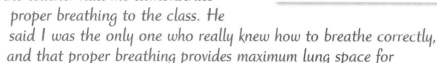

lung

diaphragm

■ **Shallow breathing,** *where only the tops of the lungs are filled with oxygen, deprives the body of vitality. With yogic breathing, the lungs are filled completely and the diaphragm is fully engaged.*

The diaphragm, a thick muscular sheet separating the chest from the abdomen, plays a significant part in breathing. As we inhale, the diaphragm moves downward into the belly, and we draw air down the trachea and into the lungs, while at the same time the abdomen and rib cage expand.

When we exhale, our diaphragm moves upward, pressing the lungs, which then expel air. As an extra treat, the diaphragm massages the organs with its up-and-down motion.

Making the involuntary voluntary

Breathing is both an involuntary and voluntary action. The key to health and awareness is in becoming conscious of the action of breathing and controlling its flow. In the following exercise, try to be present with your breath.

DEFINITION

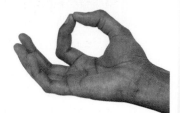

First, practice slow and deep breathing as you sit on the floor with a straight spine in Easy pose. If you like, place a firm pillow under your buttocks to straighten your lower spine. Your hands can be in *Gyan mudra*, with the thumbs and index fingers forming a circle and the rest of the fingers open. Straighten your arms, and rest them on your knees. Relax your shoulders as you breathe. Feel the natural flow of the breath.

Gyan means "wisdom." Mudra means "lock" or "seal," and is a hand position in yoga. In the yogic science, each area of the hand relates to a certain area of the brain. In applying pressure to the fingers and hands, the related brain areas are stimulated. Gyan mudra corresponds to the area that activates wisdom and knowledge.

■ **Check your breathing** *by inhaling and exhaling slowly with one hand placed on the abdomen and the other on the ribcage.*

The three-part breath

In this breathing exercise, you will inhale, retain, or suspend the breath for a few seconds, then exhale. Generally, the exhalation is longer than the inhalation. Do not practice this breath if you have serious breathing problems.

1. To begin, exhale all the breath out to clear your lungs. Then inhale. Your abdominal muscles will relax and expand outward to allow the diaphragm to drop.

2. At the top of the inhalation, suspend the breath for a second or two.

3. Exhale. Your abdominal muscles will naturally move inward to press the diaphragm up against the lungs. Some yogic techniques also pause the breath on the exhale for a few seconds.

When the breath is suspended, the body is relaxed. There should be no feeling of pressure. No part of your face, throat, or shoulders should be tight. You are merely suspending or pausing the breath for a second or two.

By taking deep, slow breaths you can expand the lungs by about eight times. If you establish a habit of breathing deeply and slowly, you will have endurance and patience. In addition, there is a strong and automatic connection between the breath and the pituitary and pineal glands. If you take your breathing rate down below eight times per minute, the pituitary starts secreting fully. If the breath rate is less than four times per minute, the pineal gland starts functioning, and deep meditation is automatic.

The three-part breath exercise is best done when sitting specifically for breath work. When you are holding yoga postures or exercises, the breath will usually be deep but may not be as slow or suspended as instructed here.

Ready, "steady"

"STEADY POSES," OR ASANAS, are the physical postures of yoga. There are a wide variety of asanas (over 200), each one with its own distinct form dictated by stretching, counter-stretching, and resistance. Alignment of the muscular and skeletal structures is a major focus of the asanas. Adding a conscious breathing pattern to the postures circulates energy and blood and brings balance to the sympathetic and parasympathetic nervous systems, which govern the automatic function of just about every other system in the body. In other words, asanas are the key to the body, which is the key to the mind, which is the key to the spirit.

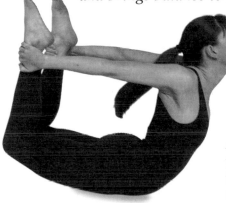

BOW POSE, ONE OF THE MANY ASANAS

Asanas are grouped according to their physical positioning. Each group works on the body and mind in a different way. When you practice an asana, be sure to read through the entire instruction for each pose before trying it.

ASANA TIPS

a Do your asanas with vigor while at the same time staying relaxed and composed.

b It is best to practice yoga barefoot.

c Turn your attention inward. Eyes will have a soft focus or be closed.

d Move slowly into the pose to avoid injury, and to increase your inner awareness.

e Stretch as far as is comfortable. Work on the edge of the stretch, but back off if there is pain. Discomfort is okay, pain is not.

f Breathe, breathe, breathe! Unless instructed otherwise, inhale and exhale through the nose. Use the breath to facilitate relaxation into the posture.

g Hold the poses for a few breaths, or for a minute, to start.

h To conclude an exercise or posture, inhale and pause the breath briefly, then exhale and relax the posture.

i A few seconds of relaxation between postures allows the energy to circulate.

j Follow your practice with a deep relaxation while lying on your back for a few minutes or longer.

■ **Most important** *is to enjoy what you're doing – a little smiling goes a long way!*

Centering

TO BEGIN YOUR PRACTICE, *set aside 15 to 20 minutes to be in your yoga sanctuary. If you don't have a particular place set up for yoga, just find a quiet spot where you will have room to move. Spread a mat or blanket that will fit the length of your body. If you are on a hardwood floor, make sure your mat does not slip. Now you are ready to begin.*

Trivia...

The sound "Om" begins with the open "o" sound then extends the "m" sound, creating a soothing hum in the throat and root of the nose. It is interesting to note that other spiritual traditions intone similarly, with an "o" sound in the beginning, and an "m" or "n" sound to end. To hear for yourself, try extending the sound of "Amen," and notice the similarity.

A centering exercise is commonly done before beginning a practice of yoga. To begin, sit cross-legged in Easy pose with a straight spine. Bring the hands either in Gyan mudra or prayer mudra, which is done by placing the palms together and pressing the thumbs into the center of the chest. Traditionally, prayer mudra (sometimes called Prayer pose) is used to create a connection between you and your inner guidance, and between you and the ancient lineage of yoga.

■ **In prayer mudra,** *the palms of the hands are brought flat together at the chest, and the thumb knuckles are pressed into the slight indentation at the sternum.*

Now take three deep breaths with your focus either at the heart center, or at the *intuitive center* at the forehead level. Feel as though each breath is entering and exiting through either the heart or the forehead.

Many yoga classes begin with a chant, usually "Om" or "Om Shanti." Om has been described as the universal sound of God. "Shanti" means peace. Chanting, or intoning, is a yogic technique to calm the heart and center the mind. If you are comfortable with chanting, do so. It is perfectly fine, though, to listen and breathe deeply instead.

DEFINITION

The sixth chakra, or the intuitive center, located between the eyebrows and about 1 in (3 cm) below the surface, is often referred to as the third eye, or the brow point. This important focal point maintains a stable focus, a higher awareness, and mental projection through that elevated awareness.

Standing poses

STANDING POSES ARE IMPORTANT *for beginners because they teach the basic principles of alignment. They also establish a firm foundation for learning other poses. Through regular practice, standing poses give strength and mobility to the hips, knees, neck, and shoulders.*

Traditionally, you would jump into these poses, but you need not jump into a pose to obtain the benefits. If you have back or knee injuries, or are pregnant, do not jump into the pose. Always come out of a pose if you feel fatigued.

Standing poses should not be practiced during the first few days of menstruation, the first 3 months of pregnancy, or by anyone with a problem pregnancy, high blood pressure, or heart problems.

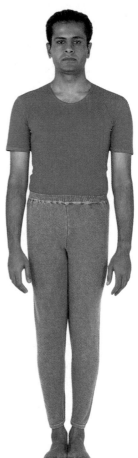

MOUNTAIN POSE

Mountain pose (Tadasana)

Mountain pose improves posture and balances the mind.

1. Stand with your feet together or slightly apart. The weight of your body should be evenly distributed between the toes, balls, and heels of your feet. Your head is centered over your legs, and your toes are spread, not gripping.

2. Keep your knees straight, but not locked. Without tensing your stomach muscles, move them up and slightly inward.

3. Raise your breastbone while keeping your shoulders and arms relaxed and straight. Arms are at your sides. Your head should face straight ahead, with the chin level.

4. Relax your facial muscles, especially the muscles around the eyes. Your breathing should be full but natural.

5. Keep your body relaxed and in line as you breathe for 1 minute.

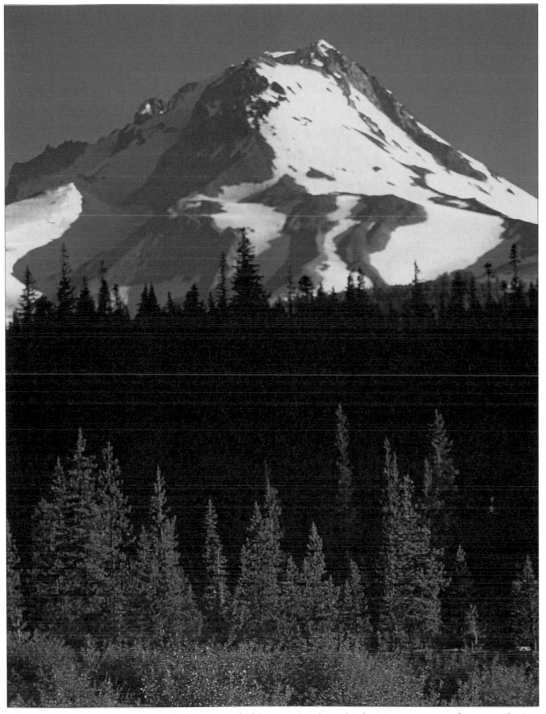

■ **Many yoga poses** *are named after natural objects, animals, or birds. Mountain pose, for example, is Tadasana: Tada means "mountain," and asana is "pose" in Sanskrit.*

Sitting poses

SITTING POSES ARE GOOD FOR ALIGNING *the spine and focusing the mind. They are considered calming and help regulate blood pressure and promote restful sleep. There are two categories of sitting poses: Upright seated postures and forward bends. Here we will focus on forward bends.*

Open angle pose (Upavista Konasana)

Forward bends, such as the Open angle pose, stretch the lower back, lengthen the hamstrings, and tone the abdominal muscles. They are considered passive poses that encourage introspection. They soothe the nervous system and quiet the mind. They are especially recommended during menstruation. If practiced after backbends, they serve as a counterbalance to the body.

1. Sit on the floor with your legs stretched out in a "V" shape. Your knees should be straight but not locked.

2. Place your hands at your sides and lift your buttocks slightly off the floor as you press downward with the hands. This will lengthen your spine and bring you more fully onto the sitting bones at the base of the spine. Keep your back and upper torso erect.

3. As you exhale, gently bend forward, stretching your right hand toward your right foot, and your left hand toward your left foot. Reach as far down as you can. If you can easily reach your toes, do so, but do not strain. Just reach as far as is comfortable for you.

4. Breathe deeply into the pose. Each time you exhale, stretch a bit more. Continue for 1 minute.

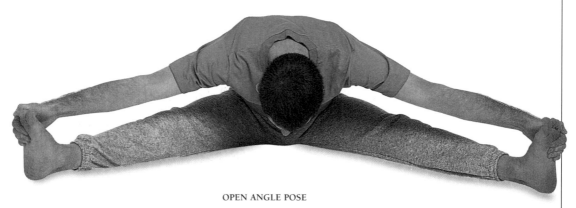

OPEN ANGLE POSE

Reclining poses

AS YOU MAY IMAGINE, reclining (also called supine) poses are relaxing and less strenuous. They are good poses during menstruation, for relieving tension and fatigue, and for recovering from illness.

Legs up the wall pose (Viparita Karani)

Reclining poses, such as this Legs up the wall pose, help to open the pelvis and strengthen the back, arms, and legs.

The least strenuous of these poses are traditionally done at the end of a session in order to cool down the body and restore energy.

1. Lie down on your back so that your buttocks are close to a wall. Then stretch your legs up on the wall.

2. Adjust your position so that your buttocks are close to the edge of the wall, and the entire length of your legs is pressed against the wall.

3. Relax your arms at your sides with the palms facing downward. Or rest them on the floor above your head with the elbows slightly bent.

4. Breathe for 1 minute, relaxing and stretching the spine and legs. To come out, bend your knees and place your feet on the wall. Roll to your side and come up slowly.

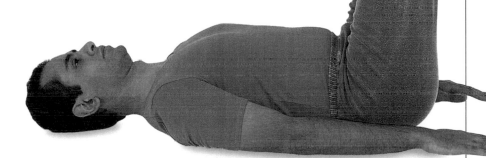

LEGS UP THE WALL POSE

You can also do this exercise with a blanket, which adds a deeper arching and stretching of the mid- and upper back. This is an example of restorative yoga.

(1) Place the long side of one folded blanket (2–3 in/ 5–8 cm thick) close to the wall.

(2) Lie down with your pelvis resting on the blanket, and continue as instructed above.

(3) For a deeper stretch to the back, add another blanket. But remember to maintain a curve in your neck, supporting your neck with a thin blanket or towel if necessary.

Backward bending poses

THESE POSES ENERGIZE *and open the body, particularly the upper spine and chest area. They are great for the nervous and digestive systems, and they strengthen the arms and shoulders and increase the flexibility of the spine. Backbends help develop courage and mental energy, as well as lift depression.*

In general, backbends are strenuous, and should be introduced gradually to a steady yoga practice. You should rest for a minute in Corpse pose or Child's pose after practicing a backbending pose.

Backward bending poses should not be done if you have serious knee injuries, high blood pressure, or heart disease, or if you are pregnant or menstruating.

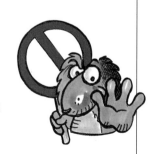

Bridge pose (Setu Bandhasana)

Bridge pose stretches the abdominal and lumbar spine muscles. It adds strength to the thighs, and opens the chest and pelvis. This pose is energizing and rejuvenating.

1. Lie on your back on the floor with your knees bent and feet hip-distance apart. Your feet should be close to your buttocks and your arms at your sides with the palms facing downward.

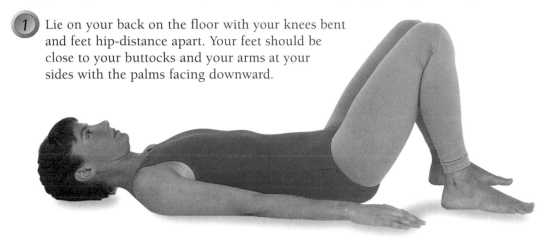

STEP 1

2. Press your feet down firmly. Tuck your chin in slightly. Lengthen your spine and lift your pelvis off the floor as high as is comfortable. Your weight should be evenly distributed between your shoulders and feet.

3. For extra support, you can place your hands on your mid-back, close to the waist, with your elbows on the ground. Or you can continue to have your arms on the floor, pressing downward.

4. Breathe and continue to lengthen the spine. After 30 seconds to 1 minute, gently relax the spine down. To release your lower back area, clasp your hands around your knees and bring the knees into your chest for a few seconds.

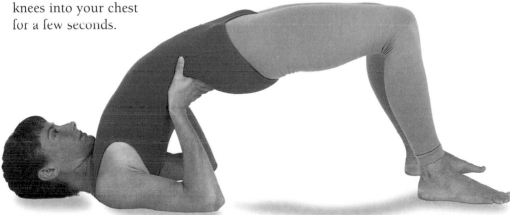

STEP 3

Inverted poses

INVERTED POSES REVERSE GRAVITATIONAL PULL, *bringing fresh blood to the head and heart, and revitalizing the whole body. They tone the internal organs and improve circulation. Some of them work to refresh tired legs.*

Do not do inverted poses if you're pregnant, menstruating, or if you have high blood pressure, headaches, heart problems, or neck or spinal injuries.

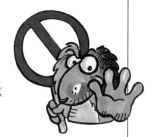

Downward-facing dog pose (Adho Mukha Savasana)

Downward dog stretches and releases tension in the upper spine and neck. It strengthens the hamstrings and arms and helps relieve depression, anger, insomnia, and stress.

1. Begin on your hands and knees. Then lift your tailbone up and bring your knees off the floor.

2. Keep your arms straight and stretch your shoulders and head downward.

3. Raise your trunk, straighten your knees, and move your buttocks upward toward the ceiling. Your weight should be evenly distributed between your hands and heels.

4. Work to bring your heels to the floor, but do not overstrain the calves or the Achilles tendons. The focus is to stretch your back fully, not to get your heels to the floor.

5. Stretch and breathe for 1 minute. Then lower your knees back down to the floor, and come out of the pose.

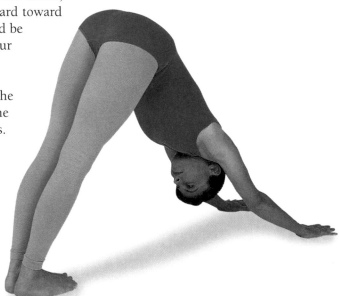

DOWNWARD-FACING DOG POSE

Wall yoga

If you found it impossible to reach the floor and straighten your legs in downward dog, there is a simple solution called wall yoga. Stand about 3 ft (1 m) from the wall and lean forward, placing your hands on the wall in front of you. You may have to adjust your standing position so that you reach comfortably while keeping your knees and arms straight but relaxed. Begin to walk your hands down the wall. Continue walking down the wall until you are stretching deeply, but not overstretching. Stay there for 1 minute, then walk your hands back up the wall and relax.

Twisting poses

TWISTING POSES ARE CLEANSING. *They energize the body and increase the range of motion and spinal flexibility, as well as massaging the internal organs. The natural focus on the neck and shoulder areas relieves joint stiffness and headaches.*

Pregnant women should avoid spinal twists.

Spinal twist (Ardha Matsyendrasana)

This pose alleviates tension in the spine, neck, and shoulders, and helps the alignment of the spinal and cervical vertebrae.

1. Sit on your buttocks with your legs crossed and your spine straight. Raise your right knee and place your right foot flat on the floor. Your left leg is tucked under your right leg with your heel close to your right hip.

2. Place your right foot on the floor to the outside of your left thigh. Place your right hand flat on the floor behind you, close to your body. Keep your spine straight. Raise your left arm straight up overhead.

3. Bring your left arm over the right side of your right knee, so that it is pressing against your knee. Reach around to catch hold of your right ankle. Keep your chest lifted and your shoulders parallel to the floor. Your head is turned over your right shoulder and your eyes look to the right.

4. Breathe deeply for 30 seconds to 1 minute.

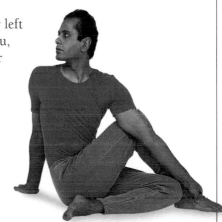

SPINAL TWIST

Balancing poses

THESE POSES DEVELOP LIGHTNESS, *strength, and agility. They also help develop muscle tone, coordination, and mental concentration.*

Tree pose (Vrksasana)

Learning how to be balanced and focused is important not only in Tree pose, but in life, too!

1. Begin in Mountain pose. Shift your weight to your right leg.

2. Bend your left leg. Clasp your left ankle with your left hand and place your left foot on the inside of your right thigh. Ideally your heel will fit snugly against the inner thigh at the groin. If this is too much of a stretch, place your foot on the highest point possible at the inner thigh, even if it is just above the knee. Your left knee will extend out to the side.

3. Bring your hands to the center of your chest in Prayer pose. Focus your eyes on a point in the distance that is unmoving.

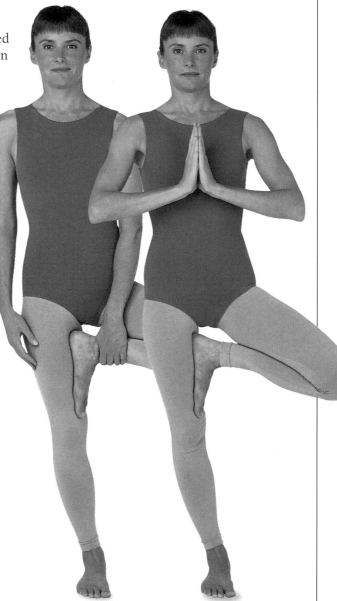

STEP 2　　　　　　　　STEP 3

(4) When you feel steady, slowly raise your arms overhead, keeping the palms together. Stretch your entire body upward, using your upper back muscles.

(5) Once you are stable in the pose, you can straighten the lower spine further by gently pressing the bent knee downward and outward.

(6) Maintain a grounded strength. Keep your foot firmly against the floor, your knee straight, and your thigh firm.

(7) Make sure your shoulders, neck, and face remain relaxed.

(8) Hold the posture for 1 minute with deep breathing. Then relax out of the posture, return to Mountain pose, and switch sides.

If you don't want to be a swaying tree, concentrate on your internal center, which is located just below the navel. Eastern teachings call this the Hara and consider it to be the source of willpower. Keep a soft focus on a point in the distance while maintaining your connection with the Hara.

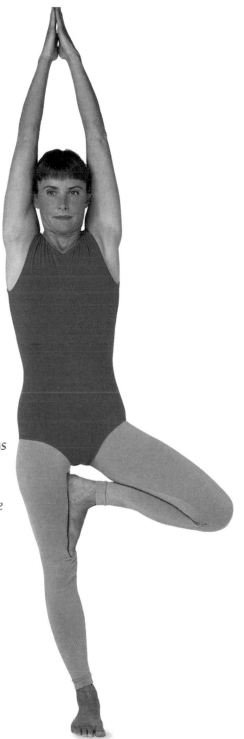

STEP 4

Relaxation poses

THE MOST COMMONLY USED RELAXATION POSE is Corpse pose. Another that is important for resting is called Child's pose, or Baby pose, which I'll show you below. Relaxation poses are healing and rejuvenating to the body and mind.

Child's pose (Mudhasana)

Child's pose relaxes the body between poses, helps to relieve back pain, and brings clarity to the mind. It's called Child's pose because it nurtures the child within.

1. Kneel down onto the backs of your heels. The tops of your feet should be relaxed on the floor.

2. Bend forward and bring your forehead to the ground.

3. Bring your arms down along your sides, resting them on the floor with the palms facing upward and relaxed.

4. Sink deeply into the pose. Breathe deeply into your lower spine and hips.

5. A variation of Child's pose is to stretch your arms out in front of you with the palms against the floor.

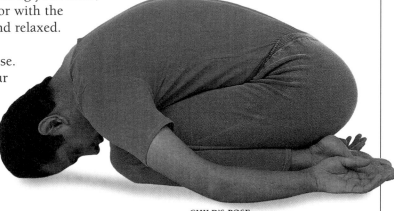

CHILD'S POSE

A word about relaxation

In any yoga class you will find a relaxation time, usually in Corpse pose, provided at the end of class. Yoga students look forward to this time, viewing it as the icing on the cake, the reward for a job well done. In a sense, that is true. But there's more to this simple practice of Corpse pose than you might think.

Not as passive as it seems

Deep relaxation, while seemingly passive, is subtly active. When you systematically wake up and cleanse your body systems through the practice of yoga, you need a relaxation time in order to assimilate the internal changes that have occurred. By putting your body and mind in a passive yet conscious state, you prepare the environment for all the body systems, including the brain, to adjust themselves. That is why you feel totally different when you return to your regular life. Words like "insightful," "calm," "centered," and "aware" are some you may use to describe your state of being. Even physical illnesses are affected. I can't count how many times I have said goodbye to a head or chest cold by the end of a good yoga session.

Try it for yourself. Compare how you feel when you go into a yoga class with how you feel afterward. Take it one step further and notice how you feel before your deep relaxation, and how you feel upon the completion of your class.

A simple summary

✔ Distinct differences between the various schools of yoga have naturally developed over time, and many types have emerged.

✔ Generic yoga is called Hatha. Most of the yoga postures in Hatha are found in almost every other school of yoga.

✔ The yoga of breathing is called pranayama. Learning to breathe properly is essential for a practice of yoga.

✔ Asanas are the physical postures of yoga. They are grouped according to their physical positions. Each grouping works on the body and mind in distinct ways.

✔ Deep relaxation after yoga is subtly active. All the internal changes that have occurred through your yoga session are assimilated during relaxation. For this reason, it is essential to have at least a few minutes, if not more, of deep relaxation after yoga.

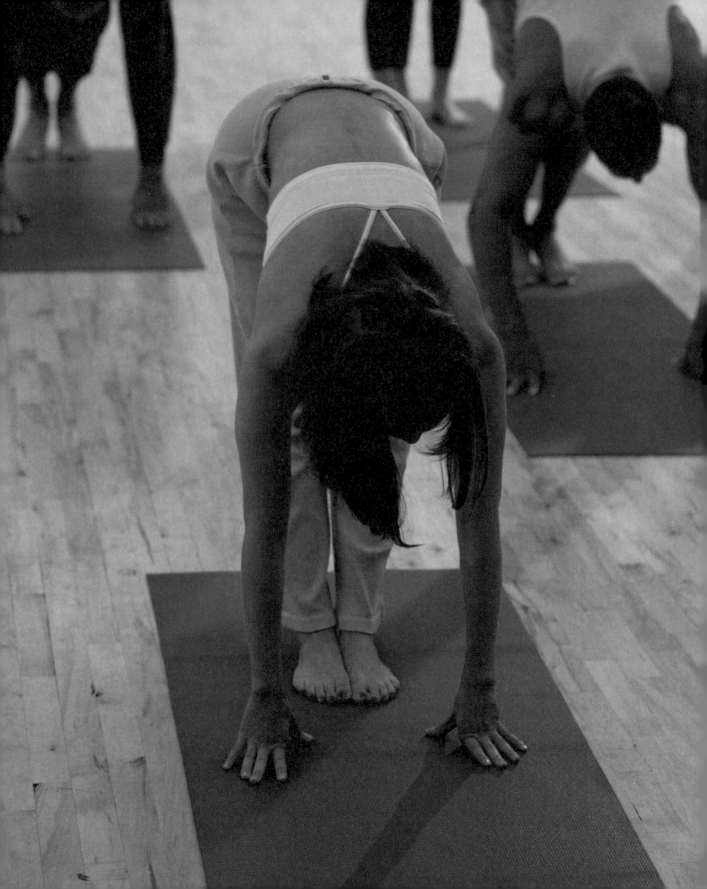

Chapter 7

Classic Yoga

WE ARE BEGINNING a very exciting journey. In this and the next four chapters we will be visiting the major schools of yoga, a few at a time. Our first stop is with two classic schools of yoga that have roots from the same master teacher: Sivananda yoga and Integral yoga.

In this chapter...

✓ Highlighting Sivananda yoga

✓ Relaxing mind and body

✓ Sun Salutation

✓ Easeful, peaceful, and useful: Integral yoga

✓ The daily postures

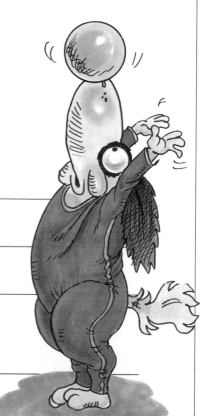

MANY CLASSIC YOGA CLASSES START WITH THE FLUID POSTURES KNOWN AS THE SUN SALUTATION

Highlighting Sivananda yoga

SIVANANDA IS ONE OF *the world's largest schools of yoga. It follows a set structure that includes pranayama, asanas, meditation, and guidelines for healthy living. If you are up for the Sivananda experience, you can retreat to their Yoga Ranch in Woodbourne, New York, to delve into the complete lifestyle of the yogis.*

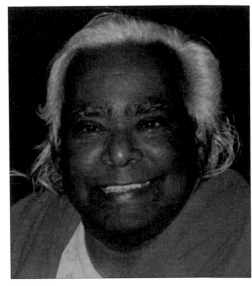

SWAMI VISHNU DEVANANDA

The 1960s and 1970s were the "Swami boom years" in the Western world. Indian spiritual teachers with 15-letter names were arriving on the shores of America and Europe by the dozens.

Several of the swamis and Eastern masters who left India and began schools in the West trained under the Himalayan master Swami Sivananda, a former physician who became a healer of the soul. Two among them were Swami Vishnu Devananda, who named his school after his teacher, Sivananda, and Swami Satchidananda, who began the school of Integral yoga.

Swami Vishnu Devananda wrote the contemporary yoga classic The Complete Illustrated Book of Yoga. First published in 1960, it is still one of the best introductions to yoga. Another wonderfully illustrated presentation of the Sivananda tradition is Yoga: Mind and Body by the Sivananda Yoga Vedanta Center.

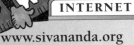

INTERNET

www.sivananda.org

Everything you want to know about Sivananda yoga can be found at their web site (including some yogic jokes!)

Simple living, high thinking

The motto of Sivananda yoga is "simple living and high thinking." The body is a vehicle for the soul, according to the Sivananda tradition, and this metaphor is extended into "the five points" of keeping your body running for as long as you need it.

The five points that every body needs

1. **Lubrication.** The asanas lubricate the body. They keep the muscles and joints running smoothly, tone all the internal organs, and increase circulation.

2. **Cooling system.** The body is cooled and recharged by complete relaxation.

3. **Electrical current.** Pranayama, or yogic breathing, increases prana, which is the electric current inside the body.

4. **Fuel.** A healthy, meat-free diet enables the body to obtain the maximum benefit from food, air, water, and sunlight.

5. **Good driver.** Meditation stills the mind, which is the driver of the body. Through meditation the mind will become clearer, wiser, and more peaceful.

Trivia...

The lengthy Indian names used in yoga may seem mind-boggling to pronounce. Do not despair! These long names can roll off your tongue if you just understand this one little key: Many of the names have "ananda" (pronounced ah-NUN-dah) on the end. If you imagine that there is a hyphen before the ananda, then you can focus on pronouncing just the first part of the word, and then add "ananda." (Generally, the letter "a" is pronounced like "ah," as in "a tree," "a bird," etc.)

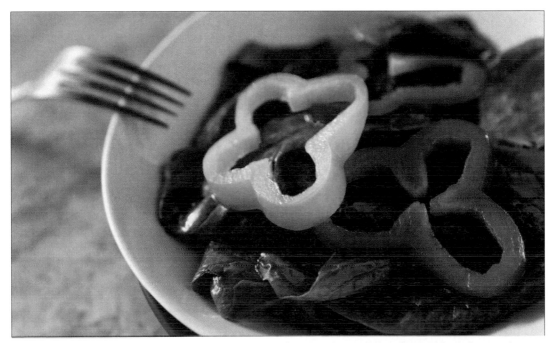

■ **According to the Sivananda tradition,** *a meat-free diet that includes plenty of fresh fruit and raw or lightly cooked vegetables will improve your health, as well as calm the mind and sharpen the intellect.*

Relaxing mind and body

BECAUSE A RELAXED BODY and mind function more efficiently, it is important to prepare yourself for the asanas with at least 5 minutes of complete relaxation. Cover yourself with a shawl or blanket to keep chill away. Learn how to relax with Corpse pose and use breathing and upper body exercises to relieve any physical stiffness.

Corpse pose (Savasana)

1. Lie down on your back and stretch and relax your muscles.

2. Rotate your legs in and out, then let them fall gently out to the sides. Do the same with your arms.

3. Feel stretched out, as though you were being pulled upward and downward at the same time. Your shoulders move down, away from your neck. Your legs move down, too, away from your pelvis.

4. Let gravity embrace you. Feel your weight pulling you deeper into relaxation, melting you down into the floor.

5. Breathe deeply and slowly from the abdomen, sinking deeper with each exhalation. Feel sensations of melting down, of expansion, lightness, and warmth.

6. Continue to relax deeply for 5 minutes.

7. Move your fingers and toes. Take some deep breaths. Turn to your side and sit up.

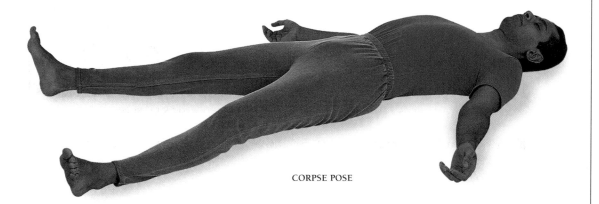

CORPSE POSE

Breathing exercise

Classic yoga such as Sivananda and Integral uses several basic pranayamas that are recommended for everyday use. One of the most common is Kapalabhati, or "skull-shining breath," so named because it increases the amount of oxygen to the brain, clearing the mind and improving concentration.

1. Sit with a straight spine. Bring your hands into Gyan mudra, or rest them on your knees. Your breastbone is raised, your shoulders are relaxed down, and your head is in line with your spine and your chin level.

2. Inhale deeply and exhale sharply, drawing your navel in toward your spine. Your abdominal muscles contract sharply, your diaphragm rises, and air is forced out of your lungs in much the same way you would exhale to clear your nasal passages.

STEP 2

3. To inhale, relax the muscles, allowing your lungs to fill with air. The exhalation should be brief, active, and audible. The inhalation is longer, passive, and silent.

4. Practice 20 pumps of Kapalabhati. Then inhale and exhale completely. Inhale fully and hold your breath for as long as you comfortably can. Slowly exhale.

5. Repeat the sequence once or twice more.

STEP 3

You can relieve any stiffness in the upper body by practicing the following exercises before moving on to asanas.

Neck exercise

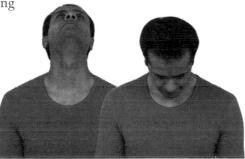

1. Let your head drop back gently, then drop forward. Do this five times.

2. Turn your head slowly to the right then left five times.

NECK EXERCISE

3. Bring your head forward, chin to the chest. Then bring your right ear toward your right shoulder. Come back to the center. Bring your left ear toward your left shoulder. Continue five times.

Eye exercises

People tend to move their heads, rather than their eyes. As a result, the muscles in the eyes are in need of exercise as much as the rest of our body. These exercises, done daily, will keep your eyes healthy.

a Keep your back and neck straight and your head still. Look up as high as possible and then look down. Do this ten times. Close your eyes and relax them for 30 seconds before moving on to the next exercise.

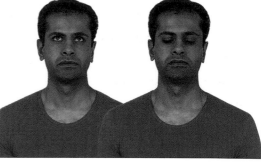

EXERCISE A

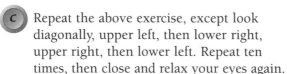
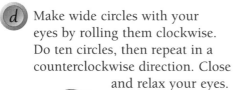

EXERCISE B

b Look as far to the right as possible, and then to the left. Keep your eyes wide open. Repeat ten times, then relax with your eyes closed for 30 seconds.

c Repeat the above exercise, except look diagonally, upper left, then lower right, upper right, then lower left. Repeat ten times, then close and relax your eyes again.

d Make wide circles with your eyes by rolling them clockwise. Do ten circles, then repeat in a counterclockwise direction. Close and relax your eyes.

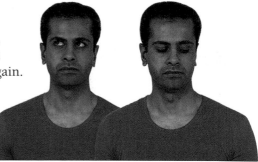

EXERCISE C

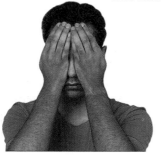

e Rub your hands vigorously until the palms are very warm. Gently cup your hands over your closed eyes, without touching the eyelids. Hold them and breathe for about 30 seconds to warm and relax the eyes.

EXERCISE E

Sun Salutation

SUN SALUTATION (SURYA NAMASKAR) is one of the most beloved and well-practiced series of postures known to yoga. Yoga styles of almost every tradition incorporate Sun Salutations, often as the beginning warm-up series. The Sun Salutation consists of a sequence of 12 positions that move the spine in various ways and promote flexibility in the limbs. It is of special benefit to beginners, to those who have stiff joints, and to the elderly. It helps the body gain flexibility, regulates the breath, and focuses the mind.

Once you become fluid with the Sun Salutation, it is important to focus on the rhythmic breathing pattern. Try to do 6–12 cycles every day.

Starting position: Stand erect with your head and body straight but relaxed. Your feet are together, your knees straight (not locked), and your arms are relaxed by your sides. Inhale deeply to begin.

1 As you exhale, bring your hands together at your chest in Prayer pose. Place your palms flat against each other at the center of your chest. Your elbows are pointing out to the sides.

2 Inhale and stretch your arms up over your head. Arch your body backward, keeping your arms alongside your ears and your knees straight. Allow your head and neck to stretch back with your body.

3 Exhale as you bend forward and bring your hands down to the floor next to your feet. Fingers and toes are in a straight line. Your head is tucked in toward your knees. If you cannot put your hands on the floor with your knees straight, bend your knees slightly.

STEP 1   STEP 2   STEP 3

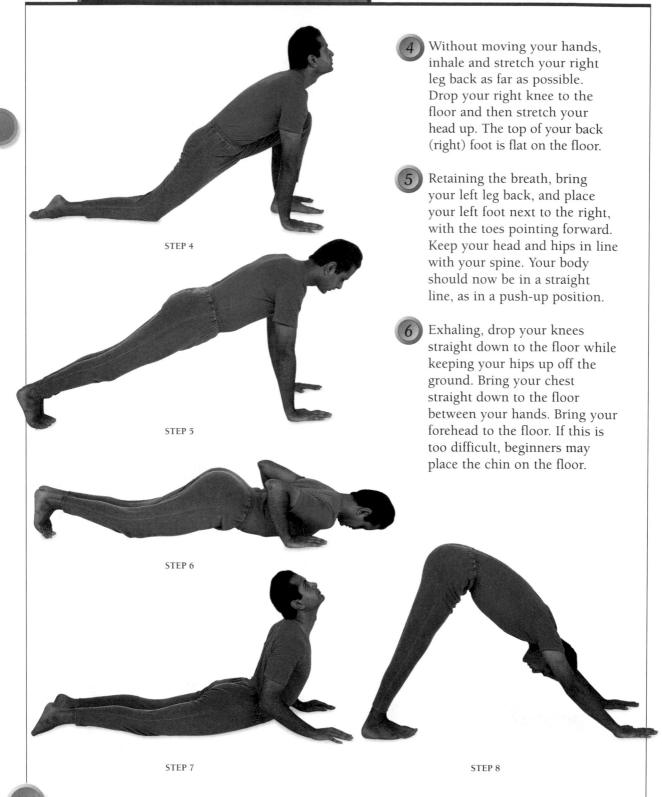

4 Without moving your hands, inhale and stretch your right leg back as far as possible. Drop your right knee to the floor and then stretch your head up. The top of your back (right) foot is flat on the floor.

5 Retaining the breath, bring your left leg back, and place your left foot next to the right, with the toes pointing forward. Keep your head and hips in line with your spine. Your body should now be in a straight line, as in a push-up position.

6 Exhaling, drop your knees straight down to the floor while keeping your hips up off the ground. Bring your chest straight down to the floor between your hands. Bring your forehead to the floor. If this is too difficult, beginners may place the chin on the floor.

STEP 4

STEP 5

STEP 6

STEP 7

STEP 8

7 Inhale as you slide your body forward until the hips are on the floor. Arch your chest up and bring your head back into Cobra pose (see p. 122). Do not move your hands. Your elbows are slightly bent, with your shoulders down and back, so that there is no tension in the neck or shoulder area.

8 Exhale as you tuck your toes under. Without allowing your hands or feet to move from their positions, bring your hips up. Push your heels toward the floor and keep your knees straight. Drop your head down between your arms.

9 Inhale and bring your right foot forward between your hands so that the fingers and toes form a straight line. Drop your left knee to the floor and stretch your head up (same as step 4 but with opposite legs).

10 Without moving your hands, exhale as you bring your left foot forward next to your right foot. Your forehead is down toward your knees (same as step 3).

11 Inhale as you slowly bring your arms up over your head and stretch back, as in step 2.

12 Exhale as you stand upright and bring your arms down alongside your body, returning to the starting position. You are now ready to begin the next Sun Salutation cycle. For the next cycle, you should lead with the left leg, because you led with the right one previously.

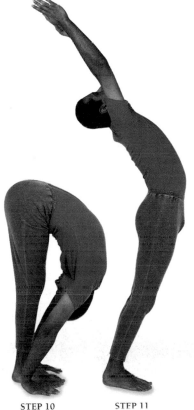
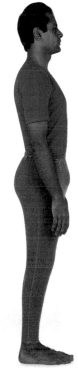
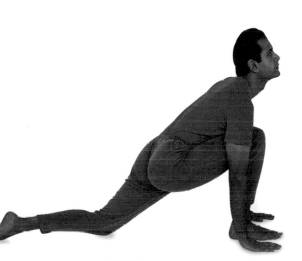

STEP 9   STEP 10   STEP 11   STEP 12

TENSE–RELAX TECHNIQUE

The final relaxation in Sivananda yoga is basically the same as the initial relaxation, except you tense and relax the muscle groups. You will first tense then relax each part of the body in turn, starting with your feet and moving to your head. It is only by knowing how tension feels that you can be aware of how relaxation feels!

In everyday life your mind instructs the muscles to tense and contract under stress. By practicing this relaxation, you can use autosuggestion to tell the muscles to relax. Sivananda yoga tells us that with practice you can learn to use your subconscious mind to extend this control to the involuntary muscles of the heart and organs.

As Swami Vishnu Devananda so aptly put it, "An ounce of practice is worth a ton of theory." In any practice of yoga, no matter what the style, this truth stands. Consistent practice, no matter how short or long, is the key to yoga.

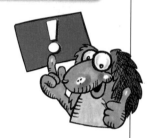

Easeful, peaceful, and useful: Integral yoga

SWAMI SATCHIDANANDA IS THE FOUNDER *of the worldwide Integral Yoga Institutes. He is often referred to as the "Woodstock Guru" because he was one of the original Eastern masters to teach yoga and chanting to a whole generation at the Woodstock Festival in 1969.*

Regarded as an apostle of peace, Swami Satchidananda has received many awards, including the Albert Schweitzer Humanitarian Award and the United Nations Interfaith Award. His credo, "Truth is One, Paths are Many," has been the inspiration behind his vision-come-true: Yogaville – a spiritual center in Buckingham, Virginia, where people of diverse faiths come together to practice the principles of Integral yoga.

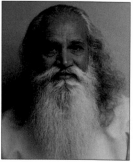

SWAMI SATCHIDANANDA

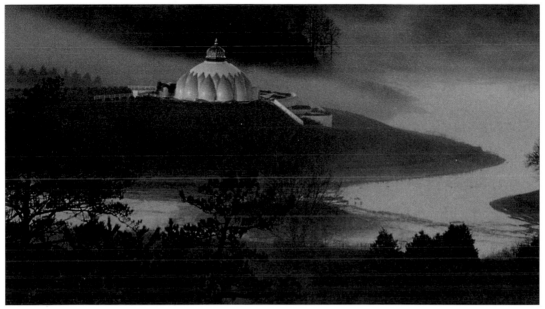

■ **The spectacular LOTUS temple** *is at the heart of the Yogaville ashram, situated in a thousand acres of woodland in the foothills of the Blue Ridge Mountains in Buckingham, Virginia.*

At the Yogaville *ashram* you can do tons of yoga, eat lots of delicious, healthy vegetarian food, chant and sing your heart out, do some Karma yoga (i.e., selfless service), and bask in the spiritual light of the spectacular LOTUS Temple. The LOTUS, an acronym for Light of Truth Universal Shrine, is a tribute to Satchidananda's rock-solid faith in the oneness of us all and the peace that comes from universal love and compassion.

Integral yoga relates to the word "integrity," which means moral excellence. Swami Satchidananda's well-known saying, "Yoga is to be easeful, peaceful, and useful," is a perfect example of Integral yoga's integrity. The goal is to live a life that is equally based on yoga and healthy diet (to be easeful in body), meditation and devotion (to be peaceful in mind), and service to humanity (to be useful to others).

INTERNET

www.yogaville.org

To find out more about Integral yoga and Yogaville, this is the site. Photos of the LOTUS temple are included.

Integral Yoga Hatha, written by Swami Satchidananda, whose words have a simple, sweet truth about them, is the best book for getting a feel for Integral yoga. Poses are demonstrated by the Swami himself.

The daily postures

THE SEQUENCE OF POSTURES *in Integral yoga follows a specific pattern, as it does in Sivananda yoga. Though the order is a little different for each, the same basic postures are recommended as a daily routine. Both also begin with a few rounds of the Sun Salutation and some eye exercises, as do many Hatha yoga classes. This specific sequence of poses is designed for gaining the maximum amount of benefit with the minimum number of poses.*

To begin, sit down on a mat or blanket. Center with three deep breaths or three "Oms."

Cobra pose (Bhujangasana)

1. Lie down on your abdomen, and bring your legs together or slightly apart.

2. Place your palms on the floor beneath your shoulders, with your elbows raised and close to the trunk of the body.

3. Stretch out your chin and, without pressing on your hands, slowly raise your head, neck, and chest, rolling the vertebrae backward one by one. Roll your shoulders back and down, opening your chest. Keep aware of lengthening your spine and moving your chest forward and upward.

Do not raise your body suddenly. Try to bring your chest up with the help of your back muscles, rather than allowing the weight to fall on your arms.

4. Stay this way for 15–30 seconds. Then exhale as you come down very slowly, lowering your trunk first, then your head. Turn your cheek to the side, and relax with your feet apart.

In this pose, your back muscles are strengthened. Your spine becomes elastic, and any slight displacements of the spinal column get adjusted. Your chest expands, and your reproductive organs are toned.

COBRA POSE

Half locust pose (Ardha Salabasana)

(1) Continue to lie face downward. Bring your chin to the floor. Tuck your arms underneath your body with your palms upward, or in fists, or clasped together underneath your body. Have your elbows as close together as possible.

(2) Bring your legs together. Inhale and stretch your right leg out, slowly raising it up as high as is comfortable while keeping the weight centered on both hips. Keep your knees straight and focus on lengthening your lower back while extending out through your raised foot.

(3) Hold and breathe for 10–20 seconds. Then lower your leg down.

(4) Repeat with your left leg. Then repeat one more time on each leg.

(5) Relax with your head turned to one side.

When you are comfortable doing this pose, do full Locust pose.

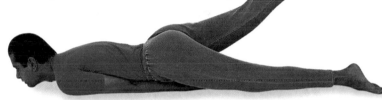

HALF LOCUST POSE

Locust pose (Salabasana)

(1) Continue to lie face downward with your chin on the floor. Tuck your arms underneath your body with your palms upward, or in fists, or clasped together underneath the thighs. Have your elbows as close together as possible.

(2) Inhale and stretch your legs back and raise them up. Keep your knees straight and your legs squeezed together. Focus on elongating your lower back while extending out through your feet.

(3) Continue for 10–15 seconds. Then slowly lower down.

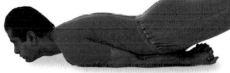

LOCUST POSE

(4) Relax with your feet apart, and your head turned to one side.

In this pose, your back, pelvis, and abdomen are exercised and strengthened, and your sympathetic nervous system is toned. This pose helps to relieve sluggishness of the liver. After a certain amount of practice, Locust pose may be retained while breathing normally for a minute.

Bow pose (Dhanurasana)

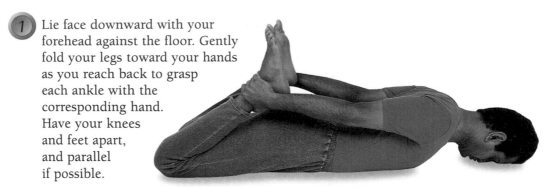

1. Lie face downward with your forehead against the floor. Gently fold your legs toward your hands as you reach back to grasp each ankle with the corresponding hand. Have your knees and feet apart, and parallel if possible.

STEP 1

2. Inhale and raise your head, chest, and thighs, arching your back and stretching up. Keep your elbows straight. Press your legs into your hands, lifting the lower half of the body. Then arch up with your head, neck, and chest, balancing on your abdomen.

3. Open your chest, relax the muscles along your spine, and look up. Keep an awareness of stretching your spine and abdominal area. Continue for 15–20 seconds.

STEP 2

Those who have high blood pressure, a hernia, or an ulcer should avoid Bow pose.

This pose gives all the benefits of both Cobra and Locust. It also reduces abdominal fat, helps the intestines to work properly, and tones up the pancreas, which helps in cases of diabetes.

Head to knee pose (Janusirshasana)

1 Sit on the floor with both legs stretched forward. Walk your buttocks back, coming onto the front of your sitting bones. Bend your left leg, bringing your left heel against the inside of your right thigh, as high up as is comfortable with your knee down.

2 Bring your arms out to the sides. Inhale and raise your arms overhead, stretching up. Exhale and bend forward from your hips, keeping your back as straight as possible.

3 Take hold of your leg or foot as far down as you can comfortably reach. Allow your head and shoulders to relax. Use your breath to continue lengthening your spine and relax more deeply into the posture. Hold for 30–60 seconds.

4 To end, exhale and stretch. Lock your thumbs, lengthen your spine, and slowly raise up. Then repeat the posture with your left leg extended.

5 Relax on your back in Corpse pose for a few seconds.

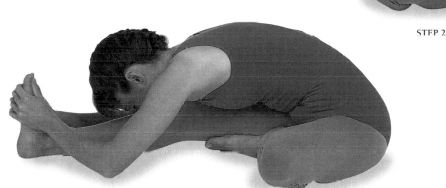

STEP 2

STEP 3

125

Forward bending pose (Paschimothanasana)

1. Sit on the floor with both legs stretched forward. Keeping both knees straight and your toes pointing upward, walk your buttocks back to come on to the front of your sitting bones.

2. Inhale and raise your arms overhead, stretching upward.

3. Exhale and stretch forward with a flat back over both legs. Take hold of your shins, ankles, or toes. Elongate your spine and lower your head. Relax your neck and shoulders while continuing to extend and breathe.

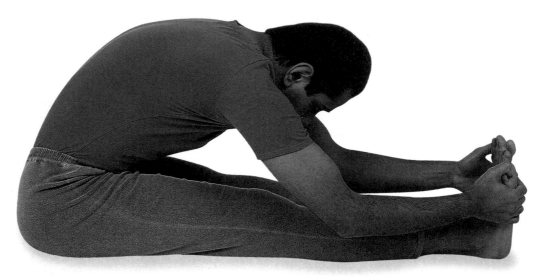

FORWARD BENDING POSE

4. Relax the backs of your legs and focus on stretching out from your lower back, lengthening your entire spine. Continue for 1 minute.

5. Lock your thumbs once again and stretch forward, then straighten your back and sit up. Exhale and, while tucking in your chin, slowly lower your back to the floor one vertebra at a time, and relax for 30 seconds.

This is an excellent stretch for all your back and leg muscles, and tones up your abdominal area. It is good for constipation, sexual or menstrual problems, and reduces fat in the belly area.

Shoulder stand (Sarvangasana)

Many people prefer to do Shoulder stand with a folded blanket under their shoulders, which eliminates extra pressure from the back of the neck. To try this, fold a blanket so that it is 1–2 in (3–5 cm) thick and place it so that when you lie on it, it comes to the top edge of your shoulders.

1. Lie flat on your back, placing your hands alongside your body. Raise your legs up to 90 degrees. Then raise the trunk of your body to a vertical position, while supporting your back with your arms. Keep your elbows on the floor in the same position they started in.

2. In Shoulder stand, your body eventually will form a straight line from the shoulders to the toes. In the beginning, though, it is fine to have your legs angled toward your head. Or you can try to straighten your torso by walking your hands closer to your shoulder blades, pressing your hips forward, and bringing your feet back so that they come more in line with your hips.

3. Relax your neck and shoulders. Feel the upward lift all the way through your feet. When you feel comfortable, try straightening up a little more in the pose.

4. Breathe normally in this pose for 1–2 minutes. To come out of the pose, slowly lower your legs overhead until they are parallel to the floor. Place your palms down on the floor for support and very slowly roll your back down without letting your head come off the floor. Lower your legs slowly and relax on your back. If your lower spine is tight, bring your knees to the chest briefly.

Shoulder stand is not recommended during menstruation or pregnancy, for those with uncontrolled high blood pressure, hiatal hernias, or neck injuries, or for anyone with headaches or other disturbances of the head area. Do not cough, swallow, or clear the throat while in the pose.

This pose regulates the thyroid and sex glands, helps with asthma, liver and intestinal disorders, heart problems, and almost anything! The name Sarva-Anga-Asana means "a beneficial pose for the whole body."

SHOULDER STAND

Fish pose (Matsyasana)

1. Lie down on the floor on your back with the palms of your hands flat on the floor under the buttocks. Resting your weight on your elbows, raise your head and the trunk of your body.

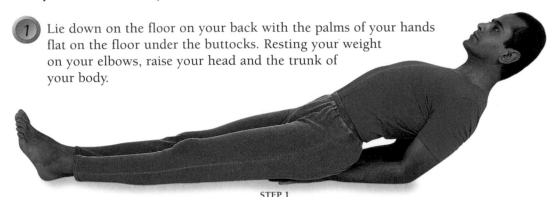

STEP 1

2. Tilt your pelvis forward, and lower the top of your head to the floor, creating a strong arch in your back. Let your chest be fully expanded and your shoulders spread wide. Breathe deeply through your nose, and have a slight smile on your face to relieve any tension in your jaws. Continue for 20–45 seconds.

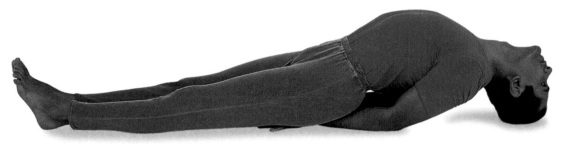

STEP 2

3. To come down, bring your weight onto your elbows, lift your head off the floor, and sit up halfway. Lower your back to the floor, vertebra by vertebra.

4. You can roll your head gently from side to side to relax the neck. Then relax on your back for 30 seconds.

This is a complementary pose to Shoulder stand, stretching your body in the opposite direction. Your chest cavity expands to its maximum, optimizing your lung capacity. Fish pose helps to prevent asthmatic conditions, gives a natural massage to your neck and shoulders, and strengthens your abdominal and back muscles.

Half spinal twist (Ardha Matsyendrasana)

1 Sit up with your legs extended in front. Bend your right leg. Cross your right foot over the extended leg, placing the sole of your foot on the floor close to your left knee.

2 Take hold of your upraised knee with both hands and stretch your spine upward.

3 Gently twist your trunk to the right, and place your right hand on the floor behind you with your fingers pointing away, to help keep your spine erect.

4 Place your left arm between your chest and upraised knee. Then, pressing against your knee, take hold of your right ankle with your left hand.

5 Stretching upward, twist a little further, looking over your right shoulder. Feel the twist in the entire length of your spine. Breathe steadily for 30 seconds.

6 To come out of the pose, turn your head back around to center. Release your back arm, then your front arm. Uncross your legs, stretching them both out in front. Relax a moment before reversing sides.

Beginners may find Half spinal twist simpler to do than Spinal twist on p. 105. All spinal twists help to balance the liver, spleen, kidneys, and adrenals. They help to tone your sympathetic nerves and ganglia, and strengthen both the deep and superficial muscles of your back.

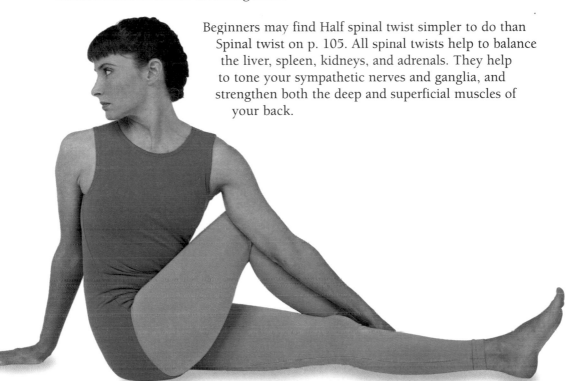

HALF SPINAL TWIST

The Yogic seal (Yoga mudra)

1 Sit in whatever cross-legged position is comfortable, with your spine erect and your eyes closed.

2 Bring your hands in back of your body and hold your right wrist with your left hand. Inhale and lengthen your spine upward. Your buttocks stay grounded on the floor.

3 Exhale and slowly bend forward, bringing your chest toward the floor. Bend forward as far as you can. Relax your head and shoulders.

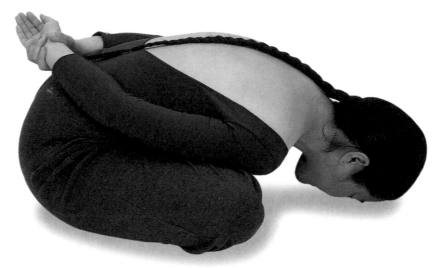

THE YOGIC SEAL

4 Relax into the pose while maintaining an inner awareness of your breath. Continue for 30 seconds.

5 Inhale and very slowly raise your head, lengthen your spine, and sit up.

The maximum benefit is obtained in Yoga mudra by maintaining an inner awareness during the pose. Yoga mudra strengthens and tones the abdominal organs and the nervous system.

Corpse pose

Always remember to leave some time at the end of your yoga session for deep relaxation on your back. When you are finished, wake your body up slowly, stretch, and roll to your right side to sit up.

Traditionally, an Integral yoga practice ends with meditation and chanting. One of the most common *mantras* used is "Om Shanti Om," which means "Peace to all."

DEFINITION

Mantra *literally means "mind projection" and is a yogic technique of focusing on an external or internal sound to create a personal transformation. Concentrated repetition (internal or out loud) produces vibrations within the individual's entire system that are in tune with the universal vibration or energy.*

A simple summary

✔ Classic yoga is practiced in the most traditional and well-known way. Sivananda and Integral yoga are two paths of yoga rooted with the same master.

✔ Sivananda yoga's teachings are compiled into five simple points: Yogic postures, breathing exercises, relaxation, healthy diet, and meditation.

✔ Many yoga classes will start with the Sun Salutation, which is a fluid series of postures.

✔ Both Sivananda and Integral yogas feature a complete lifestyle and have ashrams where yoga students and teachers can live or visit as a retreat center.

✔ Integral yoga's theme is to live an easeful, peaceful, and useful life. Yoga makes the body easeful, meditation makes the mind peaceful, and together they create a state of well-being that allows you to be useful in the service of others.

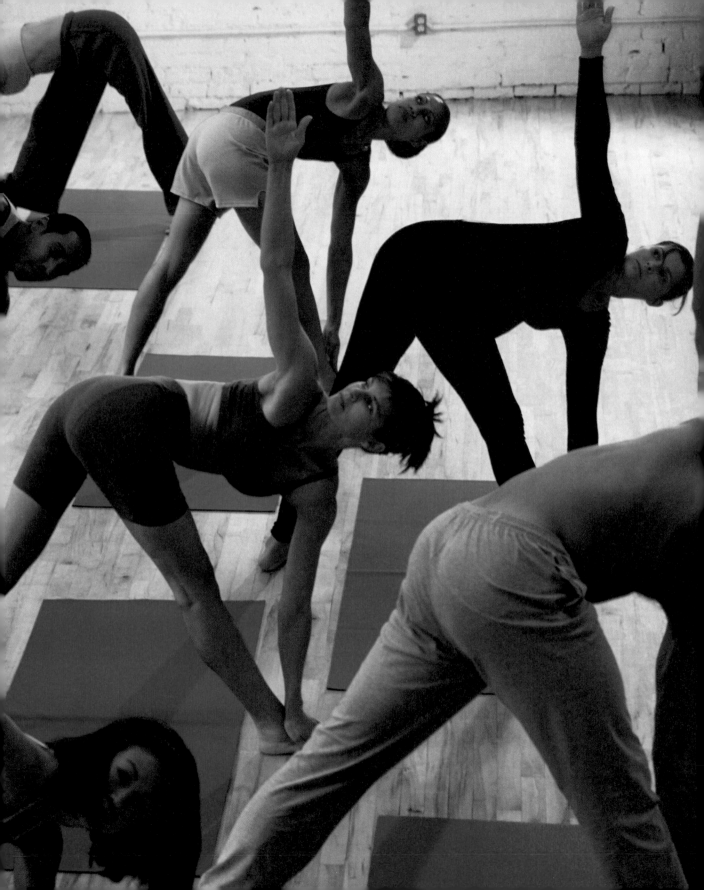

Chapter 8

Align Yourself with Yoga

How well do you line up? The two schools of yoga in this chapter focus on alignment of the physical body and, in turn, the spirit. Traditional Iyengar yoga is one of the most respected and widely practiced forms of yoga in the world. Its focus is on balance, posture, and alignment. Anusara yoga, a contemporary yoga movement, is similar to Iyengar yoga, yet distinctive. In this chapter you will gain an understanding of the bio-mechanics of yoga and try mini classes in Iyengar and Anusara.

In this chapter...

✓ Iyengar yoga

✓ The Iyengar practice

✓ Anusara yoga

✓ The yoga of grace

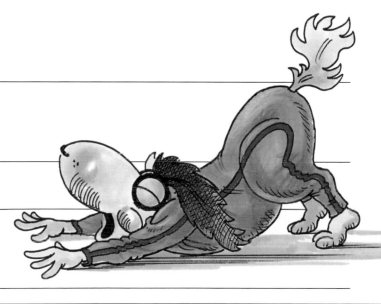

THE TRIANGLE POSE IN TRADITIONAL IYENGAR YOGA TONES THE LEG MUSCLES

Iyengar yoga

B.K.S. IYENGAR'S MUSCULAR, *pliant figure looms over the development of yoga in the West. Since first coming to the United States in 1974, Iyengar has been the inspiration behind hundreds of yoga centers with thousands of students in more than 40 countries. He is the author of* Light on Yoga, *sometimes called the "bible of modern yoga," and he continues to teach at his center in Pune, India.*

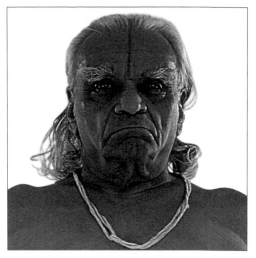

B.K.S. IYENGAR

Mr. Iyengar learned from the master-teacher Sri T. Krishnamacharya, head of the Yoga Institute at the yoga palace of Mysore, India. Krishnamacharya also taught two other well-known teachers whom we will be meeting in later chapters.

Focus on precision

The focus in an Iyengar class is on precise alignment and on meeting individual needs through the use of props. Iyengar yoga stresses the science of understanding the body and how it works. Some followers of Iyengar report that pursuing the exact alignment of each posture – instead of moving from pose to pose as practiced in some schools – is their favored method for calming the mind and strengthening the body.

Less yoga is more

In an Iyengar class, less is more. You may do only a few postures, but you will dive into them at the microscopic level. At the least, you will gain a greater awareness of the intricacies of your body's workings. Your may learn to "pull the kneecaps up" (to quote one Iyengar teacher), and do countless other feats of inner mind–body control that never even occurred to you before an Iyengar class.

INTERNET

www.iyengar-yoga.com

www.comnet.org/iynaus

The first resource for Iyengar yoga includes a chant voiced by Mr. Iyengar himself. The second includes, among other information, an international listing of Iyengar teachers.

Trivia...

Mr. Iyengar was born a poor and very sickly child. In fact, his bed was his constant companion. Rather than despairing, he was spurred on by his poor health to learn yoga and become a master of it. One of his students was the violin virtuoso Yehudi Menuhin, who recognized the greatness of yoga and Iyengar's mastery by saying, "He is my best violin teacher."

There may be so little talk of breathing that you will need a reminder, because you will be thinking so hard about your body and what it is doing. Most of the focus will be on how your sitting bones are sitting, and how your knee bone is connecting to your anklebone, the anklebone to the foot bone, foot bone to the toe bone and . . . hallelujah! You might hear the word of the Lord!

I am used to yoga being a meditative experience, so when I went to my first Iyengar class, my concept of a yoga class was turned topsy-turvy (as was I, with my legs up a wall in a modified handstand!).

Between nonstop instructions and students calling out questions, my Iyengar teacher firmly (but respectfully) tugged my legs higher into shoulder stand, making sure my props were all in place for each pose – it was more workshop than mystical experience – and I found it both enlightening and fascinating in its own way.

How to recognize an Iyengar yoga class

This one's not hard. Just look around in the corners of the room for wooden blocks, stacks of felt-like blankets, and straps and belts hanging from hooks. If this is what you find, you are most likely in an Iyengar yoga class.

Props, as these contraptions are called, are the key to most of us being able to do Iyengar yoga well. If you can't reach the floor, the floor can come to you in the form of a block of wood that has been strategically placed where you need it most. A belt can help you reach your foot while you are lying on your back with one foot in the air. Furthermore, you can stretch your leg crosswise over your body while controlling the reins with one hand. Most of us can't get a good stretch like that any other way.

■ **A chair and folded** *blanket are used here to help the Iyengar student perfect Plow pose.*

135

ALL THE PROPER PROPS

If you are new to yoga, have limited flexibility, or want to use yoga therapeutically, these are the props out there for you:

- Yoga ("sticky") mats offer a nonslippery surface for standing posture.
- Tightly woven or firm blankets are used for sitting, and for support in shoulder stand, headstand, and Corpse pose. You may need more than one.
- Wooden or dense foam blocks (approximately 4 x 6 x 9 in/ 10 x 15 x 23 cm) are used for support in standing poses.
- A strap or belt with a buckle is used for forward bends, reaching arms in back, and other poses.
- A folding chair with a back and flat seat is used for some standing and twisting poses. It's good for chair yoga, too.
- A wall is great for lots of things: Support for Plow pose, preparing for handstands, a leaning place for squatting, or arch support – for arching in Bridge pose. And you don't have to buy it (although I have actually seen yoga walls for sale in yoga paraphernalia catalogs!).

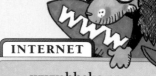

INTERNET

www.bheka.com

www.yogapro.com

www.yogaprops.net

www.huggermugger.com

www.fishcrane.com

These and other yoga toys can be found at the above web sites.

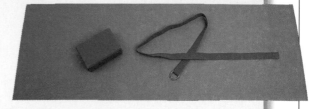

■ **Among the props** *used for Iyengar yoga are a "sticky" mat, blocks, and a strap or belt.*

The Iyengar practice

BEFORE YOU BEGIN YOUR IYENGAR JOURNEY, *there are a few good things that would be beneficial for you to know:*

1. In addition to lending energy to the pose, jumping your feet from one posture to the next serves to help you land on both feet at the same time and to keep you balanced. You might be the exception, but most people have patterns of leading with one particular leg, and following with the other.

2. You may need to make small adjustments to your feet and/or hands in the standing poses in order to do them well.

3 As far as possible, keep your mind passive, watchful, and alert. It is the body alone that will be active.

4 After completing the practice, always lie down in Corpse pose for relaxation for at least 10–15 minutes.

5 In *Light on Yoga*, B.K.S. Iyengar instructs: "In the beginning, keep the eyes open. Then you will know what you are doing, and where you go wrong. You can keep your eyes closed only when you are perfect in a particular asana for only then will you be able to adjust the body's movement and feel the correct stretches . . . . The right way of doing asanas brings lightness and an exhilarating feeling in the body and the mind. When one has mastered an asana, it comes with effortless ease and causes no discomfort."

Mountain pose (Tadasana)

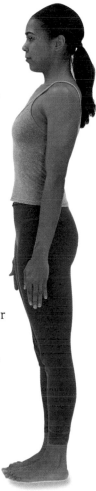

MOUNTAIN POSE

1 Stand erect with your feet together and your heels and big toes touching each other (if possible). Rest the balls of your feet on the floor and stretch your toes flat on the floor. Keep the weight of your body evenly distributed between the outsides and insides of your feet and the balls and heels.

2 Tighten your knees, then pull your kneecaps up, but do not lock your knees. Contract your hips and pull up the muscles at the back of your thighs. Tuck your tailbone into your body. Your pelvis feels light on the tops of your thighs.

3 Keep your chest out and your spine stretched up. Drop your shoulder blades downward. The back of your neck lengthens and your jaws relax.

4 Place your arms straight down at the sides of your thighs. Relax your arms, hands, and fingers.

5 Breathe normally (through your nose) for 1 minute. Keep a sense of balance, steadiness, firmness, and an uplifted feeling.

Most of us have a habit of standing and walking with most of our weight shifted to one side, or on the heels or outer edges of our feet. You can tell what kind of standing and walking patterns you have by checking the soles of your shoes.

You may be saying, "Yes, so?" If you remember that you are holistic, then you know that whatever happens to a part affects the whole. The rest of the body shifts to accommodate an imbalance in your standing and walking patterns.

Just where you are, stand with your body weight mostly on your heels. Do you feel your center of gravity changing to accommodate this action? Your hips become too loose, your belly comes forward, and your spine feels the strain. This in turn affects your brain, so that you become tired and the mind becomes dull. All because of a seemingly small shift in your posture.

Triangle pose (Uttihita Trikonasana)

1 Stand in Mountain pose.

2 Inhale deeply and, with a jump, spread your legs apart 4–4½ ft (1.2–1.4 m). Raise your arms sideways in line with your shoulders, palms facing downward. Stretch out from your fingertips. Keep your arms parallel to the floor, and your shoulders in line with your hips.

3 Turn your right foot and leg out 90 degrees to the right. Turn your left foot slightly to the right, keeping your left leg stretched from the inside and tightened at your knee. Keep your weight evenly distributed on all parts of your feet: The balls, heels, insides, and outsides.

4 Exhale, and bend your trunk sideways to the right, bringing your right palm near your right ankle. If possible, your right palm should rest completely on the floor. (If you cannot reach the floor, you can use a block, or place your hand on your shin.)

5 Stretch your left arm up, bringing it in line with your right shoulder. Lift your chest. The backs of your legs, the back of your chest, and the hips should be in a line. Gaze at the thumb of your outstretched left hand. Your right knee faces your toes, and is firmed by pulling up your kneecap.

6 Remain in this position for half a minute to a minute, breathing deeply and evenly. Then lift your right palm from the floor. Inhale and return to position 2.

TRIANGLE POSE

7　Reverse your position so that your left foot is sideways at a 90-degree angle, and your right foot is slightly to the right. Repeat the process.

8　Exhale and jump, coming back into Mountain pose.

This asana tones up the leg muscles, removes stiffness in the legs and hips, and balances them structurally. It relieves backaches and neck pains, strengthens the ankles, and develops the chest.

Warrior pose II (Virabhadrasana)

1　Stand in Mountain pose.

2　Take a deep inhalation, and with a jump spread your legs apart sideways 4–4½ ft (1.2–1.4 m), and parallel. Raise your arms sideways in line with your shoulders, palms facing down, shoulders relaxed.

3　Turn your right foot sideways 90 degrees to the right, and your left foot slightly to the right, keeping your left leg stretched out and tightened at your knee. Turn hips and chest so they are facing to the front.

4　Exhale and bend your right knee until your right thigh is parallel to the floor. This will form a right angle between your right thigh and your right calf. Your knee is directly over your ankle. Your right buttock comes in line with your right knee. Your bent knee should not extend beyond your ankle, but should be in line with your heel.

WARRIOR POSE II

5　Stretch out your hands sideways, as though you were being pulled simultaneously from opposite ends. Lift your front hipbone and your breastbone.

6　Turn your neck and face to the right, gazing at your right hand. Stretch the back muscles of your left leg fully.

7　This is Warrior pose, so be strong. Stretch out and extend through your fingers. Breathe deeply for 30 seconds.

Mastering the standing poses prepares you for more advanced poses. In Warrior pose II, the leg muscles become strong. In addition, this pose relieves cramps in the calves and thighs, brings elasticity to the leg and back muscles, and tones the abdominal organs. Keeping the bent knee directly over the ankle distributes the weight evenly, preventing the knee from overworking in this posture.

Downward-facing dog (Adho Mukha Savasana)

1. Lie down on the floor on your abdomen, face downwards. Your feet are 1 ft (30 cm) apart.

2. Place your palms by the sides of your chest, with your fingers straight. Place the underside of your toes and balls of your feet on the floor.

3. Exhale and raise your trunk from the floor. Your hips move toward the ceiling and back away from your hands. Lift your sitting bones completely up toward the ceiling. Pull your kneecaps up, and press your thighs toward the wall behind you.

4. Keep the weight on your hands evenly distributed between the insides and outsides of your hands, palms, and spread fingers. Stretch your inner elbows and your upper armpits. Stretch your spine up away from the floor as much as possible. Your head is in line with your upper spine. Pull your hips back so that your weight is drawn up away from the floor completely.

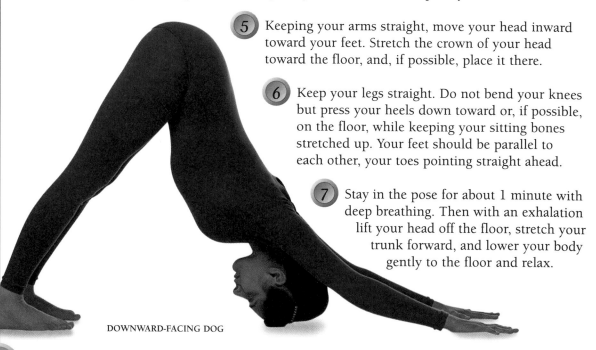

5. Keeping your arms straight, move your head inward toward your feet. Stretch the crown of your head toward the floor, and, if possible, place it there.

6. Keep your legs straight. Do not bend your knees but press your heels down toward or, if possible, on the floor, while keeping your sitting bones stretched up. Your feet should be parallel to each other, your toes pointing straight ahead.

7. Stay in the pose for about 1 minute with deep breathing. Then with an exhalation lift your head off the floor, stretch your trunk forward, and lower your body gently to the floor and relax.

DOWNWARD-FACING DOG

Downward-facing dog is especially good for runners and sprinters as it relieves pain and stiffness in the heels, strengthens the ankles, and makes the legs strong.

This is an exhilarating and rejuvenating pose because it removes fatigue and brings back lost energy. The practice of Downward-facing dog also helps to remove stiffness and arthritis in the shoulder blades and joints. The abdominal muscles are drawn toward the spine and strengthened. As the diaphragm is lifted to the chest cavity, the heart rate is slowed down.

As the trunk is lowered in this asana, it is fully stretched, and blood is circulated efficiently, rejuvenating the brain cells and invigorating the brain.

BARBARA'S STORY

A car accident in 1972 left me with two disintegrated cervical discs and trauma to my knees. As a result, I developed arthritis in both my neck and knees. I began Iyengar yoga classes in 1987 at age 60 to relieve the pain, and gain some strength and flexibility. Thirteen years later, my progress in yoga has surpassed my greatest expectations, for which I credit the guidance and encouragement of my teacher, John Schumacher of Unity Wood Yoga Center. I not only fully recovered from the car accident, but I feel younger than I used to. For example, I never dreamed that I would be able to do a headstand. Now that is easy for me.

At one point in my life, I felt like I was heading for a nervous breakdown. I was having a lot of difficulty with my son, who was drinking heavily. Through yoga and meditation I found a way to work with my feelings, and find a place of detachment and peace with him.

Four years ago, yoga helped me through another crisis. My husband was killed in an accident. I was in so much grief, and something inside of me said, "Just stay with the yoga." It has touched something so deep within me.

If you just do yoga like an exercise class, that's what you'll get out of it. If you want more, that's what you'll get. Yoga, pranayama, and meditation have changed my life. Not only does it change your life, but I feel that it prepares you for death.

Anusara yoga

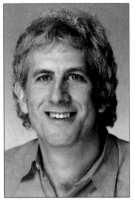

JOHN FRIEND

JOHN FRIEND, *a long-time yoga teacher, founded* Anusara *yoga in 1997. Friend, whose eclectic background in yoga has strong roots in Iyengar yoga, was inspired to develop a yoga style that would help students connect to the spiritual purpose behind the practice of Hatha yoga, while maintaining all the strong postural instruction that is the backbone of Iyengar yoga, or, in Friend's words, "both spiritually uplifting and grounded in universal principles of alignment."*

The three A's of Anusara

The central philosophy of Anusara yoga is based on the view that the body, mind, and spirit are equally divine, and therefore equally honored. These principles are expressed in the three A's of Anusara yoga: Attitude, Alignment, and Action.

THE FOCAL POINT

One more important concept that is part of Anusara yoga's terminology is the focal point, which refers to the key place of power in the body within a given asana. It can be visualized as a small orb of energy the size of a golf ball. Only one focal point is active in every asana; it's the one that is nearest to the most weight-bearing part of the pose.
For example:

● Standing and sitting poses: The active focal point is in the core of the pelvis.

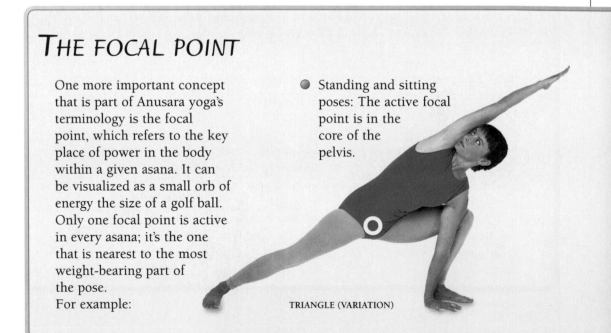

TRIANGLE (VARIATION)

1. **Attitude.** In an Anusara yoga class, the teacher will inspire you to awaken to something greater within you. This reflects the first "A" of Anusara yoga, Attitude. For inner transformation, Attitude is the most important of the three A's. A pose can have perfect alignment, and be balanced in its action, but without a pure spiritual expression from the heart, it loses its power to make changes within you.

2. **Alignment.** The second principle is Alignment. Each pose is performed with an integrated awareness between all the different parts of the body. John Friend has codified this awareness into a system he calls the Universal Principles of Alignment, which includes terms such as "energy loops and spirals," and "muscular and organic energy."

Don't let this talk about energy loops and spirals throw you for a loop! Hold on a bit, and I think you will catch on when we practice some Anusara yoga later in this chapter.

3. **Action.** Balanced Action is the final of the three A's. Here's an example: Every posture requires both muscular energy (which creates stability, strength, and physical integration) to hold it in place, and organic energy (which creates expansion in the body), to keep you relaxed and open.

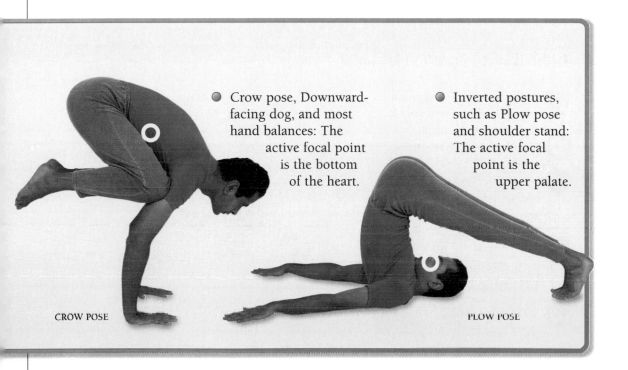

● Crow pose, Downward-facing dog, and most hand balances: The active focal point is the bottom of the heart.

● Inverted postures, such as Plow pose and shoulder stand: The active focal point is the upper palate.

CROW POSE

PLOW POSE

The yoga of grace

ARE YOU UP FOR *an Anusara experience? Get ready to "hug your muscles to your bones," as they say in Anusara. I am betting you will learn some things about yourself as you are learning about muscular and organic energy, loops, and spirals.*

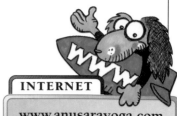

INTERNET

www.anusarayoga.com

You can find everything you want to know about Anusara yoga, including the location of teachers in your area and teacher-training sessions, at this web site.

The first few exercises that follow give you first-hand knowledge of the three A's. The second part prepares you for the well-known yoga posture called Camel pose, which will wrap up your Anusara yoga time.

Don't worry if you don't get "muscle hugging," or some of the other subtle movements, right away. I didn't. But I kept trying until I got the hang of it. I was so delighted with how well it creates good alignment while avoiding possible strains that I added muscle-hugging to my regular yoga practice.

Muscular and organic energy

Muscular and organic energy are aspects of every pose in Anusara yoga. The following exercise demonstrates these concepts.

1. Lift one arm up and hold it parallel to the floor. Stretch the arm as far forward as possible, and then bring it up overhead.

2. Maintain that arm position as you lift the other arm up parallel to the floor.

3. On the second arm, hug your arm muscles onto the bone by firming it. Draw energy from your fingertips toward your shoulder. Draw your arm bone firmly into your shoulder socket. This is an example of muscular energy.

4. Raise your arm overhead. Maintaining the firmness of your arm bone moving into your shoulder, stretch your arm up, lengthening from your shoulder to your fingertips. This lengthening is organic energy.

5. With both arms stretched up over your head, close your eyes and feel the difference between your two shoulders.

In the first shoulder you stretch, your arm bone is not integrated into the shoulder socket and stretching in that position can be damaging to the shoulder. On the second shoulder, however, your arm bone is firmly integrated into the shoulder and is in a healthier position for the shoulder to stretch. In this way, shoulder flexibility can be increased without injury.

Making an inner spiral

The challenge of back-bending poses is to do them in such a way that you create space in your back, so that there is no pinching anywhere, especially in your lower back. Doing an inner spiral of your legs can help enormously in creating and maintaining more space in your sacrum and lower back.

1. Stand with your feet hip-width apart, firm your leg muscles, and roll your thighs in.

2. Move your thighs back slightly, which moves your sitting bones apart. Feel your sacrum become broad with this action of the legs.

3. The inner spiral creates more space in your sacrum and lower back, so there is more space to then move your tailbone down and tilt it slightly inward. This is called a "cat tilt."

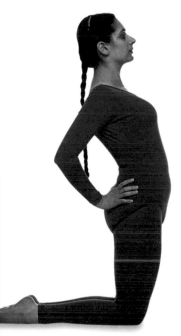

Camel pose (Ustrasana)

Read through the instructions before trying Camel pose. If you need to use blocks for resting your hands, set them up in the vertical position on the outside of each ankle before beginning.

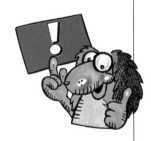

1. Kneel on a blanket with your knees and feet hip distance apart and your toes pointing straight back.

2. Bring your hands on your hips and roll your thighs in, moving the tops of your thighs back slightly. Feel your sacrum broaden. Firm the tops of your buttocks and lengthen from your waistline toward your sitting bones as you scoop your tailbone down and in. Draw your lower abdomen in and up toward your navel.

STEP 2

3 As you inhale, lift your ribcage to lengthen up through your spine. Let the fullness of your breath lift your shoulders into a slight shrug, until your collarbone is level. Press your shoulders back, taking the tops of your arm bones toward the back plane of your body. Firm your shoulder blades into your back.

4 Lift your heart straight up, and let that lift begin to bend your upper body backward from as high in your back as possible. Keep your head upright and look forward at first to keep your neck long and your head supported. Courageously feel that you are being led by your heart into the back bend.

5 Reach your hands back and place them with your fingers pointing backwards on your ankles, heels, or on the blocks. Turn your upper arms out to firm your shoulder blades into your back so that they lift and support your heart. Lengthen the back of your neck and then tilt your head back to look up. Keep lifting your spine upward so there is no pinching in your back.

STEP 4

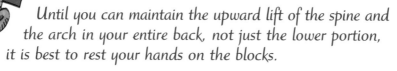

Until you can maintain the upward lift of the spine and the arch in your entire back, not just the lower portion, it is best to rest your hands on the blocks.

6 Maintain the pose for 30–60 seconds with deep breathing while you firm the tops of your buttocks to draw your tailbone down and in to support your lower back. Press your hips forward. Continue to lift through your heart to extend your spine. Relax and open up to a bigger power that surrounds you and is inside of you. Lead with your heart. Maintain an open heart.

STEP 5

7 From the core of your pelvis, stretch in two directions. Also from the core of your pelvis, extend your energy down through your legs to your knees and out through the toes. And still from the core of your pelvis, extend your energy up through your spine to the crown of your head, lifting and opening your heart. Breathe fully and evenly.

8 To come out of the pose, inhale and press down through your feet as you lift your torso from the base of your shoulder blades. Come up, releasing both hands at the same time. Keep your shoulders rolled back and let your heart lead the way up out of the pose. Keep your head back and let your head come up last.

9 After back-bending poses, do one or more poses to release your back and lengthen your spine, such as Downward-facing dog or Child's pose. Follow that with a gentle forward bend to stretch your back muscles, or tuck your knees into your chest while lying on your back. Relax with long, nurturing breaths for several minutes.

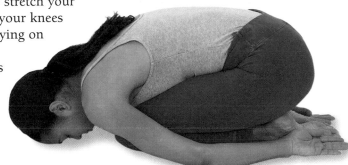

CHILD'S POSE

A simple summary

✔ Iyengar yoga and Anusara yoga are two schools of yoga that focus on the alignment of the physical body and, in turn, the spirit. Iyengar is a traditional yoga practice, while Anusara yoga is a contemporary movement.

✔ Iyengar yoga is one of the most widely practiced yogas around today.

✔ The focus in an Iyengar class is on the precise alignment of the body and meeting the needs of the individual through the use of props. Iyengar yoga stresses the science of understanding the body and how it works.

✔ Anusara yoga, which means "flowing with grace," was founded in 1997 by John Friend, who was inspired to develop a yoga style that is both spiritually uplifting and grounded in universal principles of alignment.

✔ The central philosophy of Anusara yoga is based on the view that the body, mind, and spirit are equally divine, and therefore equally honored. These principles are expressed in the three A's of Anusara yoga: Attitude, Alignment, and Action.

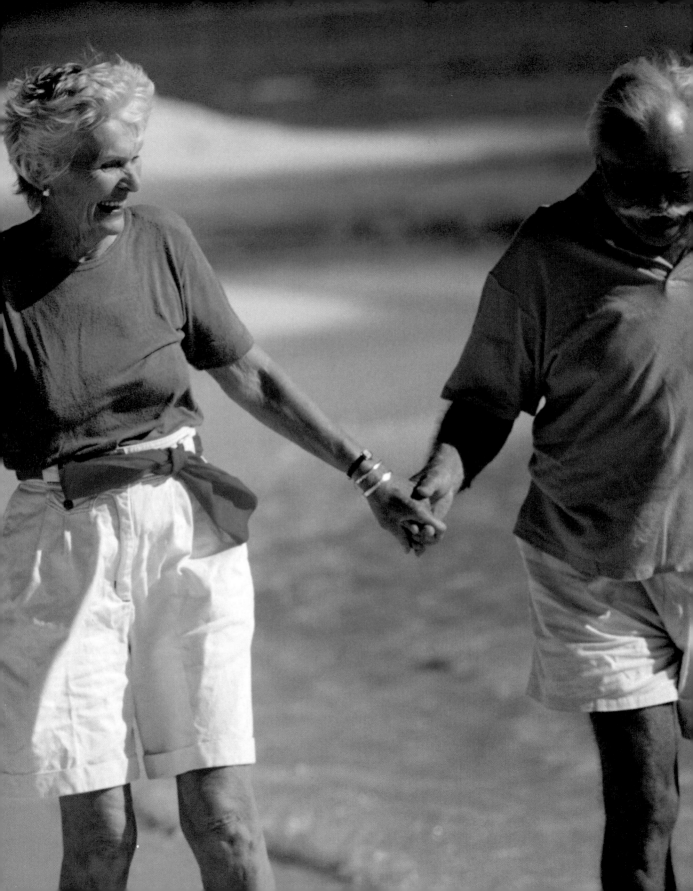

Chapter 9

Progressive Styles of Yoga

THE NUMBER ONE PRIORITY of Kripalu and Viniyoga is custom tailoring yoga to suit an individual's needs and character. Kripalu yoga and Viniyoga differ greatly in approach, but both are designed to enable each person to progress through stages in ways that are natural for him or her. Kripalu yoga has an introspective, somewhat psychological approach, progressing in stages, so that it eventually becomes a meditation in motion. Viniyoga takes a smooth, relaxing approach to yoga, and builds a practice that is both safe and progressive.

In this chapter...

✓ Connecting with Kripalu

✓ Sampling Kripalu

✓ What is Viniyoga?

✓ Breath and movement

✓ Easing into your practice

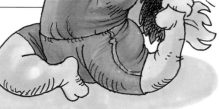

REGARDLESS OF AGE, HEALTH, AND LIFESTYLE, THERE IS A TYPE OF YOGA TO SUIT EVERYONE

Connecting with Kripalu

THE WORD "KRIPALU" comes from kripal, which means "compassion" or "mercy" in the Sanskrit language. In a nutshell, compassion is the focus of Kripalu yoga. According to Kripalu philosophy, the spirit will blossom when the body and mind are watered with the nectar of compassion. This theme is artfully woven into the class by the skilled Kripalu yoga teacher. In a Kripalu yoga class, what you are feeling is just as important as how your body feels.

The birth of Kripalu yoga

The inspiration for Kripalu's yoga program came originally from an Indian master named Kripalvananda (Swami Kripalu), who was the spiritual teacher of a yogi named Amrit Desai. Swami Kripalu's teachings were brought to America by Yogi Desai, and still serve as the foundation of Kripalu's approach to yoga and spiritual life.

Yogi Desai founded the Kripalu Center in Lenox, Massachusetts, which in the past 25 years has become one of the largest centers for yoga and holistic health in the United States. After the 1994 resignation of Yogi Desai as spiritual director of Kripalu, the center has restructured its organization so that it is now headed by a management team of long-time ashram residents and professionals.

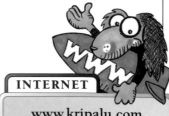

INTERNET

www.kripalu.com

The Kripalu Center serves over 20,000 guests per year and supports a network of 4,000 trained teachers. Check out the Kripalu Center's web site for program offerings and teacher directory.

Looking within yourself

How often do you look within yourself? Just for a few moments as you sit where you are, close your eyes so you can "see" inwardly rather than outwardly. Notice your arising sensations – a pang in a muscle, the rise and fall of the breath, a sound that comes from the left. Now turn your observance away from the physical to notice the mental and emotional sensations. A tightness in your forehead from straining to think, a fleeting feeling of sadness, a tension in your jaw that reminds you of the pressure of your job . . . .

When you meet these sensations consciously, you experience them fully without labeling or judging them. When you become comfortable with and accepting of these human experiences, the doorway to your inner being is opened. In Kripalu yoga, you are encouraged to look within yourself in this way. The most essential teaching in Kripalu yoga is the practice of self-observation without judgment.

THE THREE STAGES OF PROGRESSION

1 In Kripalu yoga, the very beginning stage of your yoga practice is to be willing to direct your body into postures, paying attention to body alignment, and breathing as consciously as you can. You begin to sense how far you can safely go into a stretch and how long to hold the postures.

2 In the second stage, you become attuned to the presence and flow of the life force, prana, which guides the functioning of the body and mind. You begin to develop what is sometimes called the witness, or the observer. You identify with that part of you that is neutrally and compassionately watching what is going on within you, both on physical and emotional levels. You are feeling what is present while holding a posture. In other words, you are doing yoga from the inside out.

3 As you become more tuned in to your body's sensations, you will begin to open to your own intuitive wisdom. Ask yourself, "What would feel good right now?" Prana, life energy, fills you, and you may instinctively feel like moving your body from one position to another. By allowing these movements to spontaneously come forth, you enter stage three, which in Kripalu yoga is described as meditation in motion.

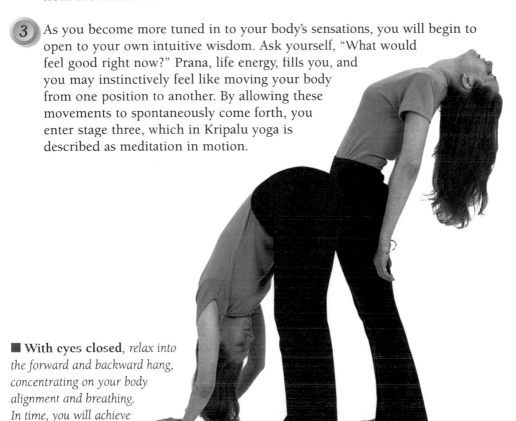

■ **With eyes closed**, *relax into the forward and backward hang, concentrating on your body alignment and breathing. In time, you will achieve meditation in motion.*

During the holding of postures, if you go too fast, have fear, or push yourself beyond your limits, your body will contract and produce additional tension. By continuing to observe yourself, you can understand how tension is created in your body. With time and practice, you can relax more fully in held postures by breathing deeply and staying kind to yourself.

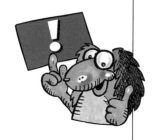

Sampling Kripalu

A KRIPALU CLASS *will consist of pranayama, stretching, postures, and deep relaxation. The following is a sampling of the Kripalu style to give you a simple and authentic experience. Find a quiet spot – your yoga space – and sit in Easy pose with a straight spine to begin. Enjoy!*

Pranayama

1. Breathe in deeply. At the same time, be aware of letting go of the outside concerns for the past and future. Allow yourself to be fully present in this breath as you exhale deeply.

2. On the next several cycles of breath, begin to focus on the breath in the following way:

3. On the inhalation, let your belly be soft. Let the breath fill your abdomen, then your heart center, and up to your collarbone. Fill each section as much as possible without forcing or straining.

4. Imagine the exhalation as water pouring out of a glass or jug. The exhalation starts at the top from your collarbone, then your heart, and finally your abdomen. At the end of the exhalation, gently pull your navel back to your spine to press out any stale air in the lower lungs.

5. Relax and soften your abdomen, letting the breath fill your lungs on another inhalation.

Trivia...

Have you ever heard of Swami Beyondananda? He's the cosmic clown who's been around as long as the yoga movement. Every once in a while I check his web site, www.beyondananda.com, for an artfully funny play on words. Today I found one that fits with Kripalu yoga's emphasis on introspection: "As we go through life thinking heavy thoughts, thought particles tend to get caught between the ears, causing a condition called truth decay. So be sure, and use mental floss twice a day." (Mental floss equals your yoga practice?)

6 Take one more breath, feeling that you are uniting all the aspects of yourself – body, mind, and spirit. Softly chant the sound of "Om," extending the "mmm" sound. Hear it, feel it, and see it as it resounds around you.

Simple pigeon pose (Kapotasana), stage 1

1 From a position on your hands and knees (table position), slide your right knee forward between your hands. Slide your left leg behind you. Depending on your hip flexibility, your foot may be underneath your pubic bone or out to the side at a comfortable angle.

2 Press outward through your back heel while lengthening your left leg. Square your hips to the front, and lay your left foot flat behind you, with the left ankle and foot in line with your left leg.

3 Begin to lower your right hip toward the floor. If there is a lot of space between your right hip and the floor (an inch or more), you may want to prop a blanket under your right hip to support it, and allow it to passively open up.

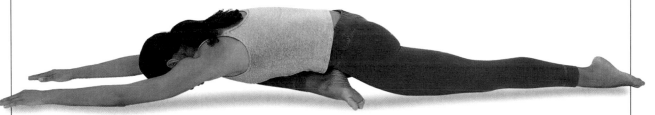

SIMPLE PIGEON POSE, STAGE 1

4 Exhale and extend from your waist, lead with your sternum, and lower your torso forward, over your right knee. Slide your hands forward on the ground and bring your forehead to rest on the floor. You can also place one hand on top of the other, and rest your forehead on your hands.

5 Breathe deeply and gently rock your hips from side to side to release any tension in the hips. Remember to keep your hips squared by gently pressing your left hip down to the floor.

The first three steps in holding any posture in Kripalu yoga are: Breathe, relax, and feel. Breathe deeply as you continue to hold. Relax every part of your body that you can. Feel all the sensations that arise. Explore the sensations for 10–20 seconds.

153

Simple pigeon pose, stage 2

1. Continue to hold the posture and begin to practice the last two steps, which are: Watching everything that arises within you without pushing away or grasping onto thoughts or feelings.

2. Be the compassionate witness of your experience, fully present in the moment. Simply watch what is happening, and allow it all to be there.

3. Allow yourself to use micro-movements to explore the posture. These are very slight movements that enable you to deepen the stretch or explore new sensations. Stay connected with your breath, holding it for 10–20 seconds.

4. You can release the pose by slowly sliding your hands back to either side of your right knee, then moving back into the table position on all fours.

Simple pigeon pose, stage 3

1. In this stage, you will be tuning in to your "inner knower." Release any mental restrictions or preconceived way of moving, and allow your body to move in accord with its own knowing.

2. When you feel ready, begin to move. Ask yourself what would feel especially good in this moment. How would your body like to move next? Go slowly and stay connected to what is happening internally.

3. Follow the urge to move. You may move into another posture such as Proud pigeon, Downward-facing dog, or Child pose. Or you may find yourself doing a movement that is not a yoga posture but one that feels like the perfect *counterpose* for you.

> **DEFINITION**
>
> *Counterposes help bring your body into balance after a strong pose or movement. For example, the Knee to chest pose is a natural counterpose for Cobra. If a pose pushes you strongly in one direction (Cobra), you may need a counterpose that moves you gently in the opposite direction (Knee to chest).*

Proud pigeon pose

This is a version of Pigeon pose that requires a certain level of flexibility in the spine. Try it as you feel ready.

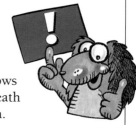

1. Be in Pigeon pose as before. Exhale and draw your upper torso upright as you place your forearms flat on the ground with your elbows bent. Your hands are flat on the floor and your elbows are underneath your shoulders. This upper body position is called Sphinx position.

2. Lengthen your spine through the crown of your head as you inhale, lifting your sternum and pressing your heart center forward. Breathe deeply in this position for 15–30 seconds.

3. If you would like to try a deeper stretch, slide your hands back to either side of your right knee. Draw your shoulders away from your ears and continue to open your chest, lifting your sternum.

4. Lengthen your spine from your tailbone to the crown of your head. Press your sitting bones down and your hips forward slightly.

5. Lift out of your waist and gently look upward toward the space where the wall and the ceiling meet. Hold for 15–30 seconds.

6. To release from Proud pigeon pose, bring your hands to either side of your front knees. Press your hands into the floor and lower your torso forward slightly as you lift your hips away from the floor. Bring your front knees back and return to table position (on your hands and knees).

7. When you feel ready, add in a practice of stages 2 and 3 with Proud pigeon.

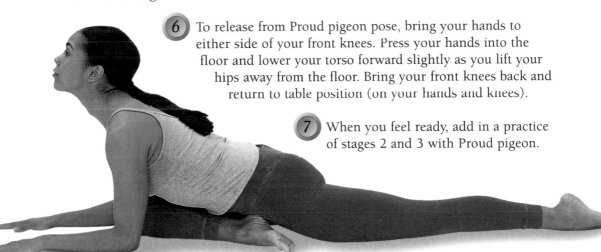

PROUD PIGEON POSE

In yoga, you generally repeat a posture on the other side, so make sure that you give both sides of your body a chance at Pigeon pose.

Pigeon pose benefits the body in many ways. It expands the chest, strengthens the lungs, and facilitates deep breathing. It strengthens the back muscles and revitalizes the kidneys and the entire endocrine system (adrenals, reproductive glands, pancreas, thyroid). Pigeon pose also increases flexibility in the hips and groin and stretches the thigh muscles.

What is Viniyoga?

FOR A PERSON WHO IS JUST BEGINNING *yoga, or who has limited flexibility or particular physical limitations, Viniyoga is a treasure beyond compare. If this describes you, read on.*

DEFINITION

Vini can be translated from the Sanskrit to mean "special" and "individual." It can also mean "step-by-step" and "gradual." It is easy to see how all of these concepts relate to Viniyoga.

Vini means many things but, mostly, it means that it meets the needs of the individual. The emphasis in Viniyoga is two-fold. It recognizes the uniqueness of each person by creating an individualized approach using all the tools of yoga – asana, mantra, pranayama, and meditation – and teaches you how to apply these tools in creating an individualized practice.

In a Viniyoga class the pace is gentle and the approach is relaxed, but, as long-time practitioners can verify, your Viniyoga practice can build to a powerful workout. Adjusting a pose so that it functions for you is more important than sticking with a form that is not working for your body. The starting point in Viniyoga is meeting your needs. This doesn't necessitate private lessons, although individual instruction is not uncommon in Viniyoga. What it means is that the teacher creates an atmosphere in which each student can find his or her own way to yoga.

A GUIDING LIGHT

The grandfather of three major paths of yoga (Iyengar, Viniyoga, and Ashtanga) was an exceptional soul by the name of Sri T. Krishnamacharya. His ancestry traces back to a famous 9th-century South Indian sage called Nathamuni.

I found it remarkable not only that Krishnamacharya's students went on to become masters in their own right, but that he taught each of them in ways that allowed each to develop his own distinctive style of yoga.

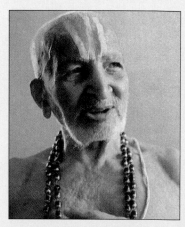

SRI T. KRISHNAMACHARYA

The inspiration behind Viniyoga

T.K.V. Desikachar, Krishnamacharya's son, is responsible for Viniyoga. In Desikachar's book, *The Heart of Yoga* (highly recommended), there are many pictures of his father at age 79 practically pulsating with vitality, stretching, and twisting in positions most of us can do only in our dreams! Krishnamacharya died in 1989 at age 100, vital to the last.

Desikachar pursued a Western-style education, and became a structural engineer. Later he realized the importance of his father's unique knowledge and left engineering to study with him for the next 27 years. As it turned out, the principle of adapting yoga to fit individual needs was a perfect match for the engineering mind of Desikachar. Each new physical or psychological challenge presented by Desikachar's students was carefully analyzed, and the right poses were adapted to help solve the problem.

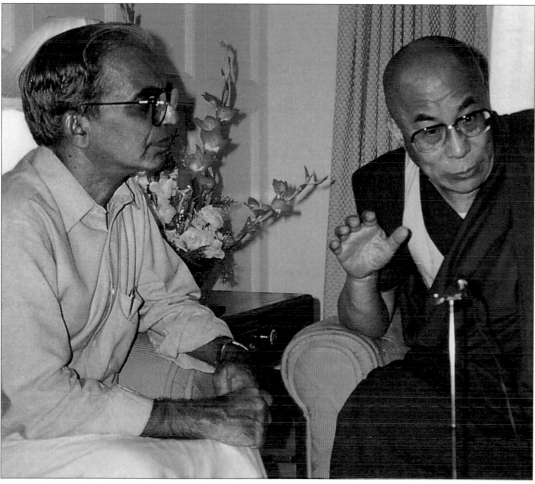

■ *T.K.V. Desikachar (left), who followed in his father's hallowed footsteps and developed Viniyoga, meets with the Dalai Lama, the spiritual head of Tibetan Buddhism.*

STUDYING WITH A MASTER

Pat Miller is a Viniyoga teacher who, in 1970, had the unique opportunity to study directly with Sri T. Krishnamacharya in India when she was 5 months pregnant. Her story:

When I first climbed the stairs to the small room of the house in Mandaveli to meet Sri Krishnamacharya, my purpose was clear. I simply wanted a program of exercise that would take me and the small life within, fit and healthy, through the remaining 4 months of pregnancy. Yet, I couldn't help but wonder what else there was to yoga, and wonder, too, what my teacher was like.

His penetrating gaze and the few gruff words he spoke were kindly, but they put me on notice that this was not to be a casual relationship. As I was to learn, I would be expected to work hard and to listen well. "How much practice this week?" The stern query, not without a glint of humor, began every session.

I had anticipated a somewhat vigorous workout, but instead had been told, in effect, to work gently within, and to take time just to breathe and to rest. Yet the feeling of energy and well-being increased as the weeks went by. My step actually felt lighter! At no time was it more so than the day my teacher said to me, "I like teaching pregnant ladies – then I am taking care of two people, not just one!" His comments on the consciousness of the baby in the womb, its sensitivity to disturbance, and the need to ease the shock of birth presage contemporary research on these subjects.

I look back and see his tender care and respect for me and my unborn son in those first months as his student, and the high expectations he had for me, along with attention to small detail in the few years that followed. I saw that the underlying principles of Sri Krishnamacharya's teaching is that the individual, who is unique, and whose circumstances change, must be the main factor in determining what should be taught and how.

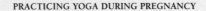

PRACTICING YOGA DURING PREGNANCY

Breath and movement

REMEMBER THE FATHER OF YOGA, PATANJALI? *In his Yoga sutras he describes an asana as having two important qualities, which are emphasized in Viniyoga. They are* sthira *(pronounced "st-heera") and* sukha.

Acknowledging your starting point

An important part of the philosophy of Viniyoga is that you must begin from where you are. If you have a stiff back, for example, you have to acknowledge this as your starting point, and work with the postures from there. Practicing postures in a progression allows you to feel the steadiness, the alertness, and the overall comfort of your yoga practice.

Joining the breath with movement

The breath is the link between the inner and outer body. The first step of your yoga practice is to consciously link breath and body. You can do this by allowing every movement to be led by the breath as you practice your postures. For example, a simple exercise of raising the arms on an inhalation and lowering them on an exhalation will help you find the rhythm of combined breath and movement.

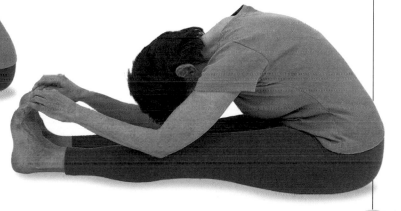

You may never have given much thought to whether you inhale or exhale as your body moves in different directions. Many times we will naturally exhale as we fold forward, for example. In Viniyoga, special attention is paid to this process of linking breath and movement.

■ **In the forward stretch**, *link breath with movement by inhaling while you expand your ribcage and lift your chest, and exhaling while you contract your chest and abdomen.*

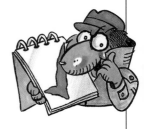

The rules of breath and movement are these: When we contract the body we exhale, and when we expand the body we inhale. Exceptions are made only when we want to create a particular effect in the asana by altering the natural breathing pattern.

Avoiding mechanical breathing

Imagine how much attention you would pay to your breath if breathing were voluntary. You might never get anything else done in life (but you might be a pretty highly evolved human!). Because breathing is involuntary, there is a tendency for it to become automatic even when doing yoga. To avoid this mechanical repetition of breath and movement, Viniyoga suggests that you introduce a short pause at the end of every movement. This means that you will pause the breath for a second or two on the top of the inhalation and the end of the exhalation.

Remember prana and apana? When you inhale, prana comes into the body, and when you exhale, apana leaves – that's the stuff you don't want anymore anyway. So it makes sense that if you extend the exhale, and make it longer than the inhale, you let go of more "stuff" – blockages and used-up mental, physical, and emotional energy. In Viniyoga, the exhale can even be twice as long as the inhale.

Consciously following the breath in and out is a form of meditation. According to yogic teachings, whoever masters this can direct his or her attention toward any activity in daily life. You can also try hearing the breath. One way to do this is through a yogic pranayama called *Ujjayi* (pronounced "oo JAH yi").

Hearing the breath

1. Let's try the Ujjayi breath. Sit straight with your legs crossed, or on a chair with your back straight.

2. Close your eyes. Make your breath calm and rhythmic. Now begin to focus on your throat. Imagine there is a valve in your throat that you close slightly in order to control your breath. The measure for this control is your sound, which becomes very gentle and ultimately should not require any effort or create any tension.

3. As your breathing becomes slower and deeper, gently contract your glottis (the opening at the upper end of your windpipe, between the vocal cords) so that a soft snoring sound like the breathing of a sleeping baby is produced in your throat. If this is practiced correctly, there will be a simultaneous gentle contraction of your abdomen. This will happen without any effort being made.

(4) The sound you make is not loud. It should just be audible to you and no one else, unless they are sitting very close by. Think of a cat purring and create a similar sound.

(5) After this technique is mastered, the sound is present during both inhalation and exhalation.

Ujjayi is a tranquilizing pranayama, and it also has a heating effect on the body. It soothes the nervous system and calms the mind. It can help to relieve insomnia, so it is good to practice before sleep.

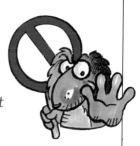

In the Ujjayi breathing exercise, there is a tendency to contort the face muscles. Relax the face as much as possible, and do not contract the throat strongly. The contraction is slight.

Easing into your practice

BREATH IN MOTION is a good way to describe the way it feels to do Viniyoga. Each of the following movements should take about 4–10 seconds, using the full length of your breath to complete the movement. When you first start practicing, your breath may be short, more on the 4-second end of things, and that is fine. It will lengthen as you continue. Allow the following set of poses to flow like a dance, and dance to your heart's content!

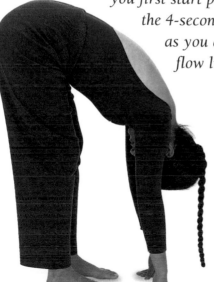

STANDING FORWARD BEND

Standing forward bend

(1) Begin by standing straight with your feet parallel, 6–12 in (15–30 cm) apart, and your arms relaxed at your sides.

(2) Inhaling, raise your arms straight up.

(3) Exhale, bending forward as far as you can, allowing your arms to hang to the floor.

(4) Repeat four times.

Upward legs and arms stretch

1. Lie down on your mat. Exhale as you bring your knees toward your chest, with your hands holding your knees or shins.

2. Inhale, and raise your legs perpendicular to the floor. At the same time, raise your arms overhead.

3. Repeat four times.

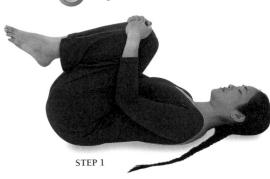

STEP 1

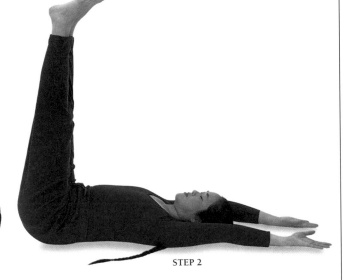

STEP 2

Bridge pose

1. Still lying down, bend your knees and bring your feet comfortably close to your buttocks. Your arms are relaxed at your sides with your palms facing downward.

2. Inhale and simultaneously raise your arms overhead, and lift your hips off the ground, arching upward. You will be resting on your upper back and shoulders and the soles of your feet.

3. Exhale as you lower your arms and hips back to the original position.

4. Repeat four times.

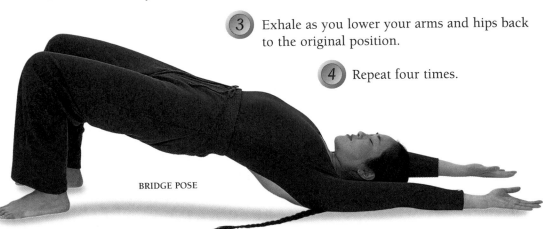

BRIDGE POSE

Cobra pose

1. Lie on your stomach with your forehead on the floor and your legs slightly apart, arms alongside your body with your palms facing upward.

2. Inhale and come up, raising your chest gradually and lifting your head slightly back. Your upper body will follow to the degree that it can.

3. Exhale and relax down to the original position.

4. Repeat four times.

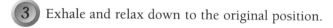

COBRA POSE

Don't strain to come up into Cobra pose. If your body is tight, you will work hard even if you come up a small amount. Avoid overworking your neck; use your back muscles instead.

ADAPTING COBRA TO SUIT YOU

If Cobra pose is too difficult, try one of these adaptations:

a. Place a soft pillow under your abdomen (optional). Bring your legs farther apart and place your arms comfortably on the floor in front of you, elbows out to the sides of your shoulders.

b. Inhale and come up onto your elbows and forearms, using your arms on the floor for support. Rest your weight on your hands, keeping your abdomen on the floor. Feel free to experiment with different arm placements to find the most effective position for you.

COBRA ADAPTATION

Knee to chest pose

1. Lying on the floor, exhale as you bring your knees into your chest with your hands on your knees or shins.

2. Inhale and allow your knees to move away from you by about 1 ft (30 cm). Your hands are still on your knees and shins.

3. Repeat 4 times.

4. Lie down in Corpse pose for relaxation time.

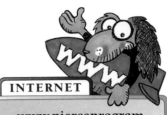

INTERNET

www.pierceprogram .com

Margaret and Martin Pierce have created a simple and clear guide to Viniyoga called Yoga for Your Life, *which can be found in most bookstores.*

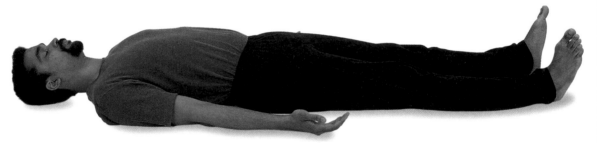

CORPSE POSE

INTERNET

www.viniyoga.com

This is the site of longtime Viniyoga teacher Gary Kraftsow, author of Yoga for Wellness.

A golden opportunity

Be sure to leave some time at the end of your practice to simply sit. You are not in the same mind that you came to yoga with, so enjoy it to the fullest. In Viniyoga, as in all styles of yoga, once you have toned and finely tuned the body and mind through yoga, it is heavenly to sit still and enjoy the fruits of your labor. In fact, it seems almost a waste of a golden opportunity not to!

A simple summary

✔ Kripalu yoga and Viniyoga are about adaptability. They differ greatly in their approaches, but both are designed so that each person can progress through stages in ways that are natural for him or her.

✔ An introspective, somewhat psychological approach, Kripalu progresses in stages.

✔ In Kripalu yoga, the very beginning stage is the willful practice of postures and breath awareness.

✔ In the second stage of Kripalu, you are encouraged to look within yourself to meet your feelings consciously, without labeling or judging them.

✔ In Kripalu's third stage, you begin to open to your own intuitive wisdom, and practice yoga from that inner place.

✔ Viniyoga recognizes the uniqueness of each person by creating an individualized approach using all the tools of yoga – asana, mantra, pranayama, and meditation – and Viniyoga teaches you how to apply these tools in creating an individualized practice.

✔ In Viniyoga, special attention is paid to the process of linking breath and movement. The postures flow, almost like a very relaxed dance.

✔ To stay aware of your breath, pause at the end of the inhalation and exhalation, or practice hearing your breath as it goes in and out, using Ujjayi pranayama.

✔ Once your body and mind have been toned and finely tuned, it is the perfect time to sit still and enjoy the fruits of your labor.

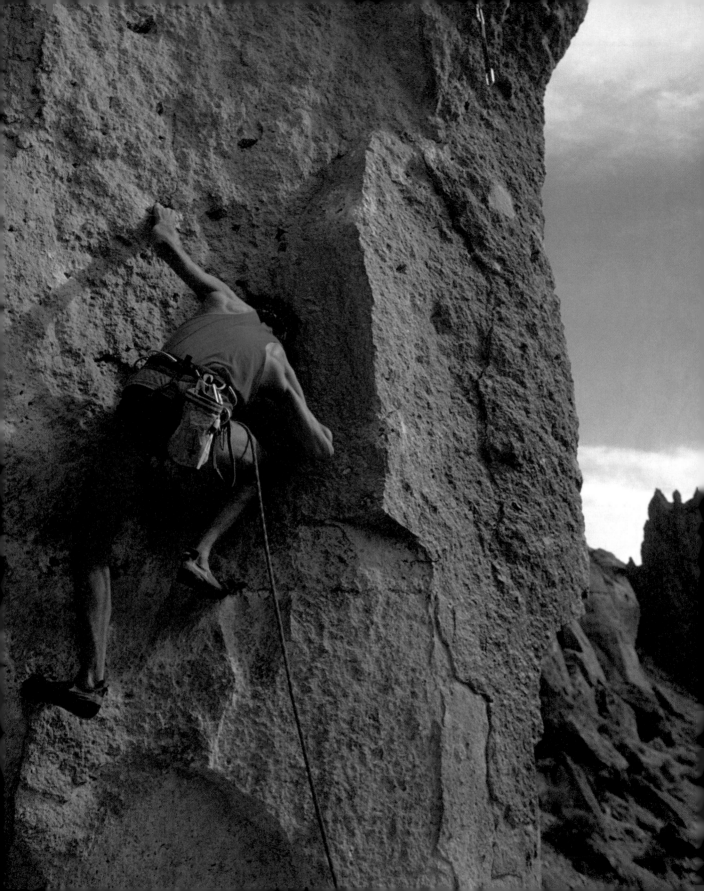

Chapter 10

Ashtanga: The Strong Side of Yoga

WHAT IS ALL THE BROUHAHA about Ashtanga yoga (Westernized as "power yoga")? Well, for one thing, this is the yoga of movie stars. Athletes love it, too, and gymnasts are right at home. This is a yoga of discipline and endurance that can at times rival Marine Corps training. Those who dedicate themselves to Ashtanga yoga say it builds flexibility, strength, and an inner freedom beyond compare. In this chapter you will get a chance to experience this exciting and powerful form of yoga.

In this chapter...

✓ A new twist to an old story

✓ The elements of Ashtanga yoga

✓ Understanding the body locks

✓ Sun Salutes, Ashtanga style

✓ Training with intention

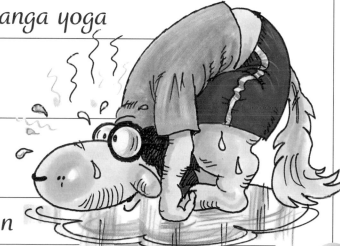

ASHTANGA YOGA IMPROVES STRENGTH, COORDINATION, AND CONCENTRATION

A new twist to an old story

THE TAUT MUSCLES, *spandex exercise wear, and sweat-glistening bare midriffs of* Ashtanga *yoga belie the ancient history of this yoga. To really understand Ashtanga, we have to go way back to Patanjali's eight limbs of yoga, for that is exactly what Ashtanga means.*

Ashtanga yoga, as taught by K. Pattabhi Jois, the third well-known disciple of Krishnamacharya, began in the early 1900s with the declared rediscovery of an ancient manuscript that described a unique system of Hatha yoga. Under Krishnamacharya's direction, Jois deciphered and collated this system, naming it Ashtanga yoga in the belief that it was the original asana practice as intended by Patanjali, involving all eight limbs of yoga. Jois, now in his 80s, still teaches at his center in Mysore, India.

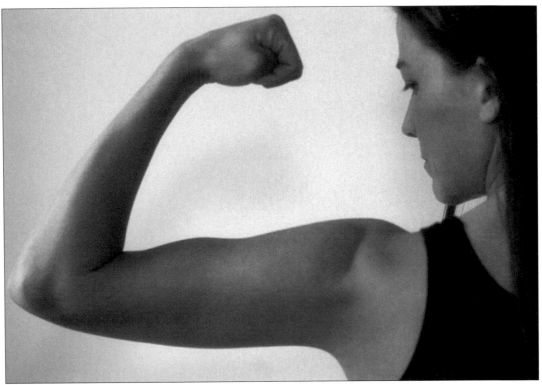

■ **Although a firm and strong physique** *is probably the most well-known benefit of practicing Ashtanga yoga, this form of yoga also improves the circulation and creates a calm mind.*

DEFINITION

The literal Sanskrit meaning of vinyasa is "breath-synchronized movement."

The ancient text emphasizes a yoga technique called *vinyasa*, a method of synchronizing progressive series of postures with a specific breathing technique. This process produces an intense internal heat and a purifying sweat that detoxifies muscles and organs. The result: Improved circulation, a light and strong body, and a calm mind.

The elements of Ashtanga yoga

AS YOU PREPARE *for your Ashtanga experience, remember, it is not what you do but how you do it that is important. Ashtanga yoga follows the following well-defined guidelines:*

- Heating the room is important to keep the muscles limber.
- Heat is generated through the vinyasas as well, to keep the internal fire stoked. The vinyasas must be followed in sequence.
- The breath and movement link and breathing patterns are very specific.
- Subtle muscular contractions, called body locks, are applied during the movement.
- The practitioner gradually learns to jump into and out of postures.

Trivia...

Here's a simple way to understand how Ashtanga, and really all types of yoga, prepare you to experience all eight limbs, or principles, of yoga: Movement through the postures (asanas) purifies the physical body, while mastering the breath (pranayama) through concentration (dharana) quiets the senses (pratyahara). This prepares you for meditation (dhyana), and eventual absorption (samadhi) in the Divine, God, Universal Oneness. A balanced yogic life rests on ethical behavior (yama) and self-discipline (niyama).

Giving attention to all of these aspects at once can be quite overwhelming for a beginner. In an Ashtanga class, the teacher will instruct beginners to start slowly, then build on the gradual changes that come with regular practice. You will focus on breath and alignment, and the body locks and jumping come with time.

Turning up the heat

Heating your room to a temperature between 70 and 75°F (21 and 24°C) for Ashtanga yoga is an important element. Just like metal is melted before it is shaped, the connective tissue in our bodies becomes heated through both external and internal heat. As it becomes more fluid, we become more pliant.

When I walked into my first Ashtanga yoga class, I noticed it was much warmer in the room than most yoga classes. My first thought was, "Oh no, am I going to get really lethargic in this class?" Once the class started, though, it was clear there was no way to be lazy. No time, nor inclination, to think about anything except what I was doing.

In an Ashtanga yoga class, you will hear the teacher say things like, "Lift the kneecaps by tightening the thighs." This lifts the quadriceps muscles in what is called a static contraction.

A static contraction, or the tightening of a muscle without accompanying movement in that body part, takes energy, i.e., heat, to accomplish.

BIKRAM YOGA

Founded by Bikram Choudhury, Bikram is the yoga of high heat and Hollywood. The temperature of the room is kept somewhere between 80 and 100°F (26 and 38°C) in order to facilitate a deeper stretch to the muscles, detoxify the body, and increase the heart rate for a better cardiovascular workout. Bikram came to Hollywood in the 1970s and taught yoga to the stars. He continues to teach at his center in Beverly Hills.

The same sequence of 26 postures, with two pranayama techniques, is followed each time in Bikram yoga. The postures include one-legged stances, backbends, twists, and other challenging positions, most of which are held for at least 10 seconds.

This approach, if you can handle it, gives you great muscle tone and strength, and builds great inner (and outer!) heat. People are drawn to Bikram yoga because the strong workout combined with extra heat produces a light, clean, energized body and mind.

INTERNET

www.bikramyoga.com

Find out more about Bikram yoga at this site. It is described as "the most exciting, hardworking, effective, amusing, and glamorous yoga class in the world."

Static contractions are important in Ashtanga (and other) yoga, not only for the toning of the muscle, but even more importantly, for the internal heat that is generated. This heat detoxifies the organs and tissues and revitalizes the entire system. It will make you sweat. Sweating is good, because it eliminates the body's "junk." That all-important energy force called apana is making more room for prana.

Your sweat during yoga may have a strong odor, but don't be embarrassed, be grateful! It means you are eliminating the residue of perhaps years of unhealthy eating habits. Eating mostly fresh fruits, veggies, whole grains, and legumes, and avoiding meat and stimulants, will take care of any unpleasant odor over time.

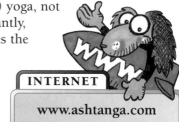

INTERNET

www.ashtanga.com

Logging on to this web site and clicking on "classes" will help you find a trained Ashtanga teacher in your area.

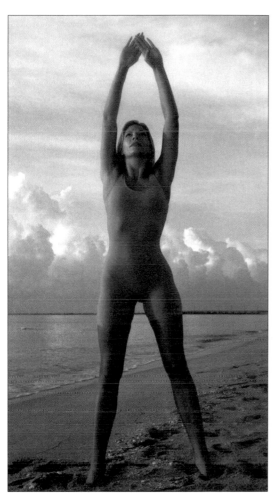

The importance of vinyasa

As you begin to practice Ashtanga yoga, remember to start slowly and carefully, moving with great awareness. As your body warms up, and as you become familiar with the postures, the movement starts to flow more easily.

In Ashtanga yoga the link between action and awareness is the most important element. But be patient: Rome wasn't built in a day, and neither is heaven on Earth.

Ashtanga yoga begins with the Sun Salutation, then, as students progress, moves into a progression of postures called the Primary Series. After years of daily practice, a practitioner may move into the Secondary Series.

■ **The Sun Salutation** *is the first pose that needs to be mastered in Ashtanga yoga. Students then slowly move on to learn more complex and demanding positions.*

What you will see in this chapter is the warm-up (Sun Salutation). Once you learn the basic alignment of these poses, and how to link them together with the breath, it will become a smooth dance. Enjoying that dance is the goal, and a very satisfying one at that.

The body's currents of energy

What makes yoga different from any other form of exercise? What is there about it that effects internal changes? Yoga's power lies in the way the movement links with the breath, which links with the consciousness, or inner awareness.

Through yoga, changes in consciousness can be brought about by setting in motion currents of subtle forces in the body. These currents are called *nadis* in the yogic science. And where the nadis cross each other forms the major energy centers, or chakras, of the body. Does this sound familiar? It should, because the nadis are also the acupuncture meridians, which we talked about in Chapter 2.

DEFINITION

The nadis *are the subtle channels within the body that prana runs through. They supply energy to every organ and cell of the body and bring about changes in consciousness.*

Breathing for effect

Think of the abdominal and intercostal muscles (these are the muscles between the ribs) as an accordion. Push them in toward the spine to press out all the air and when you relax the muscles, the air will come back in practically by itself. Eventually you will want to actively draw the breath back in, but for now, just practice actively exhaling.

"A BREATH AT A TIME"

In this practice the focus, or discipline, happens mentally a beat before it happens physically. As a result of the breathing or the strength work or the heat or the eventual stillness in a posture, some small confusion or craving will clear. But not overnight or all at once. Only a grain of sand, a breath at a time. For one instant, the clouds part, and bang, the Grand Canyon comes into full, spectacular view, and whoosh, something releases in your body, some tangled, old neuromusculature untangles, and life flows through anew. You feel it. But you can't possibly understand it until you feel it.

Beryl Bender Birch, from her book *Power Yoga*

This simple exercise is the beginning breathing pattern in Ashtanga yoga, and will eventually be replaced by the Ujjayi breath you learned in the previous chapter. The Ujjayi breath keeps you focused by allowing you to hear your breath and control it slowly. It also creates an internal heat.

Understanding the body locks

NOW THAT YOU HAVE BECOME MORE AWARE of contracting muscles on a subtle level, it is time to learn about the body locks, which are called bandhas in the science of yoga. Most yoga schools use all three locks, which can be applied separately or together.

> **DEFINITION**
>
> Bandhas, literally "lock," "bond," or "tie" in Sanskrit, are internal contractions of the muscles that are used to focus concentration, stimulate internal heat, and ultimately, control the flow of prana.

The body locks should not be practiced by pregnant women or by those with heart problems, high blood pressure, or other medical situations.

Practicing the bandhas will train your mind to be attentive because they require your complete attention in order to maintain them. In body locks, we mix the prana (which flows downward with the incoming breath) and the apana (which moves upward with the action of the body lock). The prana and apana merge, generating energy and purifying heat, which translates into vitality and health.

Please keep in mind that the bandhas are more advanced yogic techniques. It may take years with a trained teacher to learn how to practice them correctly, although some people find these contractions quite simple. In any case, approaching these potent techniques with respect is always a good idea.

The bandhas

1. **Root lock (Mula bandha).** Root lock is the contracting and lifting of the perineum and the perineal muscle, which are located between the genitals and the anus. This lock generally includes the vaginal and anal sphincter muscles as well. It is usually, but not always, applied at the end of a deep exhalation. It can also involve the abdominal muscles when specified.

   To try it, exhale all your breath out, and contract your anal muscles and the muscle of your sex organs. Hold the lock and inhale. Then relax. Try to keep the buttocks relaxed. This may take some practice to accomplish.

2. **Diaphragm lock (Uddiyana bandha).** In this lock, the navel is drawn inward and upward, usually at the end of the exhale. Uddiyana means "to fly up," and refers to the action of the navel area.

   To try it, exhale, and at the end of the exhale, tip the bottom of your rib cage in slightly toward your spine. As you do this, you will feel the muscles at your waist, just under your ribs, contract. This lock can also be applied on the held inhale.

3. **Neck lock (Jalandhara bandha).** The neck lock is applied by drawing the chin slightly in toward the throat, making sure the spine and neck are straight. You may feel a pressure at the throat, as though there is a lump there. The neck lock is usually applied at the end of an exhalation. It is often applied with the diaphragm lock.

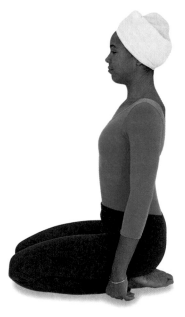

ROOT LOCK

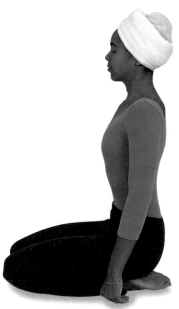

DIAPHRAGM LOCK

To try it, sit with a straight spine. Exhale completely. Contract back on your neck and throat. Your head stays level without tilting forward. Your cervical bones straighten to allow the increased flow of pranic energy to travel freely into your head. Inhale and release the lock.

(4) **The great lock (Maha bandha).** Maha means "great," and the great lock is – you guessed it – all three locks applied together. Usually this lock is applied at the end of a deep exhalation and released on the inhalation.

To try it, sit with a straight spine. Exhale completely and contract the root lock, add the diaphragm lock, and then the neck lock. Inhale and release the lock.

A word about the locks

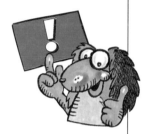

In Ashtanga yoga, beginners need not be concerned with applying body locks. Locks are boosters. When you have become familiar with the Ashtanga routine, boost the energy with the root lock (Mula bandha). This is the most commonly used lock in Ashtanga yoga.

The easiest way to focus on the Mula bandha is to try it when you are simply holding a posture. Once you are in a posture, and your alignment is good, apply the root lock at the end of an exhalation, and maintain the muscular contraction through the next one or two breaths.

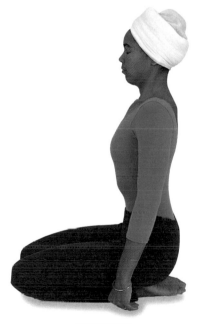

NECK LOCK

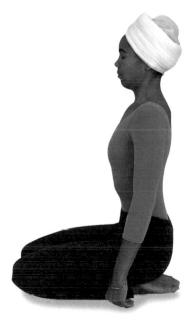

GREAT LOCK

Sun Salutes, Ashtanga style

MOST OF US LIKE TO LEARN the basics, then, with some mastery attained, we like to go for the gold. The gold in this sampling of Ashtanga yoga is to add the root lock, and use the Ujjayi breath on the inhale and exhale. Good luck!

(1) Begin in Mountain pose, with the arms at the sides.

(2) On an inhalation, bring your arms straight up overhead, with your palms together. Look up. Lift your kneecaps by tightening your thighs. Reach up as high as possible without arching your back.

(3) Exhale and bring your palms down to the floor, and your head to your knees. Tuck your head into your knees and look toward your navel. Those who need to should bend their knees.

(4) Inhale and look up, lifting your chest and extending your back. Again, keep your knees bent if you need to.

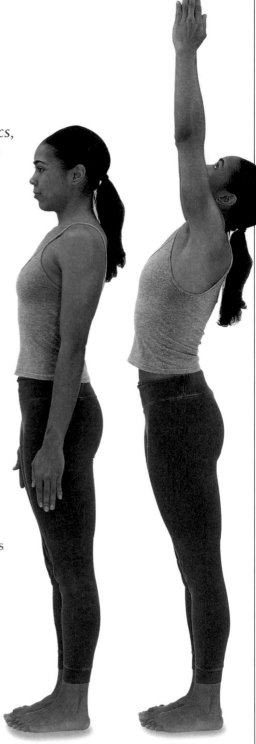

STEP 1   STEP 2

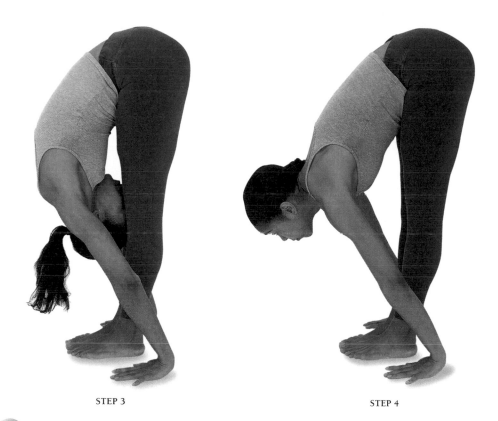

STEP 3   STEP 4

(5) Exhale and slowly lower your body to the floor by walking your legs back while stiffening your torso. (Eventually practitioners will jump their legs back.) Your feet should be parallel and about 10–12 in (25–30 cm) apart. Your hands are about the same distance apart.

Your body is resting on your hands and the undersides of your toes. Your elbows are tucked in, and you are looking straight ahead. If this is too much pressure on your lower back, put your knees down.

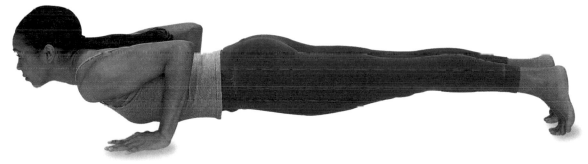

STEP 5

6 Turn your feet to point your toes back, resting on the upper sides of your feet. Inhale and lift your body, using your hands and the tops of your feet. If possible, keep your legs slightly off the ground. Look up and back. If this is too much pressure on the tops of your feet, or if it is uncomfortable for your lower back, keep your knees on the floor. This is Upward dog pose.

Do not allow your back to sag or your shoulders to hunch up around your ears. Keep your knees on the floor if there is any sense of strain or discomfort.

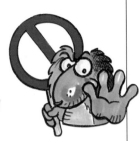

STEP 6

7 Turn your toes under so that the undersides of your toes press the floor. Exhale and push yourself up into an inverted V position. Look up toward your navel.

Flatten your hands and spread your weight out evenly between your hands and feet. This is Downward-facing dog pose. Don't worry about having your heels touch the floor; that may take time.

Take five complete breaths in Downward-facing dog pose. Listen to your breath as you count.

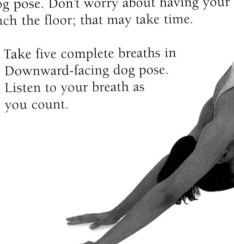

INTERNET

**www.yogaworkshop
.com**

Richard Freeman, one of the foremost teachers of Ashtanga yoga, is responsible for yogaworkshop.com. His video, Yoga Breathing and Relaxation, is highly recommended for beginners.

STEP 7

8 Inhale and return to position 4 by bringing your feet forward, one at a time. (Eventually practitioners jump their legs back to the beginning position.)

9 Exhale and return to position 3.

10 Inhale and return to position 2, and then position 1, Mountain pose, for active rest, which is a term for keeping your concentration while you recover between repetitions. You do this by keeping the mind focused so that the internal energy and heat that you are building don't drop off.

11 Begin again, and try to do at least three repetitions of the Sun Salutes.

12 At the end of your yoga practice, lie down in Corpse pose for at least 5 minutes, or more if you can.

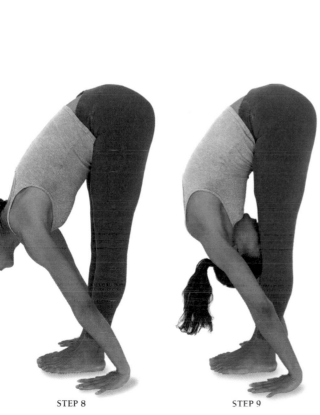

STEP 8   STEP 9   STEP 10

Training with intention

YOU CAN SEE THAT A PRACTICE *of Ashtanga yoga is great conditioning for your body and mind. It is bound to develop self-discipline and self-mastery as much as it develops a highly toned body. This is one of the reasons it has become so popular with those who train, play sports, or are fitness fanatics.*

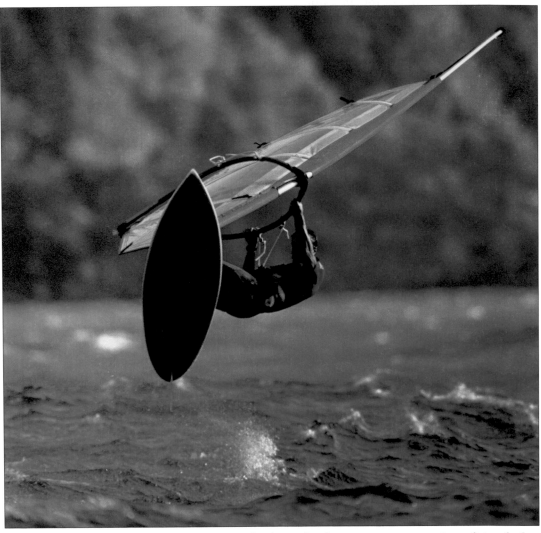

■ **Ashtanga yoga** *is an ideal training program for those who play competitive sports. It conditions both the body and mind to give you all the strength and concentration you could need.*

For those of you who train, run, bike, and play sports regularly, Beryl Bender Birch's book, Power Yoga, is the best gift you can give yourself. This is Ashtanga yoga with a straight-talking, sports-savvy master yoga teacher who unequivocally demonstrates how you can prevent and repair sports strains and injuries, as well as raise your consciousness.

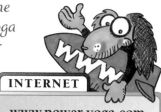

INTERNET

www.power-yoga.com

Beryl Bender Birch's web site has lots of great Ashtanga yoga information, especially for athletes.

But remember, without the intention of personal evolution for the good of all, yoga might as well be gymnastics. This intention is what sets yoga apart from every other form of physical exercise.

A simple summary

✔ Ashtanga yoga is an athletic style of yoga, building strength, flexibility, and concentration.

✔ Ashtanga yoga emphasizes a technique called vinyasa, a progressive series of postures commonly synchronized with the Ujjayi breath.

✔ The practice of Ashtanga yoga produces intense internal heat and a purifying sweat that detoxifies muscles and organs, resulting in improved circulation, a light, strong body, and a calm mind.

✔ Subtle muscular contractions called body locks, or bandhas, are applied during the vinyasa.

✔ You should start slowly in Ashtanga yoga, and build on the gradual changes that come with regular practice. Focus on your breath and alignment.

✔ What sets yoga apart from other physical exercise is your intention to grow in awareness, elevating yourself and others.

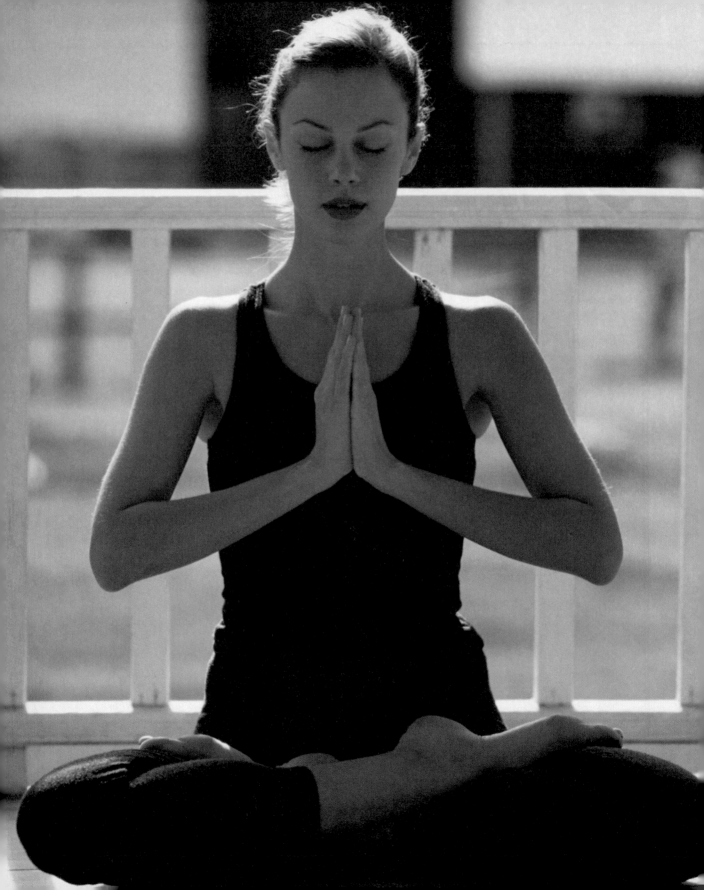

Chapter 11

Raising the Roof with Kundalini

KUNDALINI. IT SOUNDS EXOTIC. Are you curious? The kundalini energy is powerful and often misunderstood. Activating it is the ultimate purpose in all forms of yoga. And Kundalini yoga, as presented in this chapter, works directly on awakening and raising the so-called "mysterious" kundalini energy that resides in your body. In this chapter you will learn about kundalini energy, and the myths and mystery surrounding it. Then I will take you through a Kundalini yoga experience that will energize and elevate you – guaranteed!

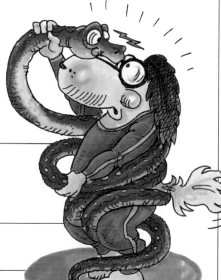

In this chapter...

✓ **The scoop on kundalini**

✓ **From secret to widespread knowledge**

✓ **Overview of your practice**

✓ **A sampler of Kundalini yoga**

GOOD PREPARATION IS NEEDED FOR THE PROPER FLOW OF KUNDALINI ENERGY

The scoop on kundalini

"SERPENT POWER" IS AN INTRIGUING but rather scary-sounding name that has been given to kundalini. Although that concept might fascinate some, the rest of us might walk away as fast as our legs can carry us from a yoga that awakens the "serpent!" This is part of the myth of kundalini that we will explore.

The easiest way to understand kundalini is to acknowledge that there is a universal spirit, sometimes referred to as God. God uncoils him/her/itself. This uncoiling process is known as kundalini. What is uncoiling and awakening is *you*, nothing more and nothing less. It is a normal capacity that most people simply are not utilizing.

Yoga is the science of the self, and kundalini is the awakening of the self. It is that simple.

The mother yoga

Kundalini yoga is sometimes called the "mother yoga." A unique and distinctive yoga form, it encompasses elements that are found in all other forms of yoga. The following are a few of the ways that Kundalini yoga shares paths with other traditions of yoga that we've talked about:

- Encompasses the eight limbs of Patanjali and all seven branches of yoga: Raja yoga, Hatha yoga, Karma yoga, Jnana yoga, Mantra yoga, Tantra yoga, and Bhakti yoga.
- Includes pranayama techniques and uses the bandhas.
- Links movement with rhythmic breathing patterns.
- Has an introspective quality of listening to the body and releasing emotions, as well as drawing on inspiration, such as holding a pose with fearlessness.
- Incorporates chanting and singing as yogic technology.
- Is directly focused on moving the energy through the chakra system, stimulating the energy in the lower centers, and moving it to the higher centers.

Activating the kundalini energy

In the physical body, the kundalini resides in the spine. Now, it is important to realize that we are talking about a super-refined energy here. If you look in an anatomy book, you will see the spine and the spinal cord, but you will not see any arrows pointing to the kundalini energy, just as you will not see diagrams of chakras or nadis.

Western science has not yet developed devices to detect these subtle life forces, though it is highly possible that it will in the future. Just remember, before the invention of the microscope, no one knew of the existence of micro-organisms either. One fact remains: Whether or not you can *see* this energy, you can *experience* its transformational effects.

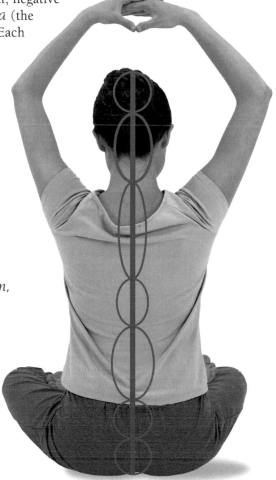

DEFINITION

The Ida is the left nerve channel, and carries the cooling, lunar, receptive energy. The Pingala is the right nerve channel and carries the warming, solar, projective energy. The Shushmana is the master nerve channel in the central column of the spine.

The two nerve channels (nadis) that intertwine around the central nerve of the spinal column are called the *Ida* (the lunar, negative energy) and the *Pingala* (the positive, solar energy). Each of them spirals upward from the base of the spine and makes 2½ turns around the central column of the spine, wherein lies the *Shushmana*.

The metaphor using a coiled snake for the kundalini is prevalent in yoga philosophy, even though the root word, as I've said, means a coiled lock of hair. Maybe it's because serpents are often associated with secret wisdom, or maybe it's because of the snakelike winding path of the Ida and Pingala.

■ **Spiraling upward** *around the spine, where the kundalini energy resides, are the two nerve channels, the Ida and Pingala. By practicing Kundalini yoga, you are conducting this energy around the body.*

Following the kundalini flow

The Shushmana originates from the first chakra, at the perineum, and ends at the crown of the head. The Ida emanates from the left side of the root chakra, spirals up the spinal cord, passing through each chakra in turn, and terminates at the left side of the sixth chakra, the third eye. The Pingala begins from the right side of the first chakra, and passes in an opposite manner to that of the Ida, terminating at the right side of the sixth chakra. The Ida and Pingala act as main conductors of the kundalini energy, feeding the entire nervous system.

Releasing the latent power

The main aim of Hatha yoga is to bring about a balanced flow of prana in the Ida and Pingala nadis. Remember that "ha" means the sun energy, and "tha" is the moon energy. So by practicing Hatha yoga, you are balancing the sun and moon of the Ida and Pingala. Once that happens, the Shushmana starts flowing, and the kundalini awakens and rises through the chakras.

In addition to the kundalini energy that is already flowing within our bodies, there is a vast reservoir of untapped kundalini stored under the fourth vertebra of the spinal column. This latent energy is activated through Kundalini yoga.

Through Kundalini yoga, this untapped energy is stimulated and allowed to rise up the spine until it reaches the top of the skull, activating the secretion of the pineal gland. Although the pineal gland has been an enigma for Western medicine, in yogic science it is the very key to life, both physical and spiritual. One of the major functions of the pineal is to vibrate and control the nucleus projection of every cell of the body.

We tend to think that how we feel has to do with our "feelings." It usually doesn't occur to us to realize that our state of consciousness is controlled by the secretion of chemicals from the higher glands. So it follows that we can affect our state of mind by working with the glandular system.

Practicing Kundalini yoga stimulates and balances the glandular system. And by doing so, it can easily change a person's whole outlook on life.

When we raise our kundalini, it causes the activation of these chemicals in the brain through our conscious, directed action. When the pineal gland is activated, a major change in consciousness is experienced. It may be subtle. It may be spectacular. It may be a gradual awakening. One thing is certain, though: Through the practice of Kundalini yoga, change happens.

From secret to widespread knowledge

THE SCIENCE OF KUNDALINI YOGA was *kept secret for thousands upon thousands of years, imparted by a master to one worthy student at a time. A student had to spend many years proving his trustworthiness and purity before receiving the guarded teachings of Kundalini yoga.*

INTERNET

www.3HO.org

The 3HO web site offers information about every aspect of Kundalini yoga, meditation, and healthy lifestyle choices.

Because of its history of secrecy and selectivity, Kundalini yoga's introduction in America met with a great deal of outrage directed toward Yogi Bhajan, a yogi and spiritual teacher from the northern part of India. Yogi Bhajan came to America in 1969 and began teaching Kundalini yoga openly to the "flower children" at Woodstock and other gatherings because he recognized the disenchantment and spiritual yearning that was felt by Western youth.

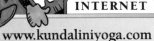

INTERNET

www.kundaliniyoga.com

In addition to providing a wealth of information about Kundalini yoga, this site can direct you to a trained Kundalini yoga teacher in your area through their link to IKYTA (International Kundalini Yoga Teachers Association).

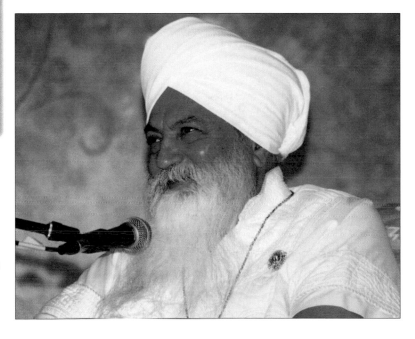

■ **Yogi Bhajan** *first introduced Kundalini yoga to the United States in the late 1960s. It has since spread all over the world.*

FROM ELITE TO EVERY PERSON

Yogi Bhajan wasn't groomed to serve the elite, but the common person. You see, many yoga masters came from an ancient lineage of masters. Many were high-caste Brahmans, who traditionally would teach only other Brahmans. By contrast, Yogi Bhajan was born a Sikh. Historically, the Sikh path rejected India's caste system, believing in equality for all.

Yogi Bhajan mastered Kundalini yoga when he was 16. Although still a teenager when India was partitioned in 1947, he took charge of leading 1,000 people from what is now Pakistan to New Delhi in India. He pursued a college education, became an all-around athlete, a family man, a commanding officer in the Indian army, and served in the Indian government. A householder with the inner discipline of an ascetic, his philosophy is that Kundalini yoga belongs to those who need it and are willing to practice it: "If you were in a desert, and I had water, wouldn't I share it with you?"

Yogi Bhajan, Ph.D., founded 3HO (Healthy, Happy, Holy Organization) in 1969, a worldwide non-profit foundation headquartered in Española, New Mexico. The community offers classes in Kundalini yoga and meditation, and incorporates teachings for all aspects of life, for example, vegetarian diet, serving others, living in spiritual communities, and yogic life skills, such as conscious parenting and partnering. In 3HO, yoga is more than a practice. It is a way of life.

Dispelling myths

For many years there has been talk that Kundalini yoga is dangerous, that it can release an energy that can cause physical and mental imbalances if a person isn't prepared for it. These claims have been founded in misunderstanding and mispractice of the technology of yoga. That is why the practice of Kundalini yoga as given by a master of Kundalini yoga is essential. Proper technique and preparation are the insulation needed for the proper flow of kundalini energy. And, of course, all yoga should be practiced with proper understanding and respect for its inherent power.

Since 1969, tens of thousands of people have been practicing Kundalini yoga as taught by Yogi Bhajan, and I am thankful to count myself among them. In 30 years I have never encountered or heard of anyone being harmed by practicing Kundalini yoga.

Another common fallacy is that your kundalini should be awakened by the physical touch of a "guru." This idea has never made too much sense to me. If you don't do it yourself, how will you maintain it? When you realize that it is your own God-given power you are working with, you can also realize that you have the ability to activate it. To me, this is the natural, organic way to higher consciousness.

Overview of your practice

A CLASS IN KUNDALINI YOGA includes centering with a mantra, warm-up yoga, practicing a specific yoga set, deeply relaxing in Corpse pose, and finishing with meditation.

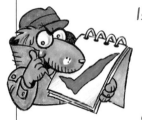

Is it kosher to recommend my own book? Try to overlook this minor detail, because Kundalini Yoga, by Shakta Kaur Khalsa, is the one basic book you will need in order to get the finer points of this chapter, and to continue your practice. You will also find around 100 (no kidding!) yoga sets and meditations, yogic health tips, and lots of yummy healing food recipes.

First things first

As with most yoga we've done in this book, Kundalini yoga begins with a centering mantra, the intent of which is to attune you to your inner teacher and the lineage of Kundalini yoga through the ages.

The tune-in mantra is "Ong Namo, Guru Dev Namo." It is chanted three times, each time on a deep inhalation. This mantra can be translated as "I call on the infinite creative consciousness. I call on the divine teacher within and without." This mantra is always chanted in the beginning of a Kundalini yoga class or practice.

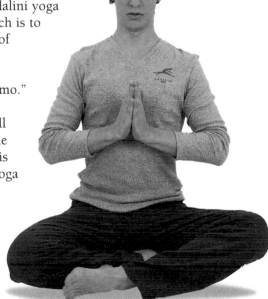

■ **When chanting** *the tune-in mantra, sit with a straight spine and your legs crossed. Press the palms of the hands together, positioning the joints of your thumbs at the sternum.*

Remember Om? Well, Ong is a variation of the cosmic syllable Om, which denotes the Unmanifested Creator. In the manifested, creative state, it becomes Ong. To chant Ong, slightly pull in the navel and vibrate the "ng" at the root of the nose. Your attention will automatically go to the third-eye center.

Breath of Fire

To many, Kundalini yoga is synonymous with strong breathing. It utilizes deep breathing, strong rhythmic breathing, and all pranayamas given in previous chapters. One of the most well-known trademarks of Kundalini yoga is a breathing technique called Breath of Fire, which is guaranteed to up your energy level a few notches, clear your lungs of old residue, and get all the neurons in your brain humming!

Breath of Fire is used consistently throughout Kundalini yoga. For example, a Kundalini yoga practitioner may perform a common Hatha yoga posture, such as Cobra pose. The addition of Breath of Fire to the pose gives a stronger effect in a shorter amount of time because of the increased efficiency of blood circulation and pranic energy.

When you first do Breath of Fire, it may be helpful to put your hand on your abdomen to feel the inward pull on the exhalation, and the subsequent relaxation of your abdomen on the inhalation.

1. As you exhale, push the air out by pulling your navel point and abdomen toward your spine.

2. As you inhale, release the pull of the navel while the breath automatically returns to your lungs.

The breath is fairly rapid (start out at one per second and work up to two to three breaths per second). It is similar to the "skull-shining breath" we did in Chapter 7, except it is speeded up and has a lighter touch. Breath of Fire is continuous and powerful, with no pause between the inhalation and exhalation (which are done through the nose, unless specified otherwise). It is said that Breath of Fire is one continuous breath moving in and out of the body.

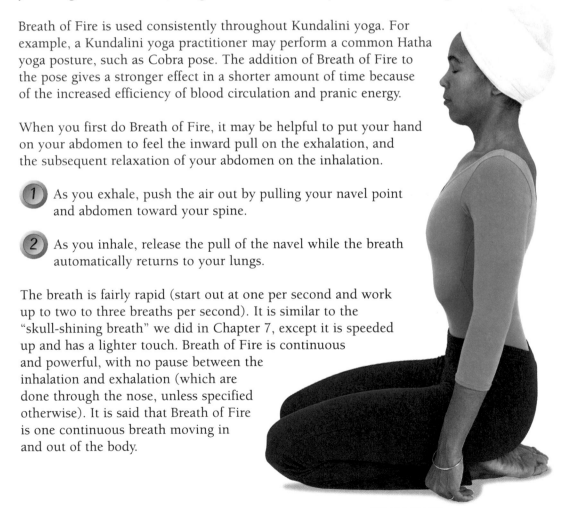

BREATH OF FIRE

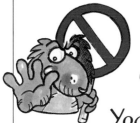

Pregnant women or those in menses should not do Breath of Fire. Nor should those with heart conditions or high blood pressure. Breath of Fire and vigorous yoga exercises should be approached with caution by those with medical conditions.

Yoga sets

Yoga sets, or *kriyas*, are one or more exercises or postures that work toward a specific beneficial outcome. When you practice a kriya, physical and mental changes are initiated that affect the body, mind, and spirit simultaneously.

Each kriya has a different effect. There are kriyas for balancing the heart and mind, for the digestion, for the spine, for becoming like angels, for developing willpower, and for strengthening your aura, just to name a few.

> **DEFINITION**
>
> *A kriya ("kriyas" in the plural) is Sanskrit for "action," and in Kundalini yoga it is considered to be a posture or a sequence of exercises that improves the well-being of specific areas of the body, mind, and spirit.*

Regulating the mind

The word mantra translates as "mind projection." It is a technique for regulating the mind and keeping it uplifted. There are many mantras, each one having its own quality, rhythm, and effect. In Kundalini yoga, an individualized, "secret" mantra is not given. All mantras can be learned and used by anyone.

In addition to using mantras in meditation, a student of Kundalini yoga is encouraged to keep the sound of a mantra on the inhalation and exhalation as he or she practices yoga.

For example, a common mantra used in Kundalini yoga is Sat Nam (rhymes with "but mom"), which means, literally, Truth–Name or "Truth is my identity." When you inhale, hear the sound "Sat," and on the exhale, "Nam." Mantras in English work, too; you can hear the words "I am" on the inhalation and "I am" on the exhalation. The double sound of "I am" will give you the understanding that "I am what I know myself to be, and I am greater than I know myself to be."

A sampler of Kundalini yoga

THERE ARE A GREAT MANY *Kundalini yoga poses, and the following are just a few of those you might want to try. I have also given some tips on how to get the most out of the poses.*

- Take about 20 seconds to breathe deeply between exercises, in order to circulate the prana throughout the body and bring it back to a state of equipoise.
- Do each exercise to the best of your ability, but if you need to, it is perfectly okay to shorten the time of an exercise.
- Once you are able, add the sound of "Sat Nam" or "I am, I am" to the inhalation and exhalation.
- Keep your eyes closed during yoga, except when you need to focus outwardly for balance. Then keep a soft gaze, and keep an inward focus.
- As you move through these exercises, be aware of changes in your mind, your physical body, and your internal energy centers.
- Call on your breath to help you through a challenging pose or exercise.

Warming up

1 **Tune in.** Sit on a mat, blanket, or sheepskin, in Easy pose with a straight spine. Bring your hands into Prayer pose at the center of your chest. Close your eyes, and inhale deeply. Chant "Ong Namo, Guru Dev Namo" three times, once per deep inhalation.

2 **Stretch pose.** Lie down on your back. Stretch your legs forward, pointing your toes, while stretching your arms overhead, and stretch deeply. Then tip your pelvis forward, bring your feet together, and raise them 6 in (15 cm) from the ground,

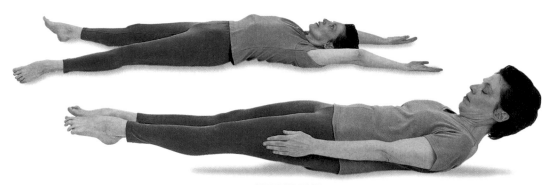

STRETCH POSE

keeping your legs straight. Raise your head 6 in (15 cm) and fix your eyes on your toes, which point away from you. Arms are held straight at your sides, palms facing your thighs but not touching. Hold this position for 30 seconds to 1 minute with Breath of Fire. Inhale and hold the pose briefly. Exhale and relax down.

Stretch pose adjusts the navel point, setting the navel pulse so it is balanced and strong, which strengthens your willpower and physical health. Stretch pose tunes up the whole nervous system as well as the digestive and reproductive systems.

EGO TRANSFORMER

3 **Ego transformer.** Draw your knees into your chest, wrap your arms around your shins, and rock on your spine a few times. Then sit either in Easy pose or on your heels. If sitting on the heels is difficult, try placing a firm pillow between the thighs and calves. Raise your straight arms to a 60-degree angle from the horizontal. Stretch your thumbs up toward the sky. The rest of your fingers are curled onto the pads of your hands. Begin a powerful Breath of Fire for 1 minute.

This exercise energizes the entire body system. In the science of yoga, each area of the hand relates to a certain area of the body or brain. In this hand position, the thumb, which represents the ego or personal psyche, is the focal point for transformation.

4 **Lower spine flex.** Start by sitting on the floor in Easy pose. Take hold of the outside ankle with both hands. Inhale and flex your spine forward, chest out and shoulders back. Exhale and slump your body. Your shoulders curve forward, your chest caves in, and your spine is rounded. Continue in a rhythmic forward and backward manner, one movement per second. Focus on rocking your pelvis forward and back, as well as moving the mid- and upper spine. Feel each vertebra of the spine curl and uncurl. As you continue, pick up the pace. Go for 1 minute. Then inhale deeply, holding the breath briefly. Exhale and relax the breath and the pose.

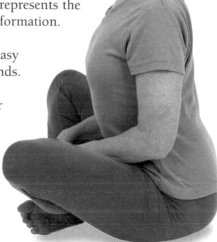

LOWER SPINE FLEX

(5) **Upper spine flex.** Still sitting in Easy pose, grasp your knees with your hands and straighten your elbows. Inhale and stretch your body forward. Your chest will be lifted, your shoulders will come down, and your chin will be level. Exhale and slump your spine as far as possible, shoulders rounded forward. Your elbows are mostly straight throughout the exercise. Focus your awareness on the areas from your mid-spine up through your shoulder blades. Again, feel each vertebra flexing. Begin slowly and pick up the pace as you go for 1 minute. Inhale deeply and stretch. Then exhale and relax the breath.

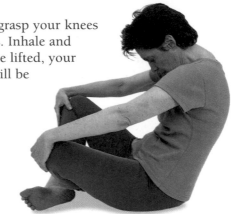

UPPER SPINE FLEX

Kriya to balance the head and heart

This yoga set helps to bring a balance between logic and feeling, between ideas and the "fire" to put them into action, between overly sensitive emotions and an overly intellectual mind. It aligns the head and heart, so you can be great and graceful, aware and loving.

(1) **Arm twists.** Sit in Easy pose, arms straight out to the sides from your shoulders, with your wrists bent so that your palms are flat, as though you were pressing them against two walls. There will be a pressure on your wrists, since you keep them pulled back in this position throughout the exercise. Begin with your fingers facing straight up. This is the inhale position. Now exhale, and rotate your entire arm so your fingers face forward. Inhale and return to the original position. Then exhale again, and twist your arm so your fingers point backward. Then inhale in the original position. Continue, keeping all four movements distinct and separate. Your elbows will rotate. Move in a rhythm of one full cycle per 4 seconds. Continue for 1–4 minutes, then inhale, exhale, and relax. Massage your arms and shoulders for a few seconds.

This exercise activates meridians in the arms and hands that create changes in the chemistry of the brain fluid through the hypothalamus and pituitary.

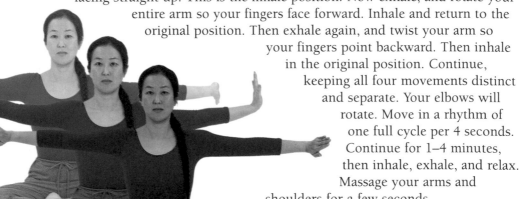

ARM TWISTS

2 **Arm arcs.** Still in Easy pose, extend your arms straight out to your sides, palms facing out, as in the previous exercise. Inhale and raise your arms overhead to form an arc, with your palms crossing each other slightly in front of the crown of your head. Exhale and lower your arms straight out to your sides once more. Then inhale again and raise your arms, crossing your palms as before, but this time slightly to the back of the crown. Continue the four-part motion powerfully, keeping your palms flat and a pressure at the wrists the entire time. Continue for 1–2 minutes.

This and the following exercise stimulate the thymus gland and activate the heart center. Crossing the arms above the head activates the higher centers of the brain through the pineal gland.

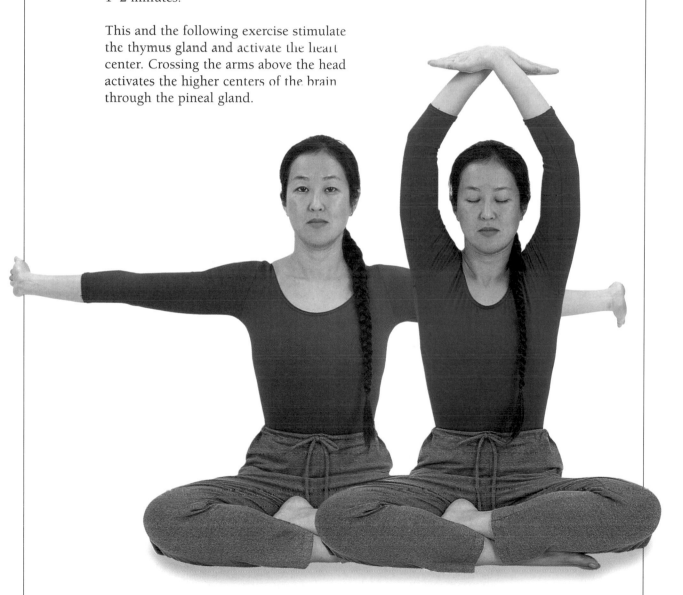

ARM ARCS

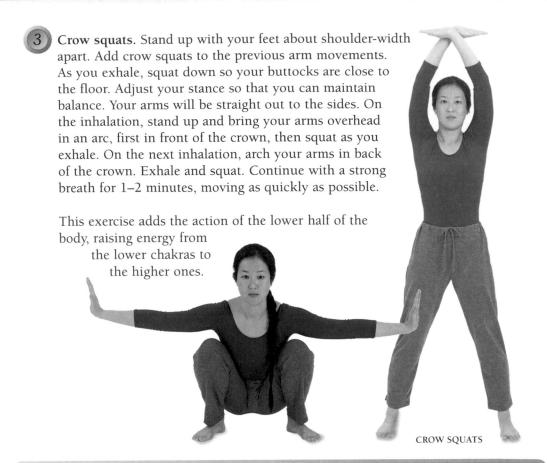

3 **Crow squats.** Stand up with your feet about shoulder-width apart. Add crow squats to the previous arm movements. As you exhale, squat down so your buttocks are close to the floor. Adjust your stance so that you can maintain balance. Your arms will be straight out to the sides. On the inhalation, stand up and bring your arms overhead in an arc, first in front of the crown, then squat as you exhale. On the next inhalation, arch your arms in back of the crown. Exhale and squat. Continue with a strong breath for 1–2 minutes, moving as quickly as possible.

This exercise adds the action of the lower half of the body, raising energy from the lower chakras to the higher ones.

CROW SQUATS

KUNDALINI YOGA AND THE CHAKRAS

The following quote is from one of my favorite books on Kundalini yoga and the lifestyle teachings of 3HO, *Kundalini Yoga: The Flow of Eternal Power*, by Shakti Parwha Kaur Khalsa:

We practice Kundalini yoga in order to balance and coordinate the functions of the lower chakras and to experience the realms of the higher chakras. After the kundalini energy rises and becomes accustomed to flowing freely through all the chakras, there is a definite change of consciousness, a noticeable transformation in the character of an individual. The person looks at life differently, feels different and therefore acts differently. The real "proof" that someone's kundalini has risen lies in the upgrading of that person's attitude toward life, his relationships with other people, and with himself.

4 After completing the set of exercises, relax on your back in Corpse pose. Cover yourself with a light shawl to maintain an even body temperature while resting. Continue with deep relaxation for 5–10 minutes. Generally, meditation is recommended to follow a Kundalini yoga practice.

A simple summary

✓ Yoga is the science of the self, and kundalini is the awakening of the self. It is that simple.

✓ Kundal means "the lock of hair of the beloved." The uncoiling of this "hair" is the awakening of the kundalini, the unlimited potential that already exists in every human.

✓ The kundalini energy is already flowing in our bodies to a degree, and there is an untapped potential residing in the nerve channels of the spine, which can be activated through Kundalini yoga.

✓ Kundalini yoga was brought to the West in 1969 by Yogi Bhajan, who openly taught this yogic science that had previously been sequestered for thousands of years. From his teachings came the creation of 3HO (Healthy, Happy, Holy Organization), a way of life that incorporates and teaches yoga, meditation, healing foods, and healthy life choices.

✓ Kundalini yoga incorporates elements from all forms of Hatha and Raja yogas, and is sometimes referred to as the "mother yoga."

✓ Kundalini yoga focuses on movement linked with strong breathing. Breath of Fire, a powerful pranayama, is one of Kundalini yoga's most well-known trademarks.

✓ Practicing Kundalini yoga is energizing and elevating. It concentrates the pranic energy in the lower chakras (root, sex organs, and navel), raises it to the higher chakras (heart, throat, third eye, crown center), then balances all the chakras.

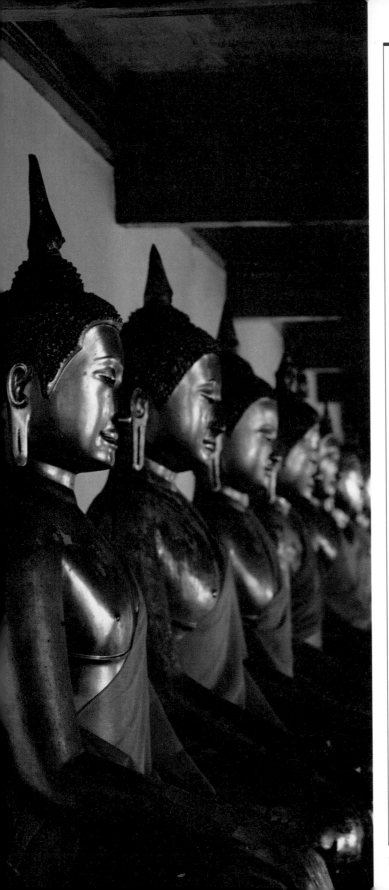

PART THREE

LEARNING TO MEDITATE IS A VITAL PART OF YOGA

THE ART OF MEDITATION

MANY PEOPLE MEDITATE to release tension and establish a sense of calm. Others report that meditation helps them at work, bringing clarity to their thoughts and sharpening their intellect. Still others use meditation as a way to express devotion and live from their hearts. Meditation is all this and more.

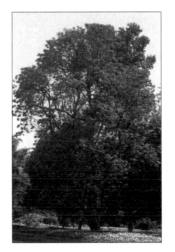

Yoga and meditation go together like the proverbial hand and glove. Yet, it may seem hard to put your finger on what meditation really is. The bottom line in meditation is that it's about becoming aware and *sensitive* to your inner environment, and is a highly individualized process. In a *simple* and *straightforward* manner, this next part of the book will help you understand and experience the art of meditation.

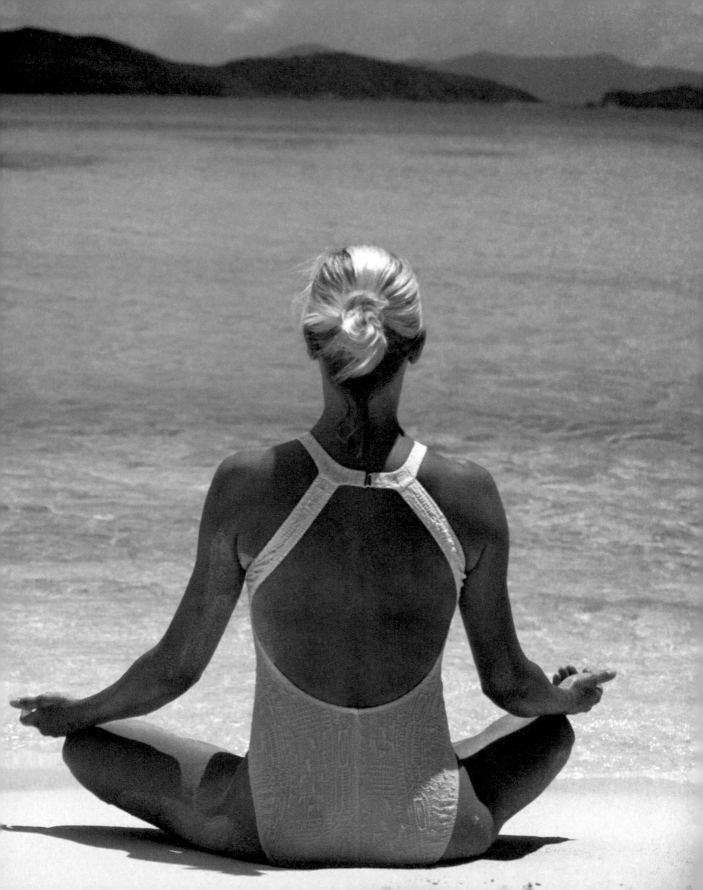

Chapter 12

The Importance of Doing Nothing

A WISE SAGE ONCE SAID, "You can go outside to get what you want, or you can go inside and let it come to you." "Going inside" is meditation – the energy-efficient solution to high-quality living. Yoga wakens you to yourself, and meditation settles you into yourself. After you've had enough experience with yoga, you will probably feel that you want to meditate. In this chapter you will learn about the many benefits of meditation, and how to maximize your meditation experience.

In this chapter...

✓ **How do I know I'm meditating?**

✓ **Don't just do something – sit there!**

✓ **Meditating to relieve stress**

✓ **The tools of the trade**

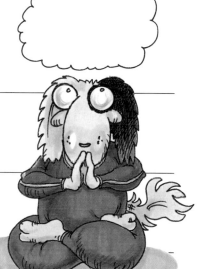

THROUGH MEDITATION, DEEP LEVELS OF STILLNESS CAN BE ATTAINED

How do I know I'm meditating?

WHEW! THIS IS A HARD ONE. *Meditation means different things to different folks. To a religious person, meditation may mean contemplation of God, in prayer or study. To a Zen practitioner, it is entering a space of "sacred emptiness." To a Transcendental meditator, it could be the mental repetition of a sound to the exclusion of all else. And that's just for starters. There are infinite roads to that intangible state called meditation, yet there is a commonality running through all its forms.*

What the yogis of old tell us about meditation is that, according to the Yoga sutras, meditation is the process of stilling the thought waves of the mind. This is kind of a Catch-22 because you can't really try to stop your mind by force. Like a needy child, it will make such a fuss. The more you try to stop it, the more it clamors for your attention.

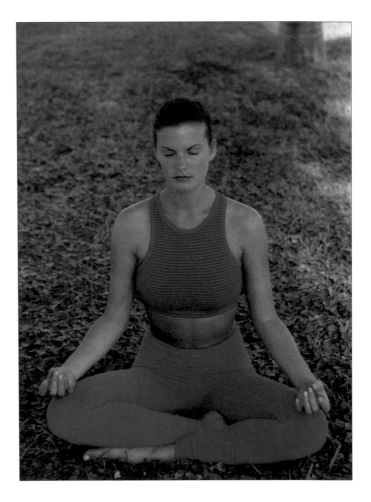

■ **Yogic meditation** *is the disciplining of the mind until it becomes still. Although it is not something you can learn to do in a day, the feeling of well-being and peace it creates is worth the time and commitment required.*

THE STAGES OF MEDITATION

As you develop your practice of meditation, you will most likely find yourself moving through progressively deeper levels of stillness.

When you first meditate, you will get drawn into the mind's drama, then you will realize you've been drawn in. Little by little you begin to watch the mental activity. As would a benevolent observer, you just watch the mind. This is the process of the fifth of Patanjali's eight limbs, pratyahara, or inner focus.

With practice, your mind will eventually settle down and behave itself. By aligning the breath and the inner focus, you experience one-pointed concentration. You find that you are able to direct your mind with your will and imagination. This is the realm of dharana.

As you go deeper, you will open into an inner space of awareness that changes constantly, yet you are solid and sitting, aware of all your thoughts without being involved in them. This is dhyana.

The last of the eight limbs of yoga is samadhi, the master realm of total identification with the spirit. You live as one who is grounded in what is often called higher awareness, or your higher nature.

The process of meditation isn't learned in a day, or even a year. I don't want to kid you about that. But if you put forth a sincere effort every day, and increase the time you spend in meditation as you continue, you will find welcome changes in your mind and your life.

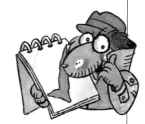

Saying goodbye to good and bad

Assuming we all have a higher nature, whether we know it or not, anyone with a mind (which, I believe, includes all of us!) can become awakened to that higher nature. In meditation, you develop a panoramic awareness of yourself, and everything you judge as good or bad about your life. In fact, you may find that those things that you label as "bad" are the very motivation for you to meditate – and so they actually have done something very good for you.

Then you can gather up all these so-called negative parts, and instead of trying to throw them away, accept them as teachers. Try to learn from these teachers. They are your compost, the fertilizer for the new soil in which your higher nature can grow.

The most important thing to realize is that you are your higher nature. It is not something unattainable, or outside of you. Your higher nature is not some angelic being – you are your own angelic being!

Every time you act in kindness, shake yourself out of negative thoughts, do what you know is best for all involved – every time you forgive yourself and others, you are in your higher nature.

And what is wrong with judging yourself as good? Well, nothing at all, if this analysis comes via neutral-minded self-assessment. But often we pat ourselves on the back one minute, then pound our heads against the wall the next, because critiquing is based on relative circumstances. Succinctly, if you puff yourself up, one day you're going to let yourself down.

Meditation goes past this seesaw of judgment, opening your mind into a panoramic mental viewpoint that allows you to remain steady through all of its fluctuations.

Picture this

Developing a meditative mind can quite possibly be the most positive, healing, and transforming act you ever do. For a couple of minutes now, simply picture yourself more calm, more relaxed, more centered, and more effective. Feel what that means to you. How would it feel to be able to be steady of heart and clear of mind? Hear your own voice expressing that attitude. Sense what it would be like to rise above pain or negativity, to look on these things with compassion and neutrality.

Meditation can do all this for you. That is why it has become a practice that hundreds of thousands of people do every day. It is an investment in your higher self, and the dividends are bountiful.

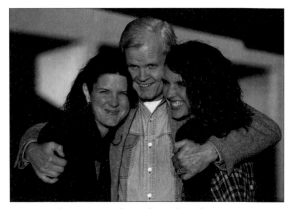

■ **One of the main benefits** *of meditation is that it will help improve relations with others, especially family and friends, and help resolve areas of conflict.*

Don't just do something – sit there!

YOU KNOW HOW IT FEELS to watch a TV or film scene that is in slow motion? You notice every subtle nuance on people's faces, every muscle flexing as they run, every curl of the ocean's waves, each leaf dancing its own dance. It seems there is wonder, a clarity, and a calmness in those actions. I love to watch people practicing Tai Chi for the same reason: I feel so calm and concentrated in a flowing way, just watching them move so slowly and subtly.

I liken a really good meditation to this feeling of slowness and subtlety. I am doing nothing, yet everything is being done. I am humming along with the universe. It is a very happy feeling, but not so much that I take myself out of the space of doing nothing and into the space of "me being happy." I am relaxed, happy, and just being.

Now and Zen

Let's "do nothing" together now. This type of meditation is traditionally associated with Zen Buddhism.

Sit in a comfortable position, in Easy pose, Lotus pose, or simply on your heels. The important part is your spine, which needs to be erect and relaxed, so that vital energy can flow through the spinal column. Bring your neck in line with your spine, so that your chin will be slightly tucked in. Your hands can be in your lap, but be aware that you are not pulling your shoulders forward when you do this. Otherwise, your hands can be in Gyan mudra, resting on the legs. Your breastbone is lifted, and your shoulders will naturally drop without rounding forward.

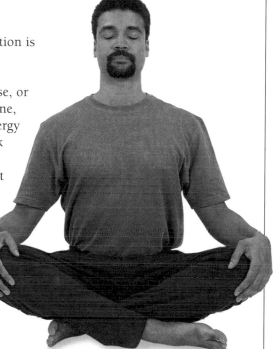

■ **To be able to meditate** *you need to be in a comfortable position, such as in Easy pose, sitting cross-legged with your hands resting on your knees.*

Begin your practice by mentally counting the breaths. While inhaling, count "one," while exhaling, count "two." On the next inhale, count "three," and so on – up to ten. Then begin again. If you lose track, just begin again with one. After all, there is no real goal you are reaching for in counting. It is just a way to give your mind something to feed on. Simply follow the breath with awareness.

Still your mind

As you will most likely find out, this "simple" practice is quite challenging. You are being asked to do virtually nothing, but your lifelong habit of mental activity doesn't simply switch off.

Remember, you are being asked not to still your mind but just to watch your mind. Look at all things alike; accept equally what you like and what you don't like. Make an effort to suspend your usual way of thinking for the time being.

Thoughts will come, and you will forget to count for moments, and even minutes. Never mind. Once you wake up and realize that you have been absorbed in thought, go back to your breath-counting process. And, this is the hard part: Do it without judgment. If you do judge, don't judge yourself about that, too! Take a deep breath, and shake yourself out of those boxes within boxes and into your neutral state of consciousness.

Eventually you will come to a point where you can leave behind the practice of watching the breaths. More and more you will find yourself in an effortless state of awareness.

At the end of your "do nothing" time, stretch your body. Be conscious of maintaining a semblance of your meditative mind as you go about your day.

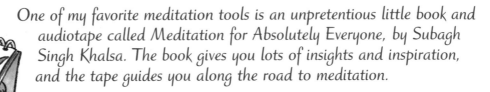

One of my favorite meditation tools is an unpretentious little book and audiotape called Meditation for Absolutely Everyone, by Subagh Singh Khalsa. The book gives you lots of insights and inspiration, and the tape guides you along the road to meditation.

Meditating to relieve stress

STRESS IS UNAVOIDABLE in the busy lives we lead. For better or worse, it is an integral part of being human. From our cave-dwelling days, we have been equipped with the "fight-or-flight" response, which, back then, was a vital tool for survival. But now, how many times has your life been threatened by a ferocious wild animal? Yet we still utilize the fight-or-flight response in our daily lives, which creates radical changes in our bodies: An increase in oxygen, raised heart rate, increased muscular tension, and a huge surge of epinephrine.

DEFINITION

*The adrenal glands produce **epinephrine**, a fast-acting hormone that prepares the body for dealing with stress or danger by increasing heart and breathing rates.*

Stress itself is not harmful, but our inability to deal with our bodies' response to it can be. If you can learn to cope with the changes that life presents you, or change your responses, you can handle life's stress. Toward this end, developing a meditation practice will be invaluable.

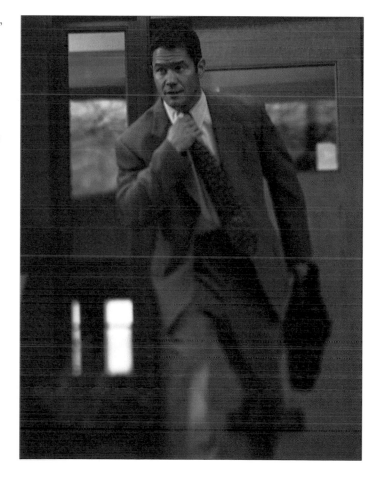

■ **Meditation helps soothe** *the mind and body, so that we are better able to deal with stress which, for most people, is an integral part of everyday life.*

KEYS TO STRESS MANAGEMENT

- Exercise regularly, including a practice of yoga.
- Set aside a relaxation time every day.
- Use a positive technique, such as meditation, a breathing exercise, or positive affirmations and visualizations.
- Be aware of your body. Notice if tension is building up anywhere and take steps to relieve it.
- Notice how your emotions affect your actions and other people.
- Find a healthy outlet for your emotions.
- Have fun with others who are positive-minded.
- Change what you can change in your life, and have patience with the rest.

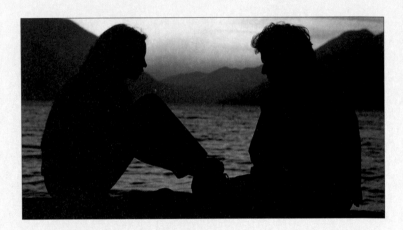

■ **No matter how** *busy you are, make sure you find time to relax and have fun.*

Some paint the picture that yoga and meditation will make life stress-free, that you will live happily ever after, and never be visited by conflict again. This vision, while attractive, is erroneous. Challenges will not go away, but yoga and meditation will give you the tools to cope with the crises of life.

When you sit in meditation, it is with the intention of exploring what it means to be aware. Your meditative mind will begin to notice in what ways your mind, body, and spirit work together and in what ways they don't. You can then explore the inner frontier of your own consciousness, using your intention, or willpower, to create the changes you want to see. Using the process of meditation, you can experiment with your mind/body/spirit connection with the detachment of a true scientist and with the heart of a true lover.

The tools of the trade

THE FIRST THING TO KNOW IN MEDITATION *is that you cannot make meditation happen. The very act of trying to make it happen pushes it away. The good news is that you can practice the means by which meditation may happen. You can approach meditation using tools such as breath awareness, eye focus, mantra, mudra, imagination, and other means.*

In meditation, the mind is focused. You may be familiar with the feeling of intense focus on your work, for example, and that can be a satisfying feeling of concentration. But in a state of meditation, you are inwardly focused – your energy is not extended outward, as it is when you are working on a project. This consolidated effort gives you a great power of concentration. It recharges your mental, physical, and spiritual batteries.

If you are engrossed in a conversation with someone, do you notice snow falling outside? Do you hear the cars passing by or smell the flowers on the table? As long as you are absorbed, you do not. This is the entry port into meditation. The senses are capable of responding, but they do not because they are withdrawn into an inner awareness.

GAZING AND MANDALAS

Two important meditation techniques that involve using the sense of sight are candle gazing and gazing at a circular design called a mandala.

Tratak is the Sanskrit name for using a visual technique for improving concentration. It requires the eyes to be partially closed as they gaze upon one object intensely for a period of time. One of the best ways to try tratak is by gazing at the flame of a candle that is placed at eye level in a semi-dark room. After a few minutes of gazing, close your eyes and see the glow of the candle in your mind.

Mandalas are colorful, complex designs that draw the eye to the center of the circle in order to strengthen awareness and concentration. The mandala is profoundly symbolic in certain cultures, such as the Tibetan Buddhist culture. Many cathedrals display mandalas of stained glass or marble.

Spine check

In order to meditate, we prepare the body physically with the tool of maintaining a straight spine. Just as water gets dammed up inside a bent hose, our pranic energy is limited by kinks in the spine.

Straight spine checklist

1. The position of preference is to sit on the floor with the legs crossed, forming a triangular base for the body. The drawn-in legs allow for more energy to be collected and used for the inward process of meditation.

2. When you sit with your legs crossed, your knees should be lower than your hips. If you need to, raise your hips with a 3- to 4-in (7- to 10-cm) cushion under your buttocks to straighten the lower spine.

3. Align your upper body and shoulders directly over your pelvis.

4. Rest your hands on your knees.

5. An alternative for those who have great difficulty sitting on the floor is to meditate sitting in a chair. The same rule still applies: Keep your spine straight. If your feet are not solidly on the floor, place a cushion or phone book under them.

6. Another alternative for those who have trouble with Easy pose but who would still like to sit on the floor is to sit on a meditation bench or a thick cushion. In both cases you kneel and place the cushion or bench between your buttocks and calves. The bench will allow your knees, lower legs, and heels to be free of pressure. Remember to straighten your spine.

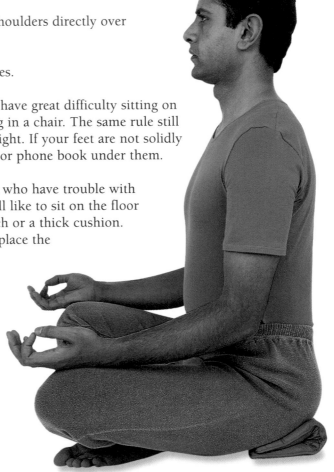

■ **You may find it easier** *to keep your lower spine straight by sitting on a cushion. This will also put less pressure on your knees.*

Using mind-guiding sounds

Mind-guiding sounds, or mantras, serve two distinct purposes. The obvious one is that they give the mind something it can hold onto while the usual mental chatter recedes into the background.

The second purpose relates to those mantras that are in the original language of Sanskrit. According to yogic knowledge, when a sound's innate vibration corresponds to or in some way reproduces what it refers to, it is a sacred language. This is the principle underlying languages such as Sanskrit and Gurmukhi (which is rooted in Sanskrit). *Chanting* these ancient syllables is the fastest possible vibratory union between yourself and the universal consciousness. In other words, the sounds that are made resound with your energy centers in a way that activates and balances them.

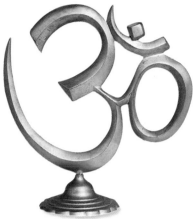

THE OM SYMBOL

Have you ever heard a Tibetan singing bowl? I use one in my children's yoga class to demonstrate how sound affects us. While the children are in a deep relaxation, I make the bowl "sing" through the friction of the wooden stick circling against the side of the bowl. It sends out a vibratory sound current that relaxes the children even more deeply. They always ask for more!

Some meditations use the technique of silent mantra, in which the practitioner hears the mantra internally, often linked with the breath. Other forms of meditation use chanted mantra. When we chant, we are consciously directing the intonations and are invoking the positive power contained within those sounds. We also tend to use the breath more fully when we extend the sound of the mantra out loud. And hearing ourselves chanting helps to keep the mind focused as well.

Positive affirmations spoken in one's own language are also highly effective tools of transformation. Affirmations are a form of mantra that affects the mental level in a positive way. Even such simple concepts as the words "peace" or "relax" on the inhalation and exhalation can have a profound effect. In the next chapter, we will explore a tradition of yoga, called Ananda yoga, that uses affirmations as an integral part of its yoga practice.

IT'S ALL IN THE HANDS

Hand positions, or mudras, are an important part of meditation. Thousands of years ago, yogis mapped out the hand areas and their associated meridians, or nadis. Mudras are hand positions that apply pressure on the different areas of the hands and fingers. Each mudra is a technique for giving clear messages to the mind/body energy system.

Each of our fingers relates to a planetary energy and to the quality that each planet represents. The thumb relates to the persona, the psyche of the individual. Touching the thumb to each of the other fingers creates a specific result. As you press each finger, you are like a musician who fingers the strings of his or her instrument to create internal notes that change brain patterns.

a Gyan mudra (passive)

For wisdom. Uses the index finger, which is represented by the planet Jupiter, planet of expansion. This mudra is used with most meditative postures.

To form passive Gyan mudra, put the tip of your thumb together with the tip of your index finger. This stimulates knowledge and wisdom within you. It gives receptivity and calmness.

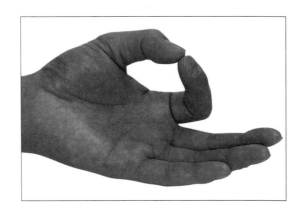

b Gyan mudra (active)

To form active Gyan mudra, curl your index finger under your thumb so that the fingernail is on the second joint of the thumb.

This gives all the same qualities as passive Gyan mudra, but with a more active, or projective, energy.

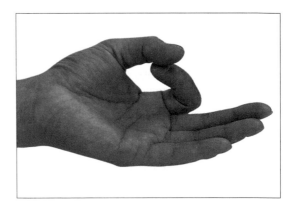

c **Shuni mudra**

For patience and self-discipline. Uses the middle finger, which is represented by the planet Saturn, planet of responsibility, sometimes called the taskmaster.

To form Shuni mudra, place the tip of your middle finger on the tip of your thumb. This gives patience, discernment, and commitment.

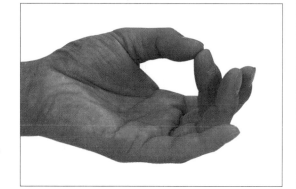

 d **Surya mudra**

For energy and creativity. Uses the ring finger, which is represented by the sun or Uranus.

To form Surya mudra, place the tip of your ring finger on the tip of your thumb. Practicing this mudra gives revitalizing energy, nervous strength, and strong creativity.

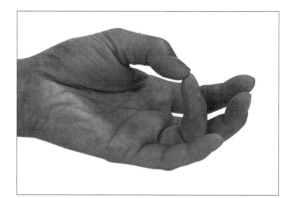

 e **Buddhi mudra**

For communication. Uses the little finger, which is represented by Mercury, the planet of mental power and communication.

To form Buddhi mudra, place the tip of your little finger on the tip of your thumb. Practicing this mudra opens the capacity to communicate clearly and intuitively.

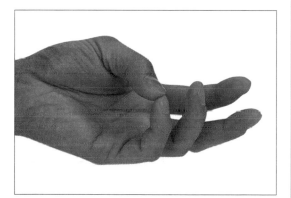

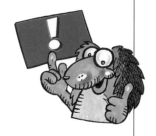

Meditation is a highly individualized process. Some meditation techniques from other traditions may not suit you. Try to stay open-minded, but it is also perfectly fine to settle with a form of meditation that really fits with your belief system. Remember, the bottom line is that meditation is about becoming aware and sensitive to your inner environment.

Focal points

A common meditation tool that is used to draw energy into different chakras and stimulate the higher glands is to focus your attention on different parts of the body. One of the most common focal points for meditation is the sixth chakra, the third-eye point. By gently rolling your closed eyes upward and imagining you can see out through the space between your eyebrows, 1/4 in (0.5 cm) deep, you not only feel centered but also stimulate the sixth energy center, your intuitive center.

Another strong focal point for meditation is to open your eyes a fraction and gaze at the tip of your nose. If you have trouble locating the tip of your nose, touch your finger to the tip and look at your finger. Then take your finger away and maintain a relaxed gaze at that point. This focal point creates a subtle, downwardly relaxing feeling in the body, while activating the pineal and pituitary glands.

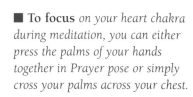

■ **To focus** *on your heart chakra during meditation, you can either press the palms of your hands together in Prayer pose or simply cross your palms across your chest.*

Many people like to focus on their heart chakra while meditating. You can bring your hands into Prayer pose, pressing the thumbs into the sternum, or simply cross your palms over your chest. Not only are you more aware of your heart center when you touch it, but the pressure points activated by the thumbs at the sternum help to open the meridians to and from the heart center.

When focusing on my heart chakra during meditation, I also like to chant or sing, imagining the sound is coming from my heart center. One definition of imagination is mental creativity, so mentally create what you want to experience!

A simple summary

✔ After you've had enough experience with yoga, you will most likely come to a point where you will want to meditate. A practice of yoga and pranayamas is the perfect preparation for meditation.

✔ According to the Yoga sutras, meditation is the process of stilling the thought waves of the mind. This idea can take an infinite variety of forms, depending on the inclination of the meditator.

✔ When you meditate, you usually focus on the breath, a mantra, or an affirmation. You may also have an internal point of focus. The sixth chakra, or third eye, is a common point of focus for meditation.

✔ Another way to meditate is to neutrally observe passing thoughts and sensations in full awareness. This is called mindfulness.

✔ A practice of meditation teaches you how to cope with changes that life presents you and helps you respond in ways that help you handle day-to-day stress.

✔ By concentrating your energies internally, you recharge your spiritual, mental, and physical batteries.

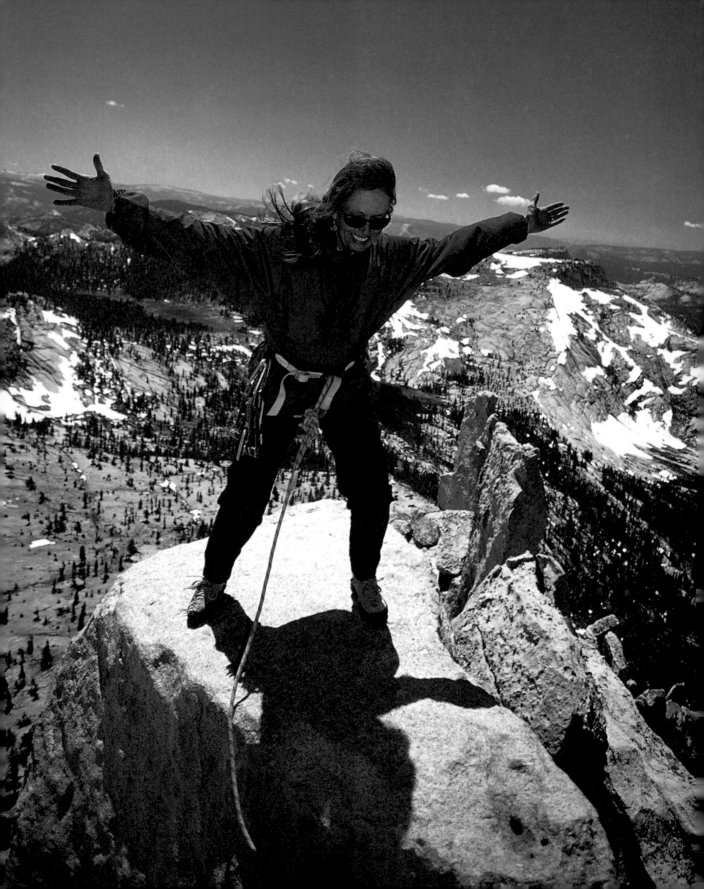

Chapter 13

The Royal Path of Raja Yoga

M AKE WAY FOR THE KING, Raja yoga! Think of Hatha yoga as the knight who aims solely to empower his king, and Raja yoga as that king. In this chapter, you will learn how meditation is essential for a happy life, and experience Raja yoga through two traditions with meditation at their core: Ananda yoga and the Himalayan Institute.

In this chapter...

✓ Straight talk about yoga

✓ Ananda equals happiness

✓ Practicing Ananda yoga

✓ From the Himalayas to America

✓ The Himalayan approach to meditation

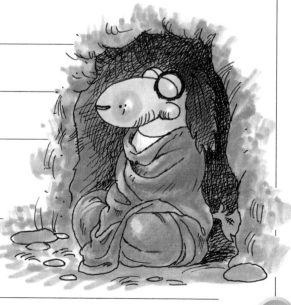

WHEN BODY AND MIND WORK TOGETHER, THE SPIRIT IS STRENGTHENED

Straight talk about yoga

WITH ITS POPULARITY GROWING RAPIDLY, *yoga has become big business. When yoga is marketed to the masses, however, it's easy to lose something in the translation, so to speak. Consider some of the stylish yoga catalogs, where happiness seems to equal having the right clothes and equipment for yoga, or magazine articles that portray yoga solely as a physical fitness program or a way to lose weight and be more attractive.*

Many people practice yoga for reasons of physical health and vitality, therapy, body toning, and stress management. All of these are wonderful benefits of yoga, but to get to the ultimate source of power within, the key is Raja yoga – the development of a meditative mind.

It's important to remember that Hatha yoga is an aspect of Raja yoga, or, in simple terms, that the physical postures are the means toward an end – awareness of your higher nature. When your body and mind work together to strengthen your spirit, the result is the meditative mind.

Moving into meditation

When you go to a yoga class, there may be little or no emphasis on meditation, except, perhaps, to maintain a meditative mood during the practice of postures. As you continue practicing, you may choose to discover the deeper levels of yoga, and that involves meditation.

Every yoga path described in this book has the ultimate goal of developing the meditative mind. For example, classic yoga, such as Sivananda and Integral, places a great deal of emphasis on meditation in a yoga practice. And Kundalini yoga offers hundreds of breath and mantra meditations.

Experience is the best teacher, so the rest of this chapter will explore two yoga paths that emphasize meditation: Ananda yoga and the Himalayan Institute.

Ananda equals happiness

ANANDA MEANS BLISS, divine happiness, so its name alone should give you a pretty good idea of what this yoga tradition is about. And when you realize that Ananda yoga is rooted with the beloved spiritual teacher Paramahansa Yogananda, the author of the classic Autobiography of a Yogi, *you can be certain this path is grounded in higher awareness.*

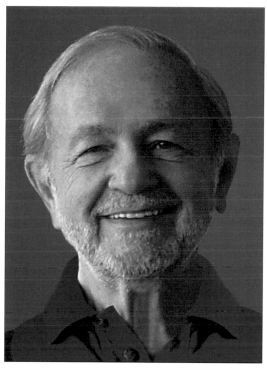

SWAMI KRIYANANDA

Ananda yoga was developed by Swami Kriyananda, an American disciple of Paramahansa Yogananda. Through his insightful practice of yoga, Swami Kriyananda realized the close connection between the yoga positions and the attitudes of the mind. He also brought into the yoga practice the powerful tool of affirmation, which Yogananda so ardently advocated as a technique for raising consciousness. Realizing the psychological and spiritual benefits that were possible in combining asanas and affirmations, Kriyananda wove them together into a system called Ananda yoga.

INTERNET

www.expandinglight.org

To find out more about Ananda yoga, teachers in your area, and teacher-training at their beautiful center in Nevada City, California, go to the Expanding Light web site.

The body–mind mirror

In every moment of any day, we can see the influence of the mind on the body. For example, sadness leads to a slumping posture. Sometimes we don't realize that the reverse is also true: Slumped shoulders and a bent spine can actually, to some extent, induce a depressed mood. The two partners of mind and body mirror each other constantly. So it makes sense that the more you are aware of your mind and body, the more they can work together for your spirit. Ananda yoga emphasizes the friendship between the mind, body, and spirit.

Tips for Ananda yoga practice

1. **Awareness.** Try your best to remain aware of energy flowing through you, empowering your movement and breath. As this awareness deepens, strive to perform the postures in such a way as to bring energy from the periphery of your body into your spine, and up your spine to your brain.

2. **Alignment.** Use correct alignment in order to avoid injury, facilitate the flow of prana, and experience the postures on the deeper levels. However, don't obsess over alignment. It is the foundation, not the pinnacle.

3. **The Routine.** Ananda yoga generally begins with pranayamas and centering. Warming-up exercises are done next, then standing poses, and seated and floor poses. Inverted poses are done to complete a practice, then deep relaxation. The practice finishes with a sitting meditation. All are done at a relaxed pace.

4. **Affirmations.** Most of the basic postures have their own specific affirmations, which are repeated (usually silently) while holding the postures. Each affirmation is designed to help you attune more deeply with the energy flows awakened by the asana. The mental affirmations are an effective, indirect way to work with the chakras.

Trivia...

Yogananda taught his students a unique method called The Energizing Exercises. This practice consists mainly of becoming aware of the body's energy through individual muscle tensing and releasing, accompanied by an energizing "double" breath. The Energizing Exercises video can be obtained through The Expanding Light Organization at their web site mentioned on the previous page.

■ **Inverted poses**, *such as the shoulder stand, feature at the end of Ananda yoga routines. They are then followed by deep relaxation and a sitting meditation.*

After settling into an Ananda yoga pose, repeat the affirmation with concentration, sensitivity, and feeling, calmly awakening yourself to a greater power within you. Keep the affirmation resonating within you during the rest between each posture as well. The amount of repetition and the manner of repeating is completely up to you.

Practicing Ananda yoga

ANANDA YOGA EMPHASIZES RELAXING into postures. It is
delightful to discover that you can perfect poses, not by straining but by
relaxing progressively deeper into the poses themselves. Think of a cat –
it never uses more of its body at any given moment than is necessary. If you
lift a cat when it is resting, it hangs limply. Yet it can leap to its
feet in an instant when it needs to. While practicing yoga,
you can learn to be relaxed, yet as ready and alert as a cat.

The two samplings of Ananda yoga given below would normally
be preceded by the warm-up routine described in tip 3 on the
previous page.

Jackknife pose (Padahastansana)

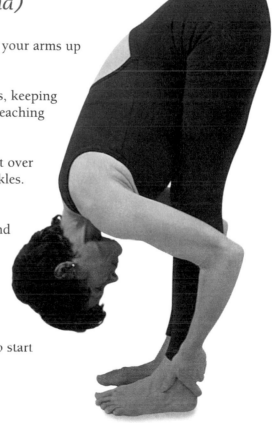

JACKKNIFE POSE

1. Stand up straight. Inhaling deeply, draw your arms up
over your head and stretch your spine.

2. Exhale and bend forward from your hips, keeping
a straight back. Feel as though you are reaching
out for the opposite wall.

3. Relax fully forward, keeping your weight over
the balls of your feet, and grasp your ankles.
Breathe normally in this position.

4. While in this posture, drop your head and
relax the base of your spine. Keep your
legs as straight as possible.

5. Affirm mentally, "What in this world
can hold me?"

6. Hold the posture for about 10 seconds to start
with, gradually increasing the time with
practice to about 1 minute.

7. Inhale and return slowly to an upright position by uncurling your back. Feel as though you are placing one vertebra on top of the next as you move up.

8. Follow Jackknife pose with Backward bend.

In this posture, the natural sense of gravity is disoriented by the half-upward, half-downward position of the body. The mind is more easily freed from its gravitational bondage, which is expressed by the affirmation. Jackknife pose helps to stretch the spine, and exercises a beneficial pressure on the abdomen.

Backward bend

1. Standing upright, put one foot in front of the other.

2. Inhale and raise your hands forward and upward, palms turned up, until you can join your palms together above your head. Stretch upward and backward.

3. Feel the triumphant freedom that is suggested by this position. Feel your energy and consciousness being swept upward to the sky.

4. Affirm mentally, "I am free! I am free!"

5. Repeat, placing your other foot forward.

INTERNET

www.crystalclarity.com

To experience more yoga with affirmations, see Swami Kriyananda's book, Ananda Yoga for Higher Awareness, *available through Ananda yoga's press, Crystal Clarity Publishers, at this web site.*

BACKWARD BEND

From the Himalayas to America

THE SPIRITUAL TEACHER *named Swami Rama was born in Northern India, and trained in the tradition of the cave monasteries of the Himalayas. Both swami and scholar, he studied Western psychology and philosophy in Europe and England before coming to the United States in 1969.*

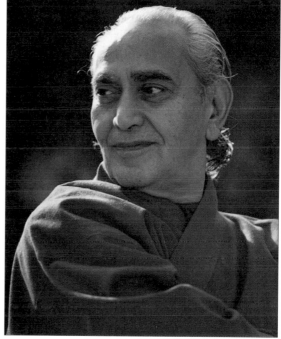

SWAMI RAMA

In 1970, the Swami assisted the Menninger Foundation of Topeka, Kansas, on a project conducted to investigate voluntary control of internal states. Using *biofeedback* under laboratory conditions, Swami Rama demonstrated his precise control of his own autonomic functions. As you can imagine, this was a real eye-opener for scientists in their understanding of a human's ability to control the body.

DEFINITION

Biofeedback is simply input applied to biological functions. A biofeedback machine is any device that makes a person more aware of an internal bodily function. The person then attempts to control the function voluntarily. Biofeedback has been extremely successful in training people to relieve muscular tension and to become aware of their ability to control their autonomic body systems.

The "possible human"

Swami Rama's demonstrations were instrumental in bringing the teachings of yoga to the attention of physicians, psychologists, and researchers, thus helping Western science understand more about the "possible human." Consider the following recorded account of what happened at the Menninger Foundation:

● Swami Rama first made the temperature of the little finger side of his hand differ from the temperature of the thumb side by 10°F (5°C). Without moving or using muscle tension, he controlled the flow of blood in the large radial and ulnar arteries of his wrist. Onlookers reported that the left side of his hand turned red, while the right side turned ashen gray.

- He stopped his heart from beating, saying "I am going to give it a shock. Do not be alarmed." His heart rate, which had been smooth and even at 70 beats per minute, suddenly, in the space of one beat, jumped to nearly 300 beats per minute. In medical terms, he created a condition in which the heart vibrates so fast that blood does not fill the chambers properly, the valves fail to work, and no blood is pumped into the body.

- After several periods of practice in the laboratory, Swami Rama announced that he would produce delta waves. Prior to this, slow delta waves had been recorded only during deep sleep. Yet he was able not only to produce delta waves but also to report accurately on what had happened in the room while he was asleep.

- When asked how he was able to demonstrate these phenomena, Swami Rama answered, "All of the body is in the mind. But," he added, "not all of the mind is in the body." In other words, each part of the energy structure of the body is found in the energy structure of the mind. The mind, however, has the ability to transcend the body.

The Himalayan Institute

Consistent with his love of merging East and West, Swami Rama then founded the Himalayan Institute in 1971 to create a bridge between the ancient Eastern teachings and modern scientific approaches.

Raja yoga is the main focus of the Himalayan Institute, which is now headquartered in Honesdale, Pennsylvania. Students at the Institute practice Hatha yoga, meditation, selfless service, and healthy lifestyle choices. Himalayan Institute-trained yoga teachers can be found throughout the world. In addition, the Institute has several locations around the world, and continues today under the leadership of Pandit Rajmani Tigunait, successor to Swami Rama.

INTERNET

www.himalayan institute.org

The Himalayan Institute's web site is a good source for learning more about their programs or finding a trained teacher in your area. It is also the source of the well-known magazine Yoga International, as well as the Himalayan Institute Press.

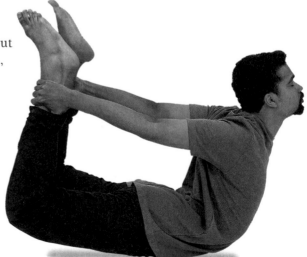

■ **Raja yoga**, *the principal form of yoga practiced at the Himalayan Institute, combines steady postures with stillness of the mind.*

The Himalayan approach to meditation

MEDITATION IS AT THE CORE *of the Himalayan Institute's teachings. Students learn the basics of meditation, then gradually are taught to individualize meditation to fit their unique needs.*

The Himalayan Institute has produced a lovely, lucid book called *Yoga: Mastering the Basics*, by Sandra Anderson and Rolf Sovik, from which I have briefly summarized two meditation practices for you to try. The first one can be used to get you ready for the second, or they can be practiced separately. Enjoy yourself, and enjoy your *Self*.

Touch of the Breath

1. To further the inward movement of awareness in preparation for meditation, you can become aware of the subtle touch of your breath as it enters and exits your nostrils.

2. Sit meditatively. Close your eyes. Bring your attention to the delicate touch of your breath entering your nostril. Feel the coolness of the inhalation and the warmth of the exhalation.

> ### Trivia...
> Christian priests understand the importance of breathing, too. Consider this quote from Rev. Ken Jenkins, a Catholic priest:
> "The union of body, mind, and spirit is mediated through the breath, the creating energy of God. Yogic breathing is meant to focus our energy and quiet our minds. When our mind is still enough, free of random thoughts, then we begin to have glimpses of our true self, the self that is the pure creation of God. For those who are beckoned to experience union of the breath of the body with the breath of the Spirit, the means are as close as a yoga class."

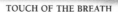

TOUCH OF THE BREATH

③ Attend to the feeling of each breath and each transition between breaths, letting your breathing flow smoothly and without pauses.

④ Your mind will vacillate between enjoyment and restlessness, but realize that this is the nature of the mind, and remain a relaxed observer. Rest in the awareness of the breath, allowing a sense of peace to come forward in you.

Continue until your effort to concentrate begins to wane. Then end the practice and open your eyes.

So ham (that I am) meditation

"So ham" (pronounced "so hum") is considered the natural sound of the breath, "so" being the sound of the inhalation, and "hum" the exhalation. The translation of so ham is, "I am that which I am." This mantra affirms that deep within you exists an identity that transcends the temporary pleasures and pain of the external world. So ham helps you to create a relationship with your deeper self.

① Sit in a meditative posture with a straight spine.

② First bring your attention to your breath touching the inside of your nostrils, as in the previous meditation.

③ Next, as you feel your breath in your nostrils, bring the sound of your breath into your mind. The sound "so" accompanies the inhalation, and the sound "ham" accompanies the exhalation. Let the two sounds quietly reverberate in your mind, flowing along with the natural movement of your breath.

WHO IS ON YOUR THRONE?

Let's go back to the initial concept of Raja yoga as the king (or, if you prefer, the queen!). In your quest to know yourself better, ask yourself at any given moment, "Who is on my throne? Is it my higher nature? My thinking mind? My emotions? Who is in charge?"

These are the questions elicited by a practice of Raja yoga. As you develop awareness, you will begin to recognize who is in charge. And as your meditative mind develops, you begin to realize that you have the power of choice – internal choice – at every moment. And that equals freedom.

(4) After a time, rest your awareness on the sound "so ham" with only the merest awareness of the breath. Continue for a few more minutes. Increase the time as you progress in your practice.

Remember to let the breath flow at its natural pace, even when the sound of the mantra is accompanying it, in much the same way that the words and music of a song flow smoothly together.

A simple summary

✓ In order to get to the ultimate source of power within, the key is Raja yoga, which means "royal" or "king," referring to the development of the meditative mind.

✓ The physical postures of Hatha yoga are the means toward an end: Awareness of your higher nature.

✓ Every yoga path that has been described in this book has the ultimate goal of developing the meditative mind. Two schools of yoga that have meditation at their core are Ananda yoga and the Himalayan Institute.

✓ Swami Kriyananda, an American disciple of Paramahansa Yogananda, realized the close connection between yoga positions and the attitudes of the mind. He began to practice yoga using the powerful tool of affirmations, developing a system that became known as Ananda yoga.

✓ The Himalayan Institute, whose main focus is Raja yoga, was founded by Swami Rama, a spiritual teacher and scholar. Students practice Hatha yoga, meditation, selfless service, and healthy lifestyle choices.

✓ As you become more self-aware and your meditative mind grows stronger, you come to realize that at every moment you have an internal choice about how you will respond to life.

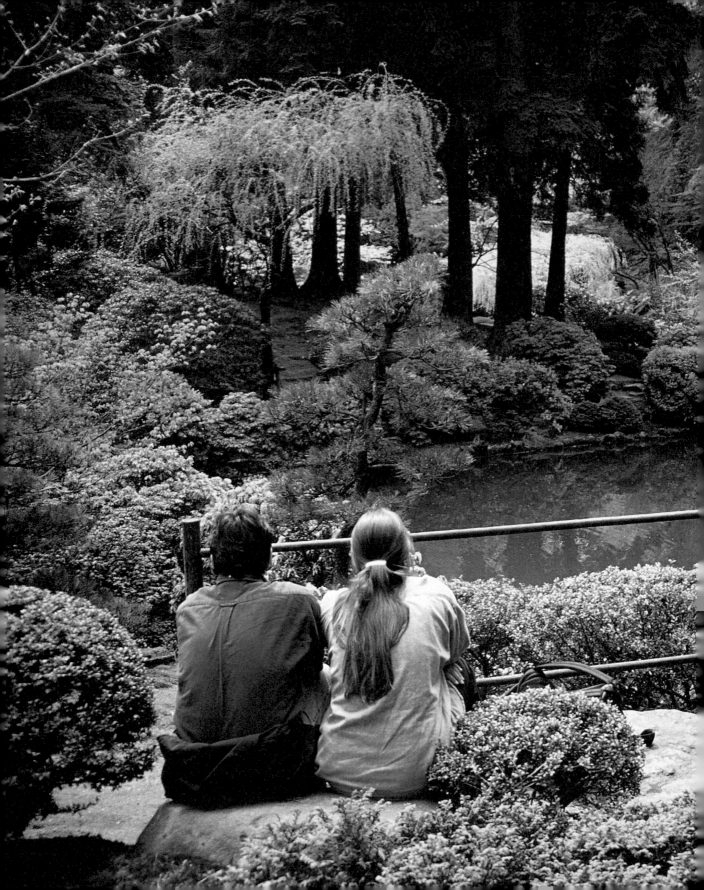

Chapter 14

How Prayer and Chanting Work

As I sat wondering how to start this chapter, I put my hands together, closed my eyes, and spoke under my breath, letting prayer, chanting, meditation, and affirmation all work together. In this chapter we will explore different kinds of prayer and chanting and their yogic connections.

In this chapter...

✓ What exactly is prayer?

✓ Blessing yourself

✓ "Yes" power

✓ Simple toning

✓ The universal sound current

✓ Using mantra to elevate yourself

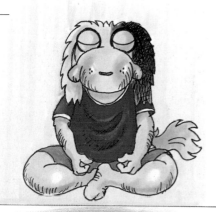

✓ The Sa Ta Na Ma mantra

USE PRAYER TO FEEL AT PEACE WITH THE WORLD AROUND YOU

What exactly is prayer?

A SAGE ONCE SAID THAT PRAYER *is a control of the self in which you can talk to the infinite. When you meditate, it's as if God is talking to you. When you pray, you talk to God.*

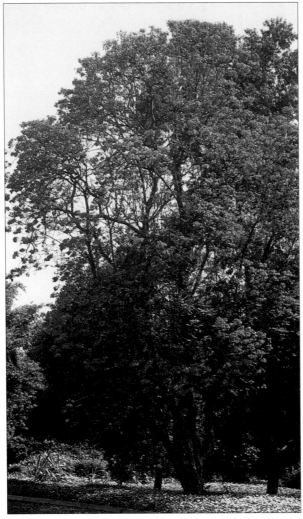

■ **The seasonal cycle of a tree** *demonstrates the three aspects of universal energy, as in the acronym GOD. A tree in blossom is the generating power (G), a tree in summer foliage symbolizes power being organized (O), and an autumnal tree represents the power of nature to destroy (D).*

The word "God" often brings up questions of religion. For the purpose of this book, "God" means whatever it means to you. Yoga, though rooted in Indian culture, is not a religion, or affiliated with any particular religion. Rather, yoga complements all faiths and philosophies.

I really like this neutral way of describing God. It is an acronym for the three aspects of universal energy:

- G – Generating power
- O – Organizing power
- D – Destroying power

Prayer is a deeply personal process. No one religion has a monopoly on prayer. Whether you believe that power comes from within or from the external power of the Absolute, the facts show that the power is there, just waiting to be accessed.

The yoga of prayer

People instinctively use prayer to get in touch with their inner selves, projecting their feelings to the universal One. This is the yoga of prayer. Viewing prayer on a purely energetic level, it is the union of body, mind, and spirit in a way that aligns the individual with the universal – and that is what makes it yoga.

Prayer is mostly thought of as something religious and mystical, and it most definitely can be. The personalizing of God as our beloved helper and friend and our passionate, heartfelt communion with that God add great power to our prayers. They fuel our prayers with the fire of the heart.

Jesus often spent hours in contemplation, adoration, and communion with God. He was anchoring himself in the presence of God. Can you imagine what kind of strength it took to live and die the way Jesus did? He used prayer and invocation to fortify Himself so that He could complete His life's mission.

Be careful what you pray for!

Some think of prayer as a verbal request to God for something that they want. But a word of caution: Be careful what you ask for! Think of Midas, who wished that everything he touched would turn to gold. That one wish did him in. Sometimes prayers are like that. You might want to acknowledge that we humans can't always see the bigger picture by saying "Thy will be done" or "May whatever is best happen."

At the same time, there is no right or wrong way to pray. When someone asked a well-known theologian how to pray, she responded, "It is simple. Ask God."

The link between health and prayer

When you live in remembrance of the preciousness of life, your entire existence can become a prayer. Living life as a prayer keeps you healthy. Blessing others through prayer can keep them healthy.

The most important factor in prayer is attitude. A sincerely compassionate and loving attitude creates prayer.

In a study that involved 393 patients in the coronary care unit of San Francisco General Hospital, prayer groups in various parts of the country were asked to pray for sick people assigned to a treatment group. No one prayed for those in the control group. Prayer was the only variable between the two groups, and no one, not even the doctors, knew who was and was not being prayed for.

The study showed that the prayed-for patients did significantly better on several outcome measures. It didn't even matter how far away the person was who was praying or what method of prayer he or she used.

THE POWER OF PRAYER

Medical doctor Larry Dossey, MD, is also the author of many books about prayer. *The Power of Prayer* is a personal journey about understanding the link between science and spirit. In this audiocassette program Dossey says, "I was actually stunned to discover that scientific evidence supported prayer. And I faced an ethical and moral decision as a doctor at that point. The evidence was so powerful that if I didn't pray for my patients, this would be equivalent to withholding a potent medication or surgical procedure."

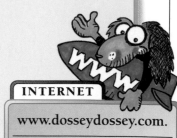

INTERNET

www.dosseydossey.com.

Visit this web site to find out more about Dossey's programs and books.

Blessing yourself

IN MY THESAURUS, the word "blessing" means everything from benediction to good wishes. In this little exercise, blessing means loving, healing, honoring, celebrating, and appreciating every part of you. Use the touch of your hands and your spoken or silent words to bless yourself. If there are other parts of your body that you wish to bless in addition to those given in this exercise, feel free to do so.

This blessing, originally given by Yogi Bhajan, was meant to be done upon waking in the morning, and in the evening. You can also use it as a deep relaxation anytime.

Upon waking:

- In the first 3 minutes that you become awake, bless your head, nose, ears, eyes, mouth, teeth, throat, chest, arms, and belly.
- Bless your good thoughts. Talk to your soul. Feel it and thank it.

In the evening:

- For 5 minutes, bless your ten toes and fingers, your earlobes, and the tops of your ears.
- Bless your good deeds of the day.
- Everything in your being is being moved by your spirit. Talk to it and befriend it.

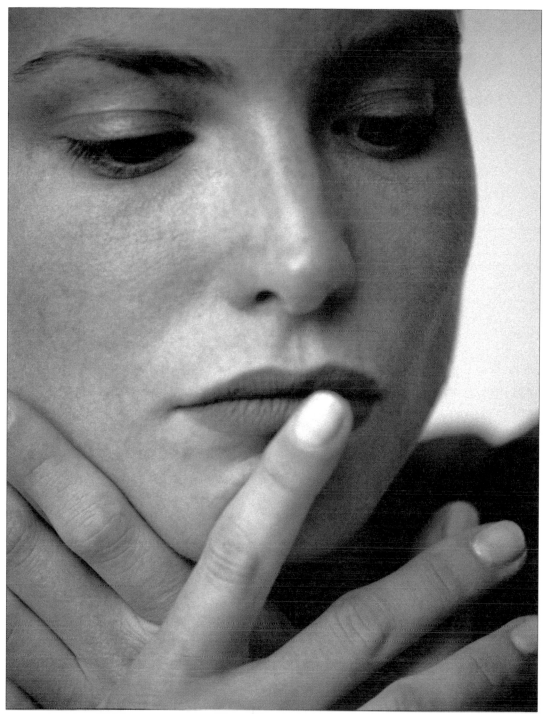

■ **Blessing yourself** is an important part of yogic practice. As you bless the various parts of your body, touch them with your hands to reinforce the love and acceptance you feel for them.

"Yes" power

WHEN PEOPLE PRAY, *they often ask for something. Affirmations work a little differently. In the science of affirmations, one of the core beliefs is that the body is pliable to human thought and feeling in both negative and positive ways. So, to affirm, you "make firm" the concept that you want to have happen by speaking about it as though it has already happened. Even in the face of contrary evidence, you assert positively that a thing is true. For example, to heal yourself you say, "I give thanks that my body is renewed and healed."*

Some simple affirmations were introduced earlier in this book, including "I am, I am," "Peace," and "One." They remind us what is important in life. Affirmations can also be highly personal statements that reinforce the highest in a person. For example, if you have a habit of worrying (which has been described as "praying for something you don't want"), you can create your own affirmations, such as "Everything I need comes to me at just the right time" or "I am safe. I am totally taken care of."

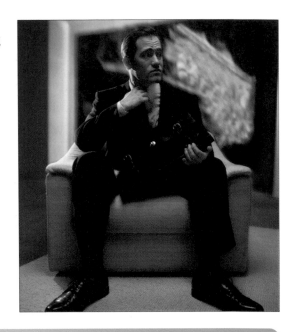

■ **When plagued by negative emotions,** *such as tension and anxiety, use affirmations to regain a positive perspective.*

WORD POWER

Catherine Ponder, a minister of the nondenominational Unity faith, is also the inspirational author of many books, including *The Dynamic Laws of Healing*, from which the following is excerpted. "The usual conversations among people create ill health instead of good health, because of wrong words . . . . When a word is spoken, a chemical change takes place in the body. Because of this, the body may be renewed, even transformed through the spoken word!"

Simple toning

MEDITATION IS LIKE OPENING UP A WINDOW to let the sun in. You don't force the sun in. You can't. The sun will come when it is ready to. In prayer you are projecting a mind–heart beam outward to invite the sun in. In chanting you open the window, and invoke – call forth. You add your voice to that beam of energy.

Toning is the beginning of chanting, the vocal foundation of a chant. In toning you extend the vowel sounds. Remember way back in first grade when you memorized the vowel sounds: "a," "e," "i," "o," "u"? You can take these simple sounds and create a wonderfully relaxing meditation by toning each one on a deep breath. Try each sound three times. As you tone, listen to where you feel the sound vibrating, or coming from within you. The different vowels will resound at different centers of your body. For example, the sound "a" is concentrated at the throat and upper chest, while "e" is in the head and sinus passages. Where do you feel the rest?

> **DEFINITION**
>
> Toning *is the utterance of an elongated vowel sound. The practice of toning uses the vowel sounds for healing and spiritual development.*

Releasing sounds

When you finally get home and can relax after a hard day, what sound do you make? Maybe "aaahhh," maybe "hhmmm," or maybe "shhhh." I call these the natural releasing sounds of the body. Try experimenting with these sounds by inhaling, then allowing "aaahhh" to escape on the exhale. Try "hhmmm" on a few exhales, then a very soft "shhhh" sound for as long as you like. Let the wisdom of your body lead the way. Perhaps there are other sounds that naturally come for you, your own releasing sounds.

The sound of your name

Just for fun, take some deep breaths, then begin to chant your own name. How does it sound? Listen to the tone. Hear how the sounds combine to create your name. How do your mouth and tongue feel while repeating your name? Listen to your name as you've never heard it before. Let it speak to you. You may feel the power of your name. You may gain insight into something about yourself through the sound of your name. You may find it strange or funny. Let yourself enjoy your response to this little experiment.

The universal sound current

CHANTING IS USED IN VIRTUALLY every cultural and religious tradition. The names of the universal One are chanted in all the varied languages of the world. Among the members of religions and cultures that use the spiritual tool of chanting are Christians, Buddhists, Jews, Sufis, Hindus, Sikhs, and the native people of North and South America.

The approach to chanting we will use in this book is the yogic system called *Naad yoga*. According to yogic understanding, sound vibration is the basic nature of the universe. In the ancient scriptures, the cosmos was said to have been created out of the ethers through the primal sound.

> **DEFINITION**
>
> *Naad means the essence of all sound. Naad yoga is the experience of how sound currents, usually chanted and linked with the breath, affect the body, mind, and spirit.*

Chants work on a purely energetic level to create vibratory changes in your state of consciousness whether you know what you are chanting or not. Because Naad yoga is a science rather than a religion, it is universally harmonious with other belief systems.

In his enlightened treatment of the inner life of chanting and celebration of chant, *Chanting: Discovering Spirit in Sound*, author Robert Gass says, "Because chanting has a direct impact on our body and our energy, as with acupuncture, chiropractic, and massage, we receive many of its benefits whether or not we 'believe in chanting.'"

THE RELAXATION RESPONSE

In the 1970s Dr. Herbert Benson, a specialist at Harvard Medical School, studied how the body responded to several practices: Christian prayer, transcendental meditation (TM), hypnosis, biofeedback, autogenic therapy (a relaxation technique), and progressive relaxation.

He found that the body showed a common response in all of them. He called this the Relaxation Response. It consisted of a lowering of the heart rate, blood pressure, and breathing rate. Benson found that our bodies did not differentiate between the different practices of prayer and meditation.

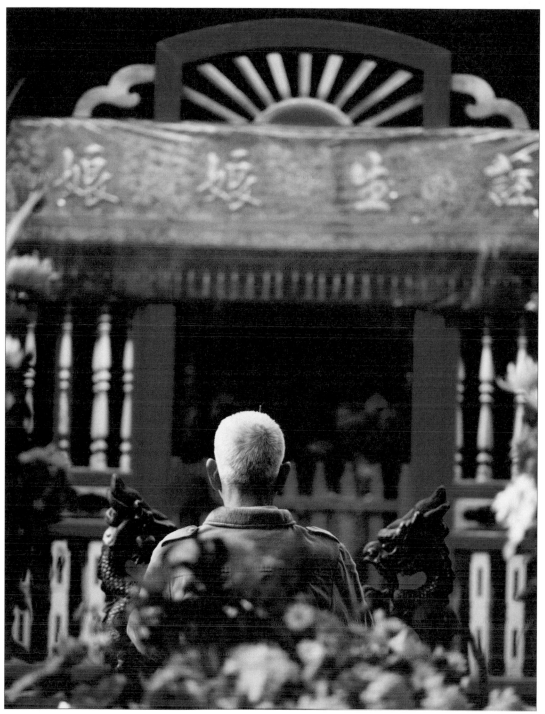

■ **Chanting is an integral part** *of many religions around the world. By chanting a mantra, you help you mind to become focused, altering the state of consciousness to foster greater spirituality.*

Using mantra to elevate yourself

IN THE REST OF THIS CHAPTER *you will have the opportunity to experience chanting that applies the yogic principles of moving energy through the body and mind for the purpose of transformation. The first mantra is "Hari om," which comes from the Integral yoga tradition. The following instructions from the booklet Meditation (available through Integral yoga) are the direct words of spiritual teacher Swami Sachidananda:*

"Om" is the basic vibration. It vibrates every cell in your body and brings peace. "Om" creates a special rhythm in your system. You are sent into an ecstatic mood just by chanting "Om." Of course, when you add "Hari" ("Ha" is pronounced as the "ho" in hot, "Ri" as the "re" in repeat), you get an added effect. "Hari" is another name for the Absolute. It means "the one that removes all obstacles, the one that purifies the entire system."

Repeating the word "Hari" makes you do a particular type of pranayama, or breathing exercise. Each syllable has its own significance. The first syllable, "Ha," requires a contraction of the solar plexus. It creates a kind of bellows-breathing vibration, and it ignites the vast storehouse of physical and emotive power at the solar plexus.

In pronouncing "Ri," the [solar plexus] system relaxes, and the throat contracts to make the force more concentrated. "Ri" brings in a special kind of heat.

Then for "O," the throat opens and the energy or sound rises upward from deep within the chest. With the prolonged "Mmm," the mouth closes, and the energy goes to the head with a strong humming vibration.

So "Hari" accelerates the system first, and the "Om"takes you to a higher level. Repeat "Hari Om" in a monotone, for as long as you feel comfortable. You can vary the pitch, speed, and intensity according to the condition of the mind, and eventually let the voice flow into silent repetition. After some time, just sit quietly and see how you are, and what you feel.

Trivia...

Prayer beads are used around the world. In some cases they are called rosary beads or "worry" beads, and in the yogic tradition they are called Japa or Mala beads. The beads are moved through the fingers as the mantra or prayer is repeated on each bead. The Mala beads are used as a physical aid to concentration. They also activate pressure points on the fingertips in much the same way as mudras.

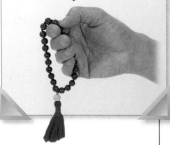

The Sa Ta Na Ma mantra

ACCORDING TO THE KUNDALINI YOGA TRADITION, *as taught by Yogi Bhajan, there are several hundred meditation practices. Out of all these meditations, there is one that is most basic to Kundalini yoga. It has been said that if you master this one meditation, you would be liberated from the cycle of birth and death (in other words, the dual nature of earthly life). This meditation is known as Sa Ta Na Ma, the seed sounds of the mantra Sat Nam.*

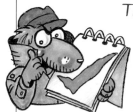

The power of Sa Ta Na Ma is compared to the energy of the atom, because dividing the mantra Sat Nam into its most basic units is like breaking the atom into its nuclear parts.

The "a" in each syllable is pronounced like "ah." Each syllable is a sound vibration with a specific meaning: Sa – the universe, totality; Ta – life, creation; Na – death, dissolution; Ma – rebirth, regeneration.

The building blocks of Sa Ta Na Ma

Sa Ta Na Ma uses every aspect of the human body that can be used to project consciousness into a meditative state: Voice, the movement of the mouth, mental projection, and hand movements.

● **Voice.** There are three "voices" used in this meditation. They are the human voice (chanting out loud), the voice of the beloved (whispering), and the inner voice (silent repetition of the mantra internally). The pattern of chanting begins with the out loud chanting for 3 minutes, then softens into whispering the mantra for 3 minutes, followed by the silent, inner voice for 3 minutes. Then the pattern reverses, so that you chant silently for another 3 minutes, whisper for 3, and come back to the out loud voice for 3. This will total 18 minutes.

● **Mouth movements.** During the chanting, your tongue touches your upper palate, pressing the many nadis, or meridian points, on your sensitive upper palate. These movements stimulate certain configurations, which activate higher brain functions, and release subconscious mind patterns.

HAND POSITIONS FOR SA TA NA MA

Remembering what you've learned about mudras, you will realize that pressing your thumb to each of your fingers stimulates a different internal quality. These qualities are stimulated in the Sa Ta Na Ma meditation as you press each of your fingertips sequentially. Coordinate the movement of your fingers with the mantra in the following way:

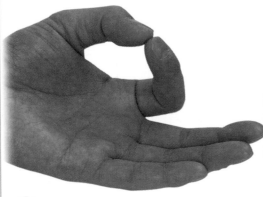

1 **Sa**

As you chant Sa, press your thumb and index finger together.

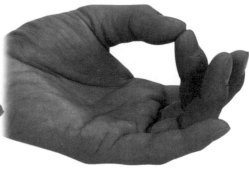

2 **Ta**

As you chant Ta, press your thumb and middle finger together.

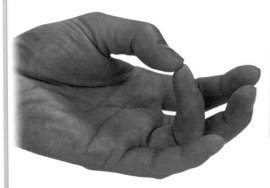

3 **Na**

As you chant Na, press your thumb and ring finger together.

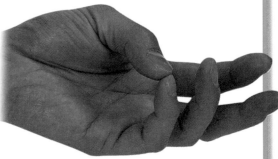

4 **Ma**

As you chant Ma, press your thumb and little finger together.

● **Mental focus.** Your eyes are closed and will gaze gently upward toward the top of your head. Imagine that the initial sound (the consonants of the mantra) comes in through the top of your head at the crown center, and the "ahh" sound flows out through your third-eye center at your forehead. You can visualize an L-shaped flow of energy in through the top of your head and out through your forehead. In other words, create an "energy loop" as you repeat each part of the mantra.

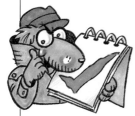

This energy flow follows the pathway called the Golden Cord, which connects the pineal and pituitary glands. Important brain areas are stimulated as you repeat the sounds, and old thoughts and feelings are released as you focus at the area between your eyebrows while extending the "ahh" sound of the mantra.

Suggestions for beginners

As you can see, Sa Ta Na Ma involves doing a lot of things at once. I would suggest you begin with chanting the mantra out loud, then add in the finger movements, and then the mental focus. When that feels coordinated, switch to whispering and then be silent for a minute or so. Before too long, you will feel in the flow of the meditation.

Eventually, you can chant each section for 5 minutes, with an extra minute in the silent part, for a total of 31 minutes, which, according to yogic teachings, is a natural cycle of completion for meditation time.

The Sa Ta Na Ma meditation can become your mind's best friend, a clearinghouse for unwanted thoughts and feelings.

INTERNET

www.SpiritVoyage.com

www.springhillmedia
.com

At the first site, you can listen to and order CDs of the Sa Ta Na Ma mantra and other mantras of the Kundalini yoga traditions, as well as eclectic mantras. The second site can give you more information about the music of Robert Gass and his chanting workshops.

Practicing Sa Ta Na Ma

1. Sit in Easy pose, Lotus, or Half lotus with your spine straight. Sit on a pillow or blanket, if necessary, to straighten your lower spine. Lift your breastbone and straighten your neck, so that your chin is parallel to the floor and slightly tucked in. Your hands will be on your knees with your elbows fairly straight. Your eyes are closed.

2. Using a clock or timer (the count-up type is best, so you are not disturbed by the sound of the alarm), begin to chant the mantra out loud for 3 minutes. Quieten the sound to a whisper for 3 minutes. And silently hear the mantra internally for a total of 6 minutes (two back-to-back 3-minute sections). Repeat the whisper, then the out loud voice to end. Feel yourself sinking into the meditation from the initial out loud voice to the whisper to the inner voice. Go deeply inward, then gently and gradually feel yourself come back out by whispering, and finally, chanting in a regular voice to return.

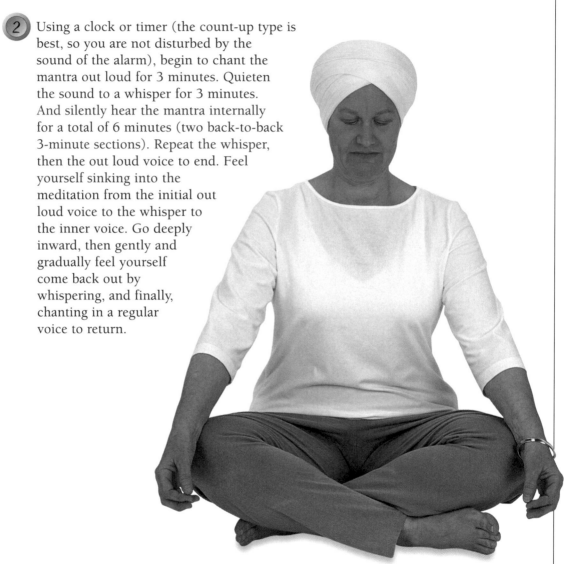

■ **Adopt Easy pose**, *as here, or the Lotus or Half lotus for the Sa Ta Na Ma mantra.*

3 Press your fingers the entire time. Keep visualizing the sound looping down from the top of your head and out through your forehead.

4 Inhale deeply and exhale. Inhale and stretch your arms up high and shake your arms and spine for 30 seconds. Exhale and relax. Stretching upward and shaking wakes up your spine and re-grounds you.

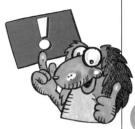

Sa Ta Na Ma meditation is designed to bring inner and outer reality into alignment, creating peace and balance.

A simple summary

✔ In meditation, God can talk to you; in prayer, you talk to God.

✔ No one religion has a monopoly on prayer. Whether you believe the power comes from within or the external power of the Absolute, prayer is a deeply personal process.

✔ Viewed on a purely energetic level, prayer is the union of body, mind, and spirit in a way that aligns the individual with the universal.

✔ Living life as a prayer keeps you healthy. Blessing others through prayer can keep them healthy.

✔ One of the core beliefs in the science of affirmations is that the body is pliable to human thought and feeling. Using affirmations, you create what you want by speaking about it as though it has already happened.

✔ According to yogic understanding, sound vibration is the basic nature of the universe. Chanting is used in virtually every cultural and religious tradition.

✔ Chants work on a purely energetic level to create vibratory changes in your state of consciousness, whether you know what you are chanting or not.

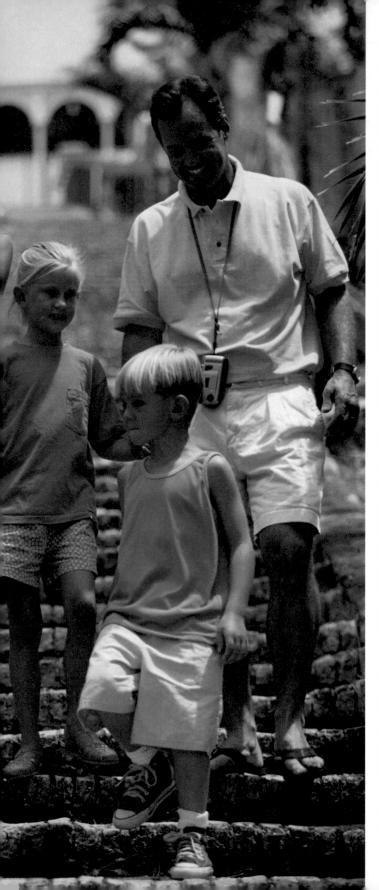

PART
FOUR

YOGA WILL HELP YOU ENJOY LIFE EVEN MORE

LIVING THE GOOD LIFE

BY NOW YOU ARE BECOMING AWARE that yoga is not really about postures, it's about life. In this part of the book, you'll learn about the simple yoga of everyday 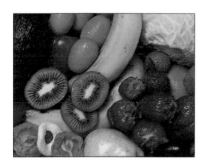 life. You will learn to make the most of the many ordinary moments of life into which you can slip some yoga to increase your energy levels, center yourself, and keep relaxed. And you'll get the whole scoop on the "health secrets" of the yogis of old.

As you build health and well-being through yoga, you will want to *simplify* and *improve* your eating habits. Through your practice of yoga, you'll most likely be attracted to the inherent flavors of pure, wholesome foods, which will in turn give you more *vitality* and *serenity* to bring to your yoga practice.

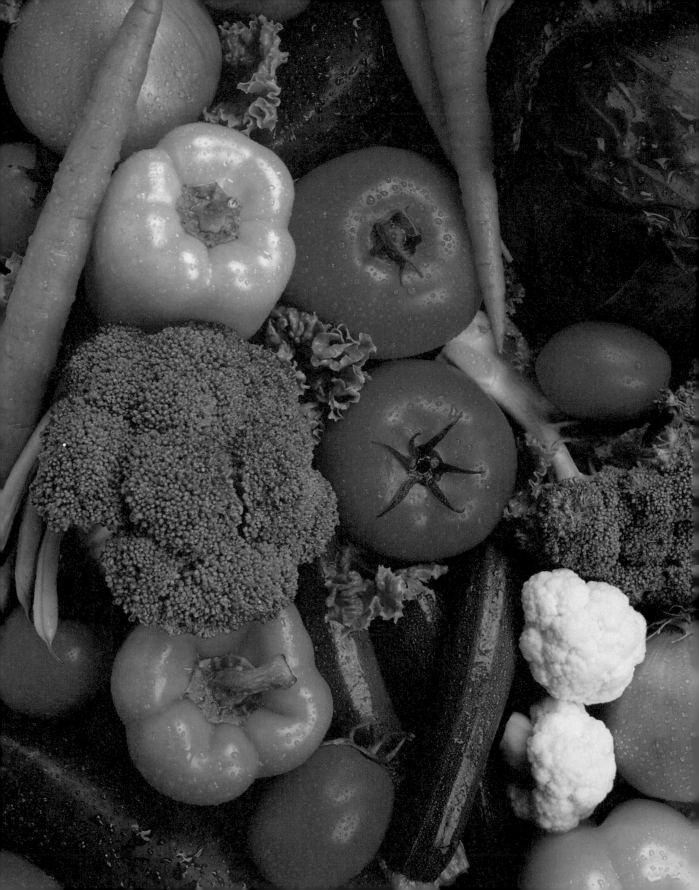

Chapter 15

Eating as Though It Matters

SOMETIMES WE EAT the wrong things by whims! "But," we say, "it *tastes* so good!" Unfortunately, it is the body that pays the price of a poor diet. Maybe you already appreciate the natural flavors of whole foods. If not, this chapter can help – plus, yoga can help. The more you sensitize your mind and body through yoga, the more you appreciate pure foods and the more vitality you gain. In this chapter you will see which foods get the thumbs up and learn some simple guidelines for good eating.

In this chapter...

✓ The three types of food

✓ Simple guidelines for healthy eating

✓ What to do with tofu

✓ The secret ingredient

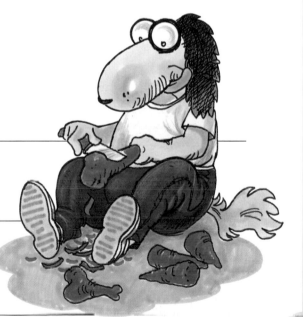

FRESH VEGETABLES AND FRUIT ARE AN ESSENTIAL PART OF A YOGIC DIET

The three types of food

NO, THE THREE TYPES OF FOOD ARE NOT pizza, cheesecake, and chocolate! Guess again. To understand the yogic way of looking at food, let me introduce you to the esteemed science of Ayurveda, a system of healing that evolved on the Indian subcontinent some 3,000–5,000 years ago. Ayurveda was established by the same great ancient sages who produced India's original systems of meditation and yoga.

The Ayurvedic system emphasizes that health is a harmonious and holistic functioning of body, mind, and spirit. It incorporates herbs, nutrition, rest, exercise, massage, yoga, meditation, and other lifestyle recommendations to restore balance and regain health.

DEFINITION

Ayurveda comes from two Sanskrit words meaning "life" and "knowledge" or "science." Together they mean "knowledge of life." The holistic philosophy of Ayurvedic medicine sees the patient as a complete individual, not just a collection of symptoms.

DEFINITION

Rajas means "overstimulating" or "overactive;" tamas "inertia" or "lethargy;" sattva "purity," "calmness," and "clarity."

In the Ayurvedic system, the universe is based on the play of two opposite forces. These forces were called yin and yang by the ancient Chinese sages, and *rajas* and *tamas* by the Ayurvedic seers, who also described a third – a balancing force called *sattva*.

Overstimulating rajasic foods

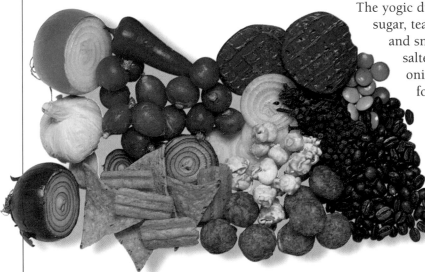

The yogic diet avoids chocolate, refined sugar, tea, coffee, soft drinks, fast foods and snacks, and foods that are overly salted. Some yogic diets also avoid onions, garlic, and heavily spiced foods. According to these traditions, rajasic foods are avoided because they overstimulate the body and mind, causing physical and mental stress and restlessness.

■ **Rajasic foods,** *such as chilies, chocolate, and fast foods, overstimulate the mind and body.*

Not all yogis avoid all rajasic food. The root vegetables, onion, garlic, ginger, and certain spices are important for enhancing the spirit of the Kundalini yoga practitioner's lifestyle.

Dulling tamasic foods

Tamasic foods are avoided in the yogic diet because they produce feelings of heaviness and lethargy. Meat, fish, eggs, drugs, and alcohol are tamasic, as well as overcooked and packaged foods. Foods that have been fermented, burned, barbecued, and fried have tamasic qualities, too. A diet high in tamasic foods makes a person dull and lazy, and contributes to chronic ailments and depression. Overeating is tamasic.

■ **Tamasic foods**, *which include meat, fish, and alcohol, are considered to be impure and lacking vital energy, benefiting neither mind nor body.*

Calming sattvic foods

The yogic diet is made up of sattvic foods that help maintain internal equipoise while nourishing the body. These are pure, wholesome, naturally delicious foods such as fresh and dried fruits, raw or lightly cooked vegetables, salads, grains, legumes, nuts, seeds, wholegrain breads, honey, fresh herbs, and dairy products such as milk and butter. A sattvic diet is easily digested and supplies maximum energy. Together, a sattvic diet, yoga, and meditation form a strong partnership that promotes health and well-being.

Yogis believe that people's food preferences reflect their level of consciousness, and that these preferences alter as they grow in higher awareness.

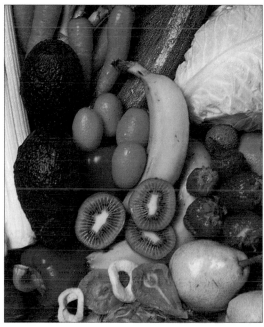

■ **As well as calming** *the mind and stimulating the intellect, sattvic foods, such as fresh and dried fruits, vegetables, nuts, and seeds, also increase energy levels.*

Simple guidelines for healthy eating

VOLUMES HAVE BEEN WRITTEN on the subject of diet and health. The few guidelines included here are simply the framework on which to build healthy food choices. To explore further, search the Web under "health" and "vegetarianism" for more information than you can ever need.

Drink water – and more water

- Nearly two-thirds of the body is made up of water. Without it, our body systems would stop working and we would die within days.

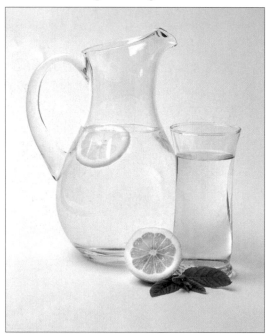

■ **Filtered or spring water**, *which should be drunk throughout the day, is vital for your physical and mental health.*

- Water is the medium by which nutrients are transported to cells and wastes are removed. It is necessary for proper digestion, and helps to bring the emotions and nervous system into balance.
- The best way to get enough water is to drink approximately 2 quarts (2 liters) every day, or enough to keep your urine pale. Drink extra water after exercising, when sweating, with fevers, and to calm emotions.
- Drink filtered water or spring water, rather than tap water, which contains chlorine and other added substances.
- Water is the only substance that quenches thirst. Thirst is quenched proportionally to the amount of water that a beverage contains.
- To avoid diluting the digestive juices, do not drink with a meal. Rather, drink water at intervals between meals.

Alcohol, tea, coffee, and colas are diuretics and actually expel more water from the system than they contain.

Hail to the plant kingdom

- Foods in their natural, preferably *organic* state provide the vitamins, minerals, and protein that the body and mind need. "Whole foods" refers to foods that have not been refined or processed, particularly grains such as brown rice and whole wheat. A large proportion of nutrients are lost in the refining process, such as vitamin E, potassium, iron, zinc, folic acid, and magnesium.

DEFINITION

Organic *produce is food that is grown without the use of harmful pesticides and artificial fertilizers. Instead, crops are grown using natural fertilizers, biological pest control, and crop rotation.*

Vegetarians come in different packages. A lacto-ovo vegetarian eats dairy products and eggs, a lacto-vegetarian eats dairy, and a vegan eats only plant-based food.

- As a practitioner of yoga and for the general well-being of your body, you would do well to eliminate meat and eggs from your diet altogether, and limit your intake of dairy to organic products or substitute soy, rice, or nut milk products. (In organic dairy products, the animals are fed grains that are organically grown without pesticides. They are free to graze, fed no hormones or antibiotics, and are treated humanely.) Not only will you feel physically and mentally fit, but you will be practicing *ahimsa* toward animals and, in a larger sense, toward the entire planetary environment.

DEFINITION

Ahimsa is the Sanskrit word for non-violence, harmlessness.

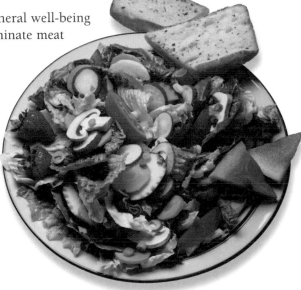

HEALTHY VEGETARIAN PLATTER

If you are a vegan, make sure to take a vitamin B$_{12}$ supplement every day. Some non-dairy beverages, such as soy milk, have B$_{12}$ added to them.

- If you are transitioning to a vegetarian diet, you may want to change your diet gradually. I would suggest that you eliminate red meat first. Gradually, over a period of a few months, begin to eliminate fish, chicken, and eggs, and limit your intake of hard cheese, as it taxes your digestive system.

THE PROTEIN MYTH

Somewhere along the line, we Westerners have bought into the "protein myth." We have gotten the idea (from those who profit from high-protein foods, no doubt!) that we need tons more protein than we actually do.

The World Health Organization has determined that the average adult requires 35–40 g of protein per day. The average American consumes 120 g per day, more than three times the amount needed! Studies have shown that the excess is converted into unhealthy fat and toxic uric acid. Excess protein in the digestive tract makes the liver and related glands overwork to the point that they may be permanently weakened.

Excess protein can add to the possibility of many debilitating illnesses, among them osteoporosis. One long-term study found that with as little as 75 g of daily protein (less than three-quarters of what the average meat-eating American consumes), more calcium is lost in the urine than is absorbed by the body from the diet. In every study, the same correspondence was found: The more protein that is taken in, the more calcium is lost. This is true even if the dietary calcium intake is as high as 1,400 mg per day, far higher than the standard American diet.

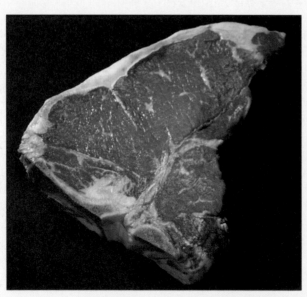

PROTEIN-HEAVY STEAK

And how does the vegetarian diet stack up with protein?

If you are getting enough calories, you are virtually certain of getting enough protein. A team of Harvard researchers who investigated the effects of a vegetarian diet found that it would be difficult to design a plant-based diet that produced an appreciable loss of body protein without resorting to "high levels of sugar, jams, and jellies, and other protein-free foods."

Vegetarian cookbooks

There is a whole world of vegetarian cookbooks to choose from. A few that I particularly like are *Laurel's Kitchen* by Laurel Robertson, Carol Flinders, and Brian Ruppenthal; the classic *Moosewood Cookbook* by Mollie Katzen; and *From Vegetables, With Love* by Siri Ved Kaur Khalsa.

I have been teaching vegetarian cooking since the mid-1980s, and for those who want to understand how our food choices affect us, and the entire planet, I always recommend my all-time favorite Pulitzer Prize-nominated book, *Diet for a New America* by John Robbins. I laughed and cried through it, and was completely inspired to fine-tune my own diet after reading this eye-opening, compassionate book.

INTERNET

www.earthsave.org

EarthSave International was organized as the direct result of the overwhelming response to the book Diet for a New America. *EarthSave leads a global movement to promote healthy food choices for the well-being of all life on Earth.*

If you can't pronounce it, don't eat it

Of course, this doesn't apply to sushi and other deliciously healthy foods that have exotic names! I'm talking about looking at labels. There are more food additives on the market than I could ever begin to mention here. The way I look at it, the farther from the natural source a "food substance" is, the more it behaves unnaturally once it gets into a body, and the less I want to ingest it in mine!

Unfortunately, many unhealthy substances are not listed on the label – chemicals used in farming, pesticides, antibiotics, antifungal additives, growth hormones, heavy metals. Can you imagine what kind of stories that cellophaned package of chicken could tell you? And I'm referring to just the additives, not the life of suffering that factory-farmed animals are subject to. (Modern science is showing evidence that the fear and pain that the animal experiences creates uric acid, which then has adverse effects on the consumer.)

Fruits and vegetables are not immune to the barrage of chemicals that are used in farming. That's where organic produce

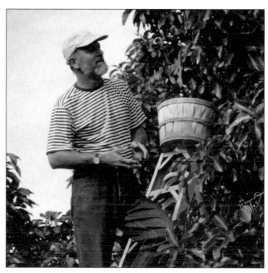

■ **Eating organic fruit,** *grown without the use of pesticides, means you can be certain you are not introducing harmful chemicals to your body.*

comes in. When that's not a viable option, you can try some of the spray washes available to remove toxic surface substances from fruits and vegetables.

Cold-pressed oils, natural sweeteners such as maple syrup or honey, and whole grains are examples of foods that provide the nutrients that our bodies need. Always know what you are eating by reading the ingredient labels on packaged food, then judge if each ingredient will help or hinder the health of your body and mind.

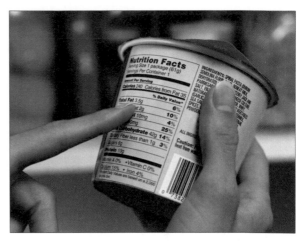

CHECKING THE LABEL

An important issue to understand is GMOs (genetically modified organisms), which, according to the environmental organization Greenpeace, we have unknowingly been eating since 1996.

Traditional plant breeding includes crossing varieties of the same species, but in the GMO process genes are exchanged between unrelated species that cannot naturally exchange genes. One example is genetically altering a tomato by putting fish antifreeze in it. (Wouldn't that make it non-vegetarian?)

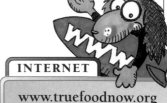

INTERNET

www.truefoodnow.org

Greenpeace's food info site is one of the best sites for information about GMOs. Check their Truefood Shopping List to find out which products have GMOs.

Miscellaneous tips

- Chew every bite at least twice as long as you think you should. Digestion starts in the mouth with enzymes from your salivary glands. And remember, you have no teeth in your stomach!
- Don't overload your system by eating until you are full. That will make you lethargic, and tax your digestion. Eat less at once, and more often.
- Try fasting for a day on water and fresh fruit and vegetable juices. Add a fasting day into your diet once a week or every two weeks.
- Eat raw foods – a salad a day – or snack on carrots and cucumber sticks.
- When you are eating, just eat. Don't read, walk around, or talk on the phone. You will feel more satisfied with your meal, and you will digest it more easily.
- When eating out, be creative. You don't have to order French fries and grilled cheese sandwiches! As a lifelong vegetarian, I know that most restaurants will be very willing to accommodate you. Ask for side orders of the vegetable parts of meat dinners. Order salad, pasta, potatoes, vegetarian burgers, or Oriental and Indian food.

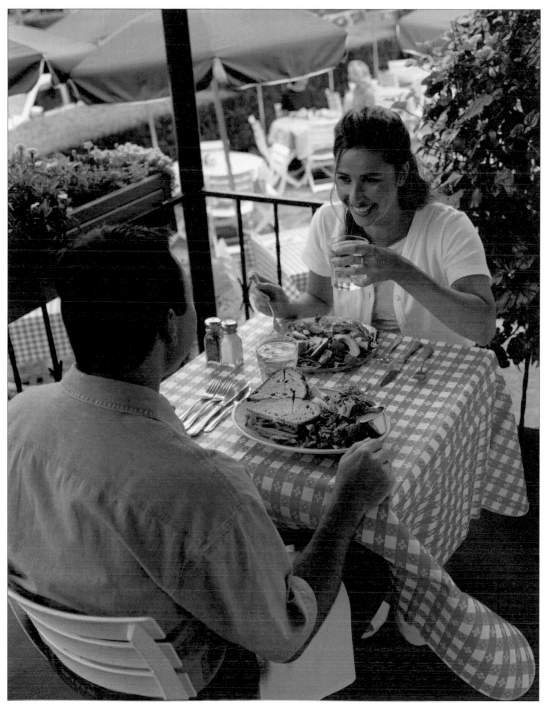

■ **Following a vegetarian diet** *while dining out is no longer the trial that it once was, and most good restaurants offer appetizing, healthful vegetarian food on their menus.*

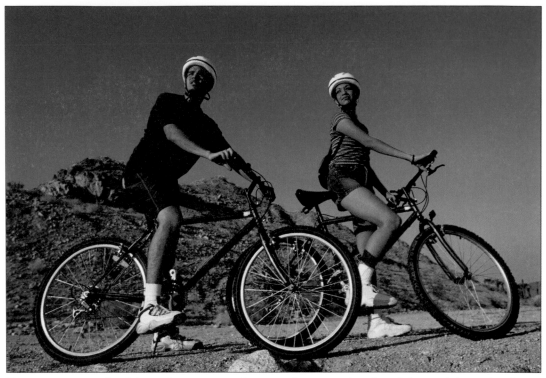

■ **Exercising, preferably in the great outdoors**, *and eating a plant-based diet, and then only when you are hungry, is the best possible way to lose those extra pounds and stay at your preferred weight.*

- Keep a bottle of water with you wherever you go. Keep several in your car. When you are not eating, drink water.
- The best weight-loss diet I have found is to eat healthy vegetarian food only when you are hungry, and only to the point of slight fullness. Have occasional small desserts. Drink lots of water, fresh fruit and vegetable juices, and banana shakes. Eat one or two meals a day. Exercise, breathe deeply, do yoga, and most of all stay happy!
- Have goals for yourself about your diet, but don't agonize over them. Trust that you can work on your health through a number of avenues: Yoga, meditation, prayer, exercise, diet, and just plain having fun! Let the hand of the universe work for you.

A comprehensive treatment of the vegetarian diet and the yogic perspective on food is given in the book Yoga: Mind and Body by the Sivananda Yoga Vedanta Center.

What to do with tofu

TOFU, ONE OF THE MOST VERSATILE *protein foods, has been a staple in parts of Asia for over 2,000 years. And tofu has been puzzling us Westerners for about 30 years now! It's no wonder. More of a texture than a taste, tofu is like a chameleon. It takes on the taste of whatever is added to it. So the clue is in knowing what to add, and how to cook tofu.*

Also called bean curd, tofu is made by curdling the mild white "milk" of the soybean.

The wonders of tofu

Tofu is high in protein, low in calories, fats, and carbohydrates, and contains no cholesterol – it's almost a perfect food. And to top it off, recent medical news shows that soy protein can help prevent heart disease, breast cancer, and prostate cancer, as well as ease menopause symptoms and help in diabetes and digestive disorders.

Whether you want to substitute tofu for the taste and effect of meat or dairy, are lactose intolerant, or want to add soy to your diet because of health benefits, here are some pointers for using tofu:

- Always rinse tofu before using, and keep any remaining pieces covered and sealed in pure water in the refrigerator.
- To minimize any gas-producing qualities, always cook tofu before eating it, and cook it with a dash of lemon juice.
- Generally, firm tofu is used for slicing and dicing. Soft tofu is for blending, and used to make sauces and puddings.

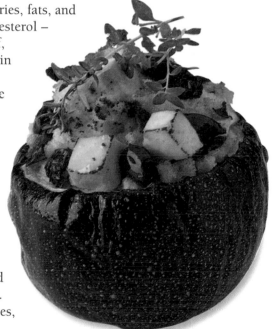

■ **Taking on the flavor** *of whatever it is prepared with, tofu is a versatile, as well as healthy, cooking ingredient. Here, a gem squash is stuffed with tofu and fresh vegetables.*

Tofu cookbooks

Tofu Cookery by Louise Hagler has tons of great recipes, such as Chili Con Tofu and Tofu Loaf. If you think you can't make elegant meals without meat and dairy, leaf through *The Whole Soy Cookbook* by Patricia Greenberg, where you will find recipes including Garden Kabobs with Orange Sauce and Soy Dessert Crepes. And check out the recipe for Spicy Pumpkin Cheesecake (*see below*) from *The Art of Tofu* by Akasha Richmond.

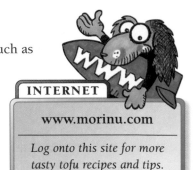

INTERNET

www.morinu.com

Log onto this site for more tasty tofu recipes and tips.

Baked tofu

1 lb (450 g) of firm or extra firm tofu
Canola oil or water
Lemon juice

Bragg's Liquid Aminos or soy sauce
Herbs/seasonings of your choice

A glass baking pan is recommended, but you can also use a baking sheet.

1. Rinse and lightly squeeze out excess water from the tofu. Slice ¼–½ in (6–12 mm) thick. Thin slices will quickly bake into chewy, hard tofu, while thicker slices will yield soft tofu, depending on how long it is baked.

2. Cover the bottom of the pan or baking sheet with canola oil, either spray or from a bottle. Water can be used in place of oil. Sprinkle lemon juice over the tofu.

3. Top with Bragg's Liquid Aminos (a broth/soy sauce substitute that is made from soybeans and water only and can be found in natural food stores) or soy sauce (tamari). You may bake as is, or add any combination of the following: Herbs, garlic/onion powder or flakes, salt-free seasonings, nutritional yeast flakes, sugar-free barbecue sauce, Japanese condiments.

4. Bake for 20–30 minutes at 350–375°F (180–190°C). The longer the cooking time, the crispier or chewier the texture will be.

Spicy pumpkin cheesecake

Canola oil cooking spray
1½ cups graham cracker crumbs
1 tbsp canola oil
4 tbsp maple syrup
1 pkg Mori-Nu Lite Tofu, puréed
8 oz (225 g) cream cheese or tofu cream cheese
1 cup canned or fresh pumpkin purée

1 cup unrefined cane sugar
3 tbsp flour
1½ tsp ground cinnamon
½ tsp ground ginger
½ tsp nutmeg
2 tbsp light molasses
⅛ tsp salt
1¼ tsp baking soda

For this recipe you will need a 9 in or 10 in (23 cm or 25 cm) round springform pan, or pie dish. Serves 8–10.

1 Position a rack in the center of the oven and preheat to 350°F (180°C). Coat the springform pan, or pie dish, with cooking spray.

2 Mix graham cracker crumbs, canola oil, and maple syrup together and press into prepared pan. Purée remaining ingredients in a food processor and pour into crust.

3 Bake for 50 minutes. Let cool for 30 minutes and refrigerate 5–6 hours or overnight before serving.

Tofu salad

1½ lbs (675 g) of firm tofu
Lemon juice

For the salad:
3 celery sticks, finely diced
a combination of radishes and carrots grated to
    equal ⅔ cup
½ cup sweet red peppers, finely chopped
⅔ cup dill pickles, finely chopped
1 scallion, finely diced

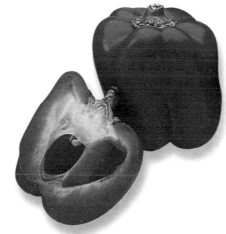
SWEET RED PEPPERS

For the dressing:
¼–½ cup eggless, sugarless mayonnaise   1 tsp lemon juice
    (this can be found in a natural food store)   ½ tsp sea salt
2–3 tsp prepared mustard   ½ tsp black pepper

The texture of the grated baked tofu is similar to chicken or tuna salad. Serves 4.

1 Slice the tofu approximately ½ in (1 cm) thick. Lightly sprinkle with lemon juice, and bake in a lightly oiled baking dish at 375°F (190°C) until medium hard (about 20–25 minutes). Grate when cooled.

2 Meanwhile, mix the salad ingredients in one bowl.

3 Mix the dressing separately.

4 Add the grated tofu to the ingredients of the first bowl, and mix well. Add the dressing, and serve with crackers or with lettuce on bread.

The secret ingredient

WHAT DOES IT TAKE to create food that is nourishing on all levels: Body, mind, and spirit? Wholesome, high-vitality food is the groundwork for a nourishing meal. But that is not the whole story.

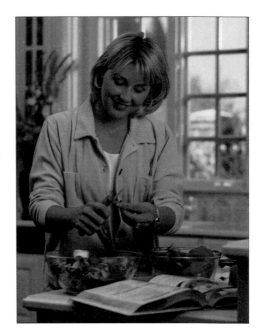

Chanting and singing, or listening to uplifting music while you prepare food also infuses it with peace and prana. Taking a few moments to give thanks for the meal, then eating in appreciation, slowly savoring each bite, produces maximum spiritual, mental, and physical nourishment.

■ **The preparation of food** *is more than just a matter of assembling the right ingredients – love, care, and commitment also play an important role.*

IT'S IN THE BREAD

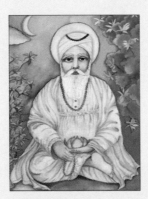

GURU NANAK

There is a story about the 16th-century Sikh master Guru Nanak, who traveled far and wide teaching of the oneness of God. In one town, he was invited to an extravagant banquet at the mansion of a mean and selfish man. He declined, eating instead a very simple meal at the hut of a humble, devoted man and his wife. Upon hearing about this, the rich man was outraged, and confronted Guru Nanak, who then requested a chapati (flat Indian bread) from the kitchens of both the rich and the poor man. Guru Nanak held one chapati in each hand and squeezed them. From the rich man's bread came drops of blood, from the poor man's bread came drops of milk. Guru Nanak said, "This bread is made from the sweat and blood of servants whom you treat as slaves. The other bread, made by hand with love and devotion, is filled with the sweetness of that love."

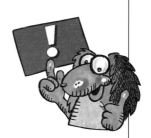

When you prepare food with a relaxed and happy heart, a meditative mind, and devoted efforts, it is subtly infused with prana beyond the vitality in the food itself. The yogic science teaches that food is nourishing proportionally to the amount of prana, or life energy, that it embodies.

A simple summary

✔ In the Ayurvedic system, health is a harmonious functioning of body, mind, and spirit. In Ayurveda, the universe comprises three qualities: Rajas, tamas, and sattva.

✔ Food that is rajasic is overstimulating. Tamasic food produces lethargy. Sattvic food is calming and vitalizing.

✔ Foods in their natural, preferably organic, state provide the vitamins, minerals, and protein that the body and mind need.

✔ A healthy diet consists of wholefoods: Fruit, vegetables, grains, and legumes. For optimum health, gradually eliminate meat from your diet, and limit dairy products.

✔ Water is necessary for proper digestion, and helps to bring the emotions and nervous system into balance. Drink at least 2 quarts (2 liters) a day.

✔ Tofu is high in protein, low in calories, fats, and carbohydrates, and contains no cholesterol. It takes on the flavor of whatever it is cooked with.

✔ According to the yogis, food is nourishing proportionally to the amount of prana, or life energy, that it embodies. You add prana to the food you prepare by being relaxed and meditative.

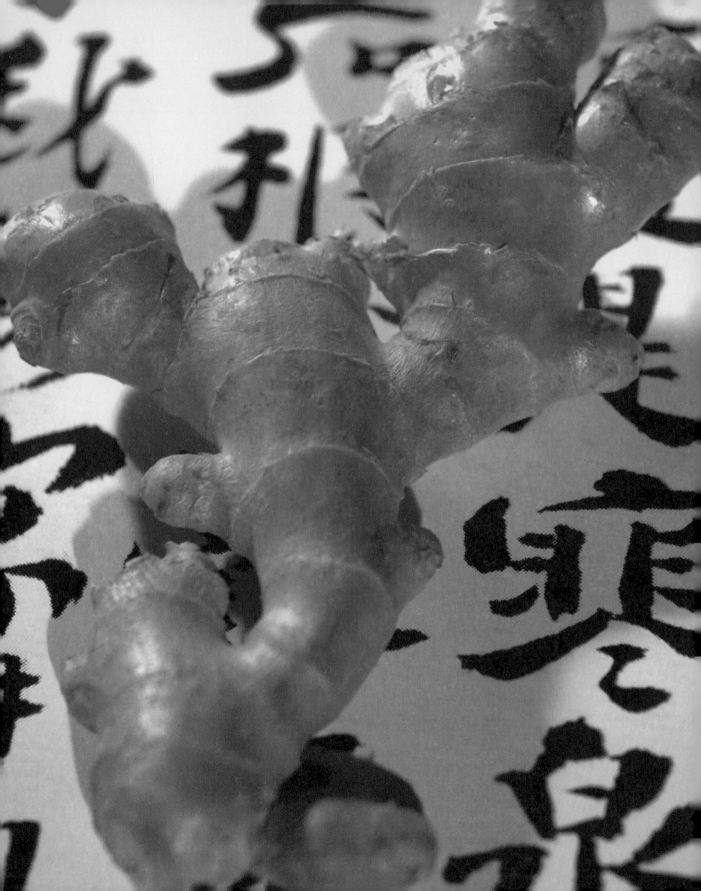

Chapter 16

Health Tips from the Yogis

LITTLE THINGS MEAN A LOT, especially in this chapter: Things like making tea, taking showers, and improving your digestion with your own abdominal muscles. This is the simple yoga of everyday life. The health tips in this chapter have stood the test of time. For centuries, wise men and women have been practicing good health by using food as medicine, and by practicing internal cleansing exercises and techniques. It's time for these sages of old to share their "health secrets" with you.

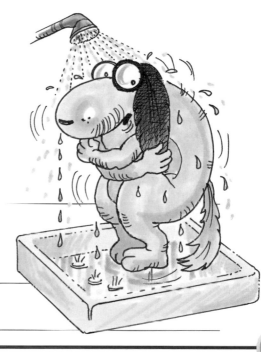

In this chapter...

✓ Food as medicine

✓ Cleaning from the inside out

✓ Cold showers rule!

GINGER, WITH ITS HEALTH-GIVING PROPERTIES, IS A MAINSTAY IN THE YOGIC WAY OF COOKING

Food as medicine

HAVE YOU EVER THOUGHT *about what people did before modern medicine? The answer is that before there were pills and surgery, healing foods and herbs prevented and cured illness. People understood the principles of healthful eating, and discovered the hidden properties of common foods and herbs that could cleanse their bodies internally, correct imbalances that brought disease, and even heal damaged tissue. Included in this section are some of the core foods used by the yogis to maintain health and remedy illness.*

The trinity roots

Onions, garlic, and ginger are so well respected in Indian cooking that they are called the trinity roots. While each of these roots is beneficial when taken alone, cooking them together causes them to interact, amplifying their effect on the body. Onions purify the blood, garlic is for the immune system, and ginger is for the nervous and reproductive systems. In the yogic way of cooking, onions, garlic, and ginger are sautéed to create a *masala*, which is then added to legumes, rice, or vegetables.

■ **Basmati rice**, *here made into a vegetable biryani, is considered a sacred food throughout Asia. It is used by yogis to keep the body healthy and cure illness.*

DEFINITION

The word masala *literally means "blend." A masala is a combination of spices and root vegetables cooked together.*

Basic masala

1 onion	2 tbsps grated (peeled) ginger
Canola oil	3 garlic cloves, minced
1 tbsp turmeric	Vegetables, cooked lentils, or beans
Salt	Soy sauce, or Bragg's Liquid Aminos

1. Sauté the onion in a little canola oil for 1 minute, then add the turmeric and sauté for another 5 minutes. Add the ginger, and after 5 more minutes, add the garlic. Cook until all is soft and blended.

2. Add the vegetables, cooked lentils, or beans. Season to taste with salt, soy sauce, or Bragg's Liquid Aminos, then serve.

Rice dishes

Basmati rice is a naturally white rice that is revered throughout Asia as a sacred food. It is also grown in Mexico. Basmati is a fragrant, high-quality white rice that is not milled or polished, so its vitamin and mineral content is intact. Basmati rice is abundant in B vitamins, iodine, and high-quality protein, and is easily assimilated. (Brown rice, although rich in vitamins, can be hard to digest unless cooked for a very long time.) Cook basmati rice in water with a two parts rice to one part water ratio for about 20 minutes, or until the water is completely absorbed.

Kicheree

Kicheree is an Indian word for a highly digestible, well-balanced food made with rice and mung beans. It is ideal for rebuilding strength during and after illness, and is a soothing, healthful addition to your basic diet.

Add more water for a soupier consistency, less for a stew-like consistency. Serves 4–6.

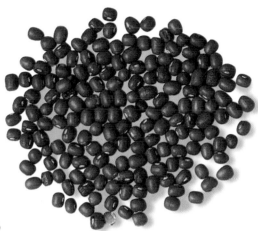

MUNG BEANS

$^1\!/_2$ cup mung beans (washed and picked through for small stones)
1 cup basmati rice (rinsed until water is mostly clear)
5 cloves garlic, finely minced
$^1\!/_4$ cup ginger, finely minced
1 large onion, finely chopped
3 cups of vegetables, finely chopped: Carrots, potatoes, zucchini, and green beans
$^1\!/_4$–$^1\!/_2$ tsp each cumin seeds, cracked red chili, and black pepper
Bragg's Liquid Aminos or soy sauce to taste
$^1\!/_2$ cup ghee

> **DEFINITION**
>
> Ghee is *clarified butter, which is butter that is cooked on a low flame until the impurities separate and are strained out, yielding a clear golden liquid.*

1. Cook the mung beans in water in a separate pot on medium high heat until the beans begin to break open. Meanwhile, pour 2½ quarts (2½ liters) of water (more or less according to your taste) into a pan, add the chopped onions, garlic, and ginger, and bring to the boil.

2. Add the chopped vegetables, Bragg's or soy sauce, and spices. When the mung beans are ready, and if there is an excess of liquid, strain them; otherwise, pour the beans and liquid into the pot along with the rice. Cook until all the ingredients are blended, stirring often. Finally, add the ghee and stir well before serving.

The benefits of turmeric

Turmeric, a root that is ground into a bright yellow powder, is one of the main ingredients in curry powder. Current research indicates that turmeric may be of value in preventing diabetes and cancer.

Best known as a lubricant for the joints, turmeric is also excellent for the skin, the mucous membranes, and the female reproductive organs. It should always be cooked for at least 5 minutes in water or oil before using.

Keep turmeric away from your clothes – it stains! If you get a stain, douse with lemon juice and set clothing in the sun, or, more traditionally, use bleach to take it out.

Golden milk

This very tasty drink is wonderful for the spine, lubricates the joints, helps to break up calcium deposits, and in general keeps yogis and yoginis flexible. Comfortingly warm in the winter and refreshingly cool in the summer – have it your way!

$1/4$–$1/3$ tsp turmeric
$1/3$ cup water
1 cup milk, dairy or non-dairy

1 tbsp raw almond oil
Honey to taste

1 Boil the turmeric in the water for about 8 minutes. Add more water if too much boils away. Add the milk, and bring to boiling point.

2 Remove from the heat and add the honey and almond oil. Drink warm, or allow the mixture to cool, and chill in the refrigerator before serving.

Almond oil taken raw in food or drink will help lower cholesterol, reduce body fat, eliminate hunger, and keep the skin healthy and lustrous. It can be found in the health food or spice section of your local supermarket.

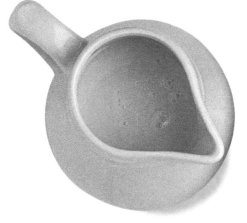

GOLDEN MILK

Yogi tea

You don't have to practice yoga to love yogi tea, but a cup after a yoga class is heaven! The benefits of yogi tea are vast – it's invigorating yet relaxing, and a great coffee substitute. The spices used in this tea are said to have the following properties:

- Black peppercorns are a blood purifier
- Cardamom pods aid digestion
- Cloves strengthen the nervous system
- Cinnamon sticks strengthen the bones
- Ginger root is healing for colds and flu, and increases energy

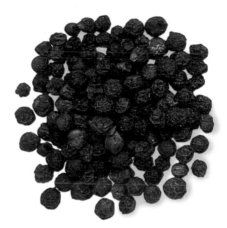

BLACK PEPPERCORNS

In yogi tea, the milk (dairy or soy) helps in the easy assimilation of the spices. A pinch of black tea acts as an alloy for all the ingredients, creating just the right chemical balance, with less caffeine than decaffeinated tea.

The ingredients below make one cup of yogi tea, so double or triple them to make more, as required. When making large quantities of yogi tea, you will not need to use as many spices per cup.

1¹/₄ cups (¹/₄ liter) water
3 cloves
4 green cardamom pods, cracked
4 black peppercorns
Half of 4-in (10-cm) stick of cinnamon

1. Cover and boil the ingredients together for 10–15 minutes. Add a tiny pinch of black tea, and let it sit for a minute or two. Then add ¹/₂ cup of milk and return to a boil.

2. Immediately remove from the heat, strain and serve with honey to taste.

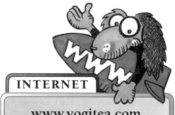

INTERNET

www.yogitea.com

Check out the Yogi Tea web site. An easier (and still delicious) way to have yogi tea is to buy it in concentrate from the health food section of your grocer. There are several varieties, but the original is called "Classic India Spice."

Cleaning from the inside out

INTERNAL CLEANSING TECHNIQUES *have been basic to yoga since times of old. We've already practiced two cleansing breath exercises: Skull-shining breath and Breath of Fire. Both clear out the nasal passages and lungs, helping the body eliminate large quantities of carbon dioxide and other impurities. Internal cleansing methods assist nature in its work, as you will see in the following simple exercises.*

Abdominal churning (Nauli)

Nauli massages and invigorates all the internal organs, and gets the intestines moving. When you practice naulis regularly, your elimination system becomes regular, efficiently moving wastes out of your body.

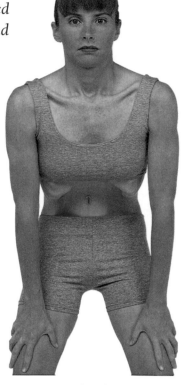

STEP 2

1. Stand up with your legs apart, knees slightly bent, and your hands resting on your thighs.

2. Take a deep breath then exhale completely as you push on your thighs. When your lungs are emptied, draw your diaphragm upward.

3. Without taking a breath, begin moving the central band of muscles in your abdomen forward and back, in and out. Relax and inhale when you need to. Then repeat the process a few more times.

4. Once you have become accustomed to this practice, try abdominal churning. Press harder on your thigh with your right hand to move your muscle to the left, then use pressure on your left hand to move your muscle to the right. Continue with this wave-like motion a few more times.

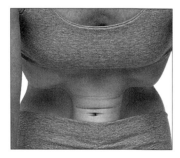

STEP 3

It is best to practice the internal cleansing techniques with a teacher. Those with medical conditions should consult their doctors first.

The neti pot

Neti is a simple nasal cleansing process. Practiced daily, this exercise helps to counteract the effects of pollution, so it is very beneficial to those with asthma, allergies, and other respiratory problems. It helps clear the sinuses, and is an aid to preventing headaches.

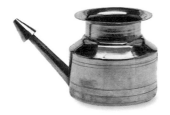

BRASS NETI WATER POT

To practice, you will need a small teapot-type pitcher. Neti pots are available through many of the yoga supply web sites listed previously.

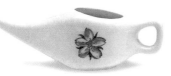

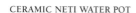

CERAMIC NETI WATER POT

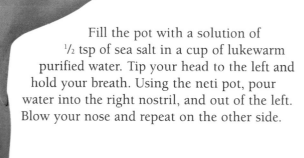

Fill the pot with a solution of ¹/₂ tsp of sea salt in a cup of lukewarm purified water. Tip your head to the left and hold your breath. Using the neti pot, pour water into the right nostril, and out of the left. Blow your nose and repeat on the other side.

■ **Cleansing the nasal passages** *through the practice of neti is simple to do and very beneficial, particularly to those who suffer from respiratory problems, including asthma and allergies.*

Putting an end to "morning mouth"

If you've ever felt like your toothpaste is coating your mouth rather than really cleaning it, this yogic technique will help.

When you wake up in the morning, you have mucous in your throat that has been collecting there overnight. This is your body's way of collecting trash, so to speak, and the most natural thing would be to throw out the trash.

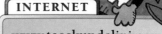

The best way to release this trash is to stimulate yourself to have a gag reflex by brushing your tongue progressively farther back in your mouth until you feel the reflex. At that point, it is important to keep the throat open, so the mucous ball can be released.

The gag reflex will cause your eyes to water, which cleanses your eyes and, according to the science of yoga, helps to prevent cataracts from forming.

The yogic teaching is to combine a mixture of potassium alum (from pharmacies) and sea salt in a ratio of two parts alum to one part salt for brushing your teeth and clearing the "junk" from your mouth in the morning. Alum (very puckery stuff!) and salt clear the coating on your tongue when you brush it and help to release the mucus from the throat.

INTERNET

www.taoskundalini.com

www.thecleanse.com

These are good sources for potassium alum. The Cleanse is also a comprehensive internal cleansing program using diet, Chinese herbs, yoga, and meditation.

Cold showers rule!

YOU MAY NOT LIKE WHAT I HAVE TO SAY, *but I have to tell you. A daily cold shower is one of the best things you can do for yourself. The yogis have known through the ages that cold water keeps you young and healthy. Can't you just imagine the yogi coming out of his hut in the pre-dawn morning and immersing himself in the glacial stream of water that runs through the Himalayan mountains? We may not have Himalayan mountain water, but on some mornings in winter it can't be too far off!*

The yoga of cold water

Why would anyone want to take a cold shower when a warm shower feels so good? Because when that cold water hits your skin, your body systems begin to do what can only be described as internal yoga.

You see, cold water opens the capillaries and strengthens the entire nervous system. When you take a cold shower, your blood rushes out to meet the challenge. This means all the capillaries open up and all toxins are cleansed out.

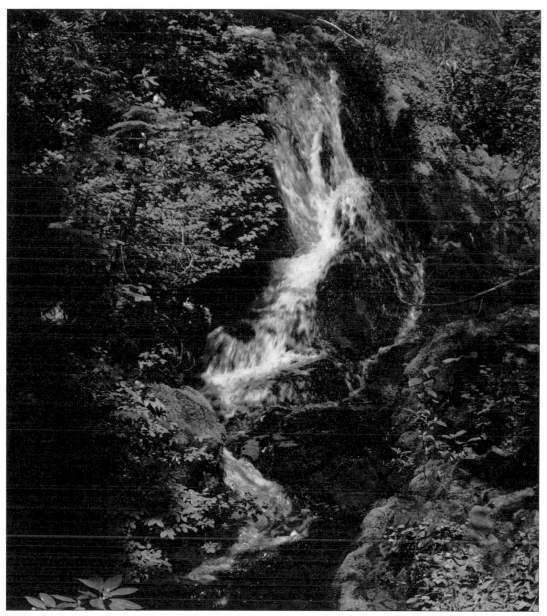

■ **The next best thing** *to a dip in a mountain stream is a cold shower. The cold water will revitalize the entire body, cleansing it of toxins and strengthening the nervous system.*

When the capillaries return to normal, the blood supply goes back to the organs. Each organ has its own blood supply. In this way, the organs get their flushing, like a beautiful rain that grows the fertile crops. When the organs get flushed, immediately the glands have to change their secretion. When the glands secrete, the entire body system is revitalized.

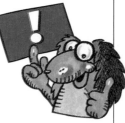

The glandular system is the key to vitality. According to the science of yoga, youth is measured by how vibrant and healthy the glandular system is.

When you are under the cold shower, your body will feel the cold. But if given enough time (30 seconds to 1 minute), your blood and capillaries will open to the maximum and your body will not feel cold.

If you bring your body to that temperature where it can meet the cold by its own circulatory power, you have won the day. You have empowered your own health and happiness.

Preparing the body

Cold showers are strictly for the purpose of internal health, and are not meant to replace warm showers or bathing.

(1) First massage your body with pure oil. Almond is preferred for its high mineral content. The oil will be driven into the skin through the pores while showering, and it will provide a protective coating to the skin.

(2) Using a pair of mid-thigh or knee-length underwear or shorts while in the shower will protect the femur bone in the thigh, which controls the calcium–magnesium balance in the body. If no such protection is available, keep the thighs from the direct hit of the water.

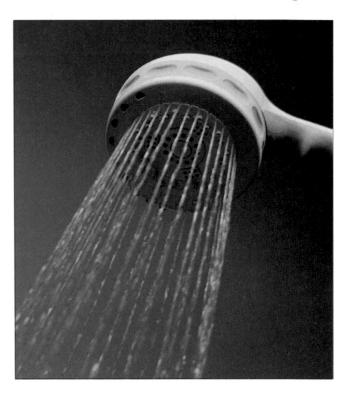

■ **Although warm showers** *can be taken at any time of the day, a brief, cold shower is best taken first thing in the morning.*

(3) Allow the cold water to hit your feet, bottoms and tops, and then the rest of your body, including your face, but not your whole head. Massage as you move in and out from the cold water. Pay special attention to the lymph nodes under the armpits to help prevent colds. Women should massage their breasts under the cold water to keep circulation strong and cancer away.

(4) Breathe deeply or chant a mantra to keep yourself going. Start at 30 seconds, and work up to 1 minute. Towel dry, rubbing the skin briskly.

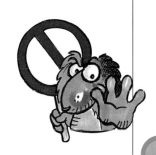

Those who have circulatory problems or other medical conditions should seek medical advice before trying cold showers. Pregnant women or those in their menses should not take cold showers.

A simple summary

✓ Before there was modern medicine and surgery, healing foods and herbs prevented and cured illness.

✓ Onions, garlic, and ginger are called the trinity roots. They work together to energize and purify the body and keep the immune system strong.

✓ Turmeric has been used through the ages to keep the joints supple and disease away.

✓ Through simple internal cleansing techniques, you are helping nature to do its job. For example, stomach pumping (nauli) strengthens the internal muscles of digestion.

✓ Cold water opens the capillaries and strengthens the entire nervous system. All the capillaries open up, and the toxins are cleansed out.

✓ When the capillaries return to normal, the blood supply goes back to the organs. When the organs get flushed, immediately the glands have to change their secretion. When the glands secrete, the entire body system is revitalized.

273

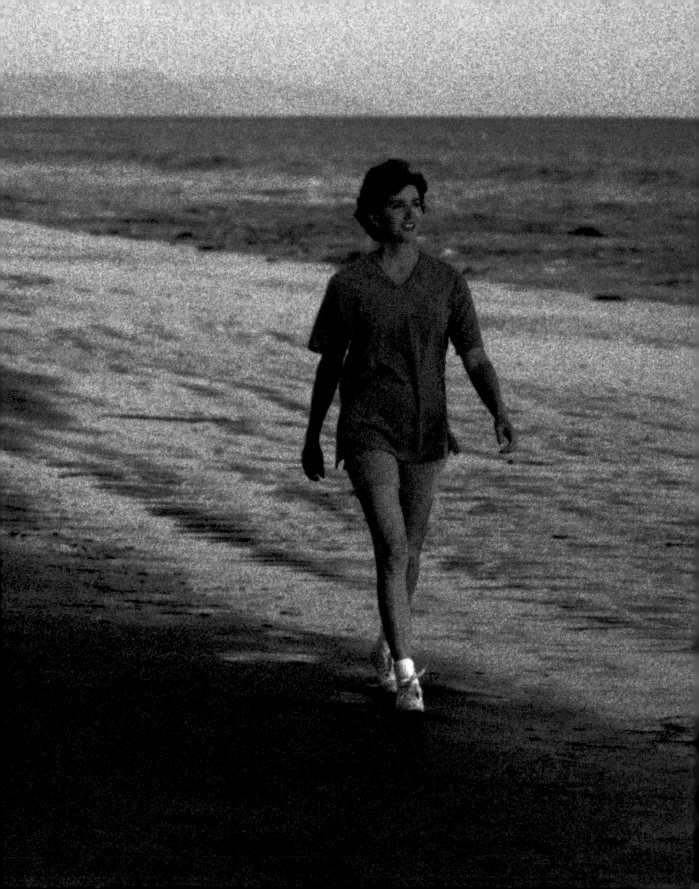

Chapter 17

Portable Yoga

AT ANY GIVEN TIME, you are totally equipped to do yoga. You have your body, your breath, and your awareness, and luckily, that's everything you need for yoga. If you have a desire to practice, and a little creativity, you and yoga can go everywhere together. In this chapter I will help you make the most of the many ordinary moments of life into which you can slip some yoga or meditation to increase your energy, calm and center yourself, and keep fit.

In this chapter...

✓ Things you can do while waiting around

✓ When you need energy

✓ Cool yoga

✓ In a state of equipoise

✓ Getting the most out of walking

A FORM OF YOGA CAN BE PRACTICED WHEREVER YOU GO AND WHATEVER YOU DO

Things you can do while waiting around

IMAGINE YOU ARE IN THE DENTIST'S CHAIR. *You've got your little paper bib around your neck, and you are just waiting for something to happen. From my many years of dental experience, this wait can go on quite a long time, so I use it as an opportunity to relax myself. The reclining chair helps quite a lot. You can practice deep breathing or consciously relax your body, starting from the feet upward – any number of yogic techniques will work.*

Here are a few more for the dentist's chair, the doctor's office, and, the ultimate test of patience, when you're on hold for so long your ear hurts and you've listened to that automated voice tell you how important your call is 20 or 30 times already. What can I say? Isn't it the perfect time to practice yoga?

Time out for yoga

1. Practice the eye exercises – up, down, side to side, diagonal to diagonal.

2. Relax your jaws by rolling your tongue around the outside of your teeth (with your mouth closed) in a circle several times, then reverse the direction.

3. Practice listening to your breath, then deepen the exhalation.

4. Hear an affirmation or mantra on your breath.

5. Improve your digestion while you wait by inhaling, holding your breath, and pumping your navel toward your spine five times. Exhale, then inhale and repeat the pumping. (Do this one on a fairly empty stomach.)

6. Shrug your shoulders up when you inhale, and down when you exhale. Roll them around backwards a few times, and then forward a few.

7. Roll your wrists and ankles to get the kinks out.

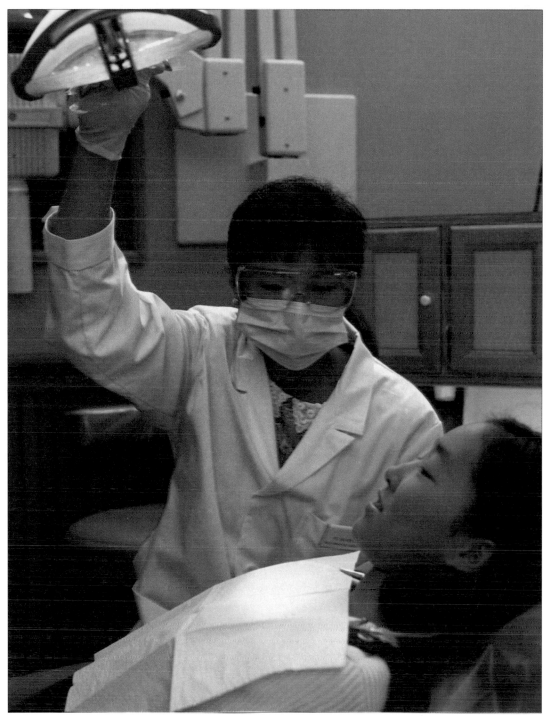

■ **Whether you're in the dentist's chair** *or some other stressful situation, practicing yoga techniques can help calm your nerves and release pain and tension from your body.*

AIRPLANE YOGA

More and more of us spend more and more time on airplanes and in airports. Cramped quarters, long lines, unending noise, flight delays, jet lag, time changes, the list goes on and on. A friend and yoga practitioner, Keith Newins, is a computer consultant who travels more than he's home. I asked him how he maintains a balanced sense of health and well-being while being subjected to countless circumstances beyond his control. His answer: Yoga and meditation – plus a little creativity. Here's how he does it:

I travel great distances every week, and mantras like Sa Ta Na Ma help me with standing in lines and waiting for services. I observe others struggling with difficult situations that I now am learning to deal with slowly – with patience, kindness, and consideration for the other side. Silently chanting while traveling in cars, taxis, trains, or planes has helped me have a greater sense of inner peace. I get a spiritual boost while enjoying inner peace.

I wear earplugs continuously in the terminal and on the plane to calm the noise of the plane engines and thoughtless chatter around me. The earplugs act as a biofeedback mechanism for breath awareness, since I can easily hear myself breathe. I try to maintain slow, deep breathing. I feel like I am slipping and gliding through the same systems that people all around me seem to strain and struggle with.

If I am on a flight longer than an hour, I might stand in the back and stretch for 30–45 minutes. This allows me to go through my whole frame, from the bottom of my feet to my head. I use the walls for support, and for isometric tensioning. In addition to stretching against the walls, I like to hang forward, either with my hands touching the floor, or with my hands clasped behind my back and stretched up. This one is great for the upper back, and brings energy to your head. Rolls work well, too – shoulder rolls, wrist and ankle rolls, waist rolls, neck rolls. Squatting relaxes the lower back. And, of course, I breathe deeply, coordinating the breath with the movements of the yoga I am doing.

I try to get an aisle seat for long flights where I will not be sleeping, so I can get up and go to the back of the plane while the beverage service is going on. The beverage cart blocks the passage back to my seat, and not too many other people are moving around then, so it is pretty private. Actually, I am not always the only person stretching. Rarely there is another person, and we sometimes chat.

If we let out these "secrets," I may be challenged to find space in the back of the plane to stretch. I will look forward to that day!

When you need energy

MANY PEOPLE THINK *of reaching for a cup of coffee when they need energy. But yogis and yoginis use their breath to energize them. It works, has no side effects or long-term health implications, and is not addictive – though you may want to do it often for the smooth "up" feeling that breathwork provides!*

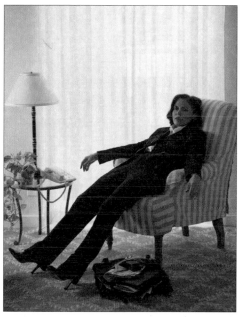

■ **Whenever you're feeling** *completely drained of energy, use yogic breathing techniques to revitalize you.*

Rapid belly breaths

Breath of Fire and skull-shining breath are enlivening because they rid the lungs of stale air and make way for fresh oxygen. Practice with a straight spine and concentration at the third-eye center ensures that energy is circulating through your entire body and into the brain centers. For quick energy, practice one or the other for 2 minutes.

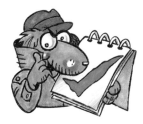

Driving long distances late at night, staring at the same black road with the yellow line snaking down the middle, can make you a little loony, not to mention sleepy! In cases like this, I like to do a light Breath of Fire, which, for me, doesn't interfere with driving at all.

If you find that you need more energy while driving, it's probably wise to pull over to the side. Get out of your car, stretch your arms up in a "V" shape, open your chest, and begin Breath of Fire for a couple of minutes. Then do a few stretches against the car.

Right nostril breathing

In the ancient science of yoga, the left side of the body is the moon side: The cooling, receptive, feminine energy. The right side is the sun side: The warming, projective, and masculine energy. This understanding applies right down to the details of the body, including the nostrils. According to yogic teachings, nostrils are not just passive portals for air to travel into and out of the body, but are gateways to the vast energy within.

The left nostril cools the air as it is drawn in. This relaxes you. The right nostril warms the air as it draws it in, which energizes you. Yoga teaches that you can control how you are feeling by breathing mostly through one nostril or the other.

Yogis say that at any given time you will breathe mostly through one nostril. The dominant nostril will switch gradually every 2½ hours. Your master gland, the pituitary, serves as the "thermostat" to control the switch in nostril dominance.

Find a place now where you can feel comfortable experimenting with single and alternate nostril breathing. You probably want a private place, where you won't have to explain what you are doing with your nose!

To energize yourself, sit with a straight spine. Make a "U" shape of the right hand and, using the side of your index finger, block off your left nostril. Inhale deeply through your right nostril, then exhale through the right only. Continue breathing through the right nostril only for a few minutes with your eyes closed.

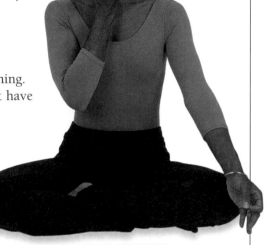

RIGHT NOSTRIL BREATHING

Cool yoga

OF COURSE, ALL YOGA IS COOL! *But I'm referring particularly to cooling off, cooling down, chilling out – all those similarly descriptive phrases that basically mean slowing down and relaxing.*

Left nostril breathing

When you need to relax, remember your "moon side," that receptive, relaxing energy that is contained within you. Activate it by breathing through the left nostril. Make the same "U" with your hand as you did previously, only this time block off the right nostril, and breathe deeply through the left nostril only. Continue for a few minutes with your eyes closed.

Practicing sitali breathing

Another pranayama, called *sitali*, is cooling and relaxing, helps to maintain alertness, and is great for cooling off anger. To practice sitali breathing, sit with a straight spine. Open your mouth and make a straw of your tongue by curling the sides up. Then inhale through the curled tongue, drawing cool air in through the mouth. Close your mouth and exhale through your nose.

DEFINITION

Sitali *is a cooling breath that relaxes the body while keeping the mind alert.*

If you cannot curl the sides of your tongue, just relax your tongue outside of your mouth, and imagine you are curling the sides. It will still work. You will feel the cool air come into your body. Exhale through your nose.

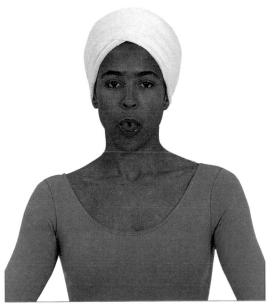

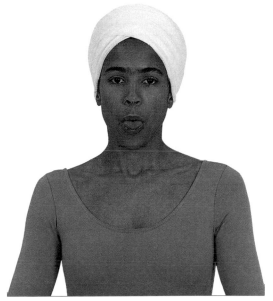

■ **For sitali breathing,** *the tongue is pushed a little way out of the mouth and the sides curled up.*

■ **If you can't curl your tongue**, *relax it outside of your mouth and imagine that you can.*

According to yogic science, sitali breath soothes and cools the spine in the area of the fourth, fifth, and sixth vertebrae. This in turn regulates the sexual and digestive energy. Often the tongue may taste bitter at first. This is a sign of detoxification. As you continue the practice, the taste of the tongue will become sweet.

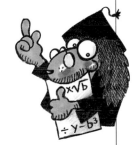

In a state of equipoise

EQUI IS LATIN FOR "EQUAL," *and poise means "composure" or "balance." To be in equipoise means to be with all things in equal balance, with equal composure. Alternate nostril breathing gives the gift of equipoise. It is one of the very first pranayama taught in yoga classes, and is an excellent preparation for meditation. Through this breathing exercise, you will harmonize the moon and sun energy within you, and create a powerful, peaceful inner balance.*

Alternate nostril breathing

This exercise, otherwise known as Analoma viloma or Nadi sodhana, may seem confusing, so remember that whichever side you just exhaled from is the same side you inhale on. Hold each inhalation briefly, then exhale on the opposite side.

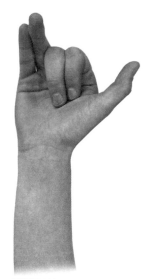

1. Sit with a straight spine. On your right hand, extend your thumb, ring finger, and little finger, then fold your index finger and your middle finger toward your palm. This is called Vishnu mudra. It may feel a little awkward to hold, but try your best. Your left hand is on your left knee in simple Gyan mudra.

2. Block off your right nostril with your thumb and inhale through your left nostril.

VISHNU MUDRA

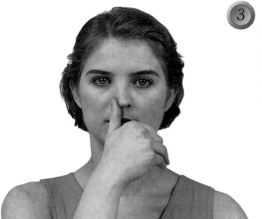

3. After you have inhaled, with your thumb still gently pressing against your right nostril, bring your ring finger on to your left nostril and hold it closed. Both nostrils are now closed. Hold them closed for a few seconds.

STEP 2

4. To exhale, lift your thumb and exhale through your right nostril. Empty your lungs, and begin again, inhaling through your right nostril.

5. Closing your right nostril, hold both nostrils closed for a few seconds.

6. Then exhale through your left nostril. Continue from step 2.

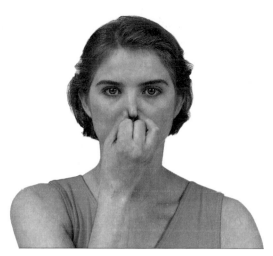

STEP 5

There is a tendency to bend the neck forward in this breathing exercise. Be aware of keeping your head and neck aligned with the spine and your breastbone lifted.

Getting the most out of walking

BESIDES SITTING OR LYING DOWN, *walking is the activity that we spend the most time doing. So in our quest for health and awareness, it makes sense that we would apply the principles of yoga to walking. There is something about swinging our bodies to the rhythm of an inner beat that gets stagnant parts of our mind moving. Coupling awareness of yoga, breathing, and meditation with your walking step raises the simple act of walking to a whole new energy level.*

Whether you are walking on a forest path, along a bike trail, in a shopping mall, or on a city street, you can breathe and meditate while you walk. A very simple walking meditation is to inhale and exhale in rhythm with your walking step. Here are a few simple suggestions for rhythmic walking.

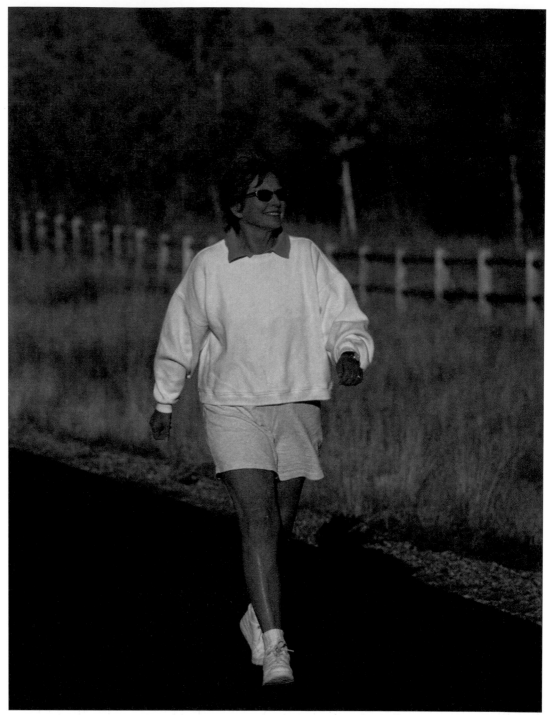

■ **No matter where you are**, *whether in the city or the great outdoors, get the most out of walking by inhaling and exhaling in rhythm with your step while you meditate or focus on your breath.*

1. Inhale to a four-step count, then exhale to a four-step count.

2. Inhale in four separate "sniffs" while taking four steps, then exhale in four separate "sniffs" as you take the next four steps.

3. Hear the sound of a mantra on each step. Sa Ta Na Ma works well for the four-step breath.

4. Hear the sound of one extended mantra for every four steps. Try "Ommmmmmm," coordinating the mantra, the four steps, and the inhalation. Then do the same on the exhalation.

5. Chant a mantra out loud or softly under your breath.

6. Create your own rhythmic patterns of breathing and walking.

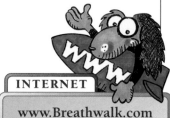

INTERNET

www.Breathwalk.com

This web site will provide you with more information about the Breathwalk program. Instructor training programs are also offered.

The book and program called Breathwalk by Yogi Bhajan and Gurucharan Singh Khalsa combines our two most simple and yet powerful actions — breathing and walking — in a meditative system that creates health on all levels. Breathwalking has been taught for many years to thousands who attend the Anthony Robbins Life Mastery University in Hawaii.

A simple summary

✔ Yoga goes with you wherever you go, because all it requires is you and your willingness to practice.

✔ Pay attention to those moments when you are just waiting around, and use them for conscious breathing, stretching, relaxing, and centering.

✔ You can use the yogic technique of alternate nostril breathing to relax, energize, and bring your mind to equipoise.

✔ By being creative, you can find simple opportunities to relax and replenish your energy while traveling, walking, or just sitting.

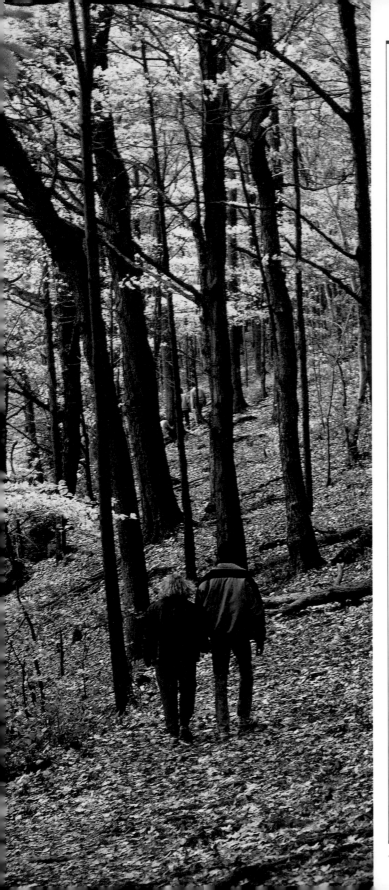

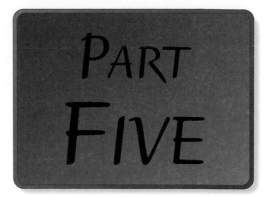

PART
FIVE

YOGA HELPS MAKE SENSE OF THE WORLD AROUND US

THE FUTURE OF YOGA

Y OGA MAY BE ANCIENT, but it is the perfect remedy for what ails our modern world. With work often being synonymous with stress, it is only natural that yoga has found its way into the corporate world. Athletes have discovered 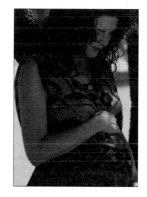 a powerful helper in yoga, too. The medical community is beginning to acknowledge the benefits of yoga. Complementary or alternative medicine is the preferred healing modality of more people than ever before.

Yoga is one of the keys to peace in our world. Peace comes piece by piece, and person by person. Through yoga, you can experience the depths of your heart and the height of your *awareness*. Then *peace* and *clarity* will naturally extend from you to everyone whose life you touch.

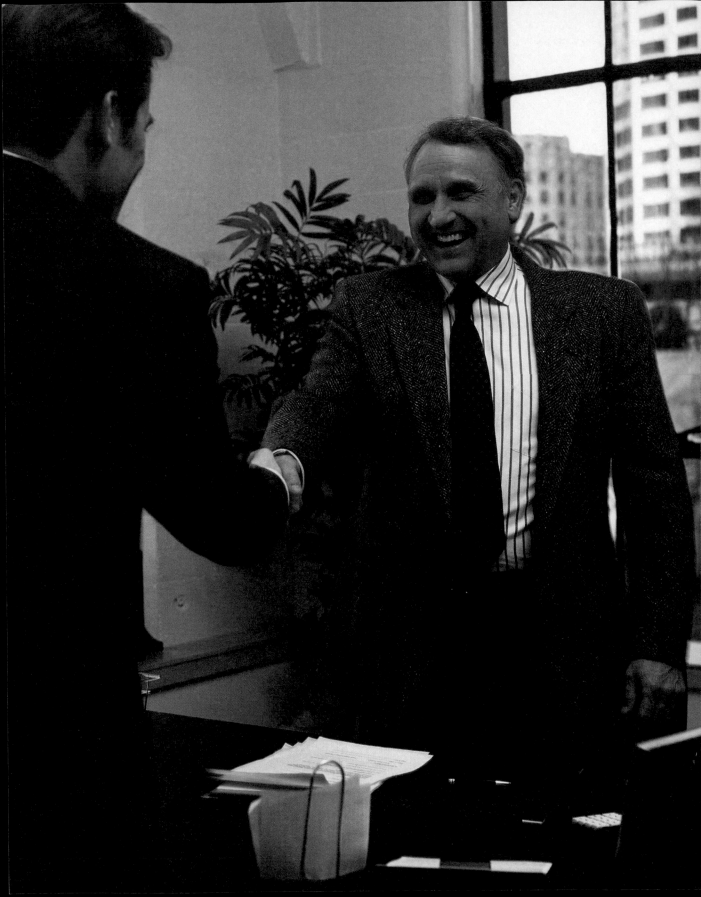

Chapter 18

Yoga at Work and Play

IN THE PAST FEW DECADES, yoga has been steadily making headway into the corporate world, with more companies offering lunch-time yoga classes. Yoga also provides the basis of good alignment, improved flexibility, and mental focus that is essential for athletes. In this chapter we will explore some simple techniques for keeping your body aligned and your mind clear – no matter what kind of work you do.

In this chapter...

✓ Addressing stress in the workplace

✓ Yoga is good business

✓ Yoga for your personal best

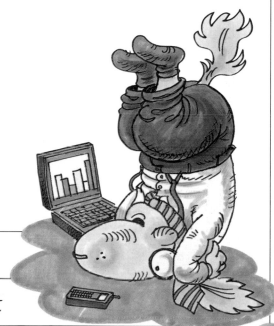

YOGA WILL GIVE YOU A MORE POSITIVE ATTITUDE TOWARD LIFE AND WORK

Addressing stress in the workplace

OFFICE FATIGUE CAN HAPPEN *to anyone.*
All day long I write about the wonders of yoga, relaxation,
alignment, breathing, and well-being, but as the day
goes on, my body begins to feel quite the opposite.
Work takes over, and the body doesn't seem to exist.

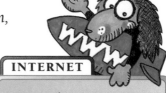

INTERNET

www.stressaway.com

Check out this web site for
software you can purchase to
exercise with. You will
probably relate to the title of
one of their books, Help!
My Computer is Killing
Me! *by Dr. Sheik N. Imrhan,*
a specialist in ergonomics.

I feel crunched and stiff, my breathing is shallow and unconscious. My eyes sting from staring at a computer screen for hours. Then, all of a sudden, the proverbial light goes on overhead. "Okay now," I tell myself. "You know what to do. Take a deep breath. Relax the shoulders down, lift the breastbone upward, keep the neck straight. Blink and look around. Get up and stretch, drink some water, then put on some uplifting music. Ahh! Much better. I'm human again!"

The good news is that the days of sitting hunched over your desk for hours, endless hours, at a time are on their way out. Ergonomically designed workspaces are becoming commonplace in the conscious workplace, and so is yoga. You can program your computer to tell you when to get up and take a stretch and a breath. You can even log on to a web site or two that will take you through a few stretches. Liberation has arrived for those of us who are "slaves to the desk."

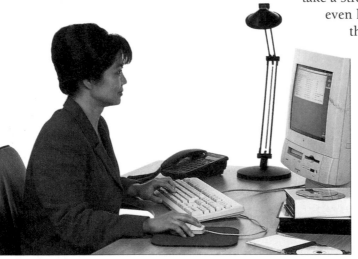

■ **If you have** *a well-designed*
workspace and take frequent
yoga breaks, you will not only
feel better physically but you will
also be more productive.

Desktop yoga

More corporations are offering yoga to their employees, and that trend will continue to grow. If lunchtime yoga is not on your company's menu, don't worry. It's pretty easy for yoga to come to you. Take a yoga break instead of a coffee break!

Yoga works to alleviate the number one work-related health problem, namely – you guessed it – stress. Through yoga, you'll be more productive as you increase blood flow to your brain, which makes it easier to concentrate and think clearly. Here are some very simple exercises you can do at your desk throughout the day.

a   Lower your head forward toward your chest. Hold for a few moments while you relax and stretch the muscles of the back of your neck. Let your shoulders drop. Keep your eyes closed. Massage the back of your neck and shoulders for a minute.

b   Slowly roll your neck in one direction, then the other. Coordinate your breathing with the movement.

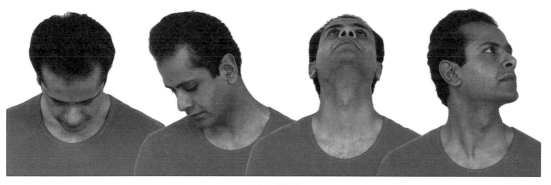

EXERCISE B

c   Clasp your hands in front of you, then inhale and stretch the arms upward. Feel the stretch in the mid- and upper back. Exhale and stand up. Repeat a few times.

d   Do some of the "waiting around" yoga exercises in Chapter 17.

Drinking water, as you know, balances your mind and emotions as it hydrates your body. Drinking water is a good excuse for getting away from your desk, too.

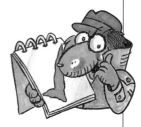

Pointers for a healthy work day

- Get up from your desk and move around every half hour.
- Once a day, move at least 8 ft (2.4 m) away from the "waves" of the computer screen and refresh yourself with a juicy piece of fruit.
- Go to the restroom and put a cool, wet paper towel over your eyes and another on the back of your neck, and rinse your hands and wrists with cool water.
- Take your eyes off the screen periodically and look into the distance. Move your eyes left and right, up and down.
- As much as possible, keep aware of your posture while sitting at your desk.
- Take deep breaths as often as you remember to.
- Do not eat lunch at your desk. During your lunch break, find some physical activity to do away from your desk.
- Check your computer monitor level. Can you see it without tipping your chin either upward or downward? Check its placement for distance also. Your screen should be comfortable to look at – neither too far away, nor too close.

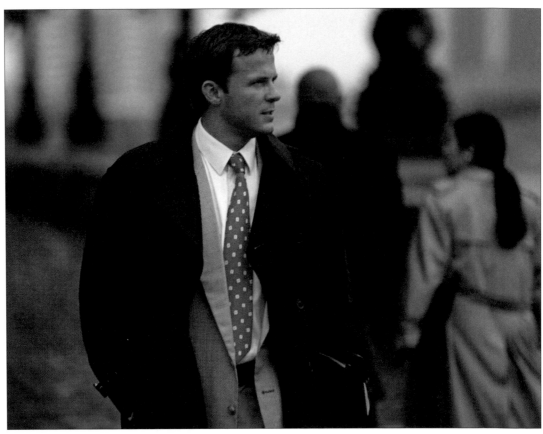

■ **Getting away from the workplace** *during your lunch break will boost your energy levels. Taking some form of physical exercise, preferably outdoors, is even more beneficial.*

Dealing with repetitive stress

Repetitive stress refers to the stress that is placed on localized areas of the body from repetitive movements over a period of time. With the advent of the computer, the wrist has become the most common target of repetitive stress injury.

Common among computer users is Carpal Tunnel Syndrome, which can be so painful that the afflicted hand cannot be used. Carpal Tunnel Syndrome and other repetitive stress disorders are preventable. Many of these disorders can be avoided by staying alert to what the body needs in order to stay healthy.

Carpal Tunnel Syndrome is a potentially debilitating nerve disorder of the hand that is usually caused by repetitive motion. It is triggered by pressure on the median nerve, which controls sensations in the thumb and index and middle fingers.

Trivia...

Yoga Therapy News on www.yogasite.com reports a recent study at the University of Pennsylvania Medical School that showed that a simple yoga program worked better than the conventional treatment of wearing wrist splints to reduce pain and improve the hand strength of those with Carpal Tunnel Syndrome. After 8 weeks, the yoga group had significantly less pain and greater hand strength. The control group experienced no significant reduction in either areas.

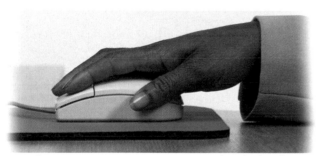

■ **When using a computer mouse**, *relax the hand, keep the wrist straight, and use a light touch.*

Carpal Tunnel Syndrome may begin with pain and burning in the wrist or numbness in the fingers. Other repetitive stress symptoms show up in the elbow, shoulder, neck, and the upper or lower back. It is important to act immediately by changing what you can in your work environment and by seeing a health care professional if you are experiencing problems.

If you work with a computer for a good portion of the day, make sure you have a good mouse pad. I highly recommend one that the Fellowes Corporation makes called the Easy Glide Wrist Rest/Mouse pad. It is designed with a wrist pad that moves in every direction, so when you move your mouse, the action stems from your arm instead of your wrist.

Yoga for your wrist

Here are some of the exercises that were part of the study done by the University of Pennsylvania Medical School.

The following exercises are for strengthening the wrist and releasing tension, but a wrist that is hurting should be given rest and gentle massage.

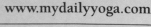

INTERNET

www.mydailyyoga.com

This is the best desktop yoga web site I have found. Using clear animation that's easy to follow, Ellen Serber demonstrates over a dozen yoga exercises that anyone can do while sitting or standing at a desk. Bookmark this one!

a Sit upright on a chair. Press your hands into the chair on either side of you. Press your shoulder blades in toward the back while moving the shoulders back and downward.

b Bring your hands into Prayer pose. Press your palms and fingers together, and stretch and bend your fingers.

c Stand up and find an empty wall. Your feet are about hip-width apart and about 3 ft (1 m) away from the wall, so that your hands will reach the wall when you bend at the waist. Inhale and stretch upward, then exhale and bend so that your palms are completely on the wall, and your upper body is parallel to the floor. Stay there for a minute and breathe deeply.

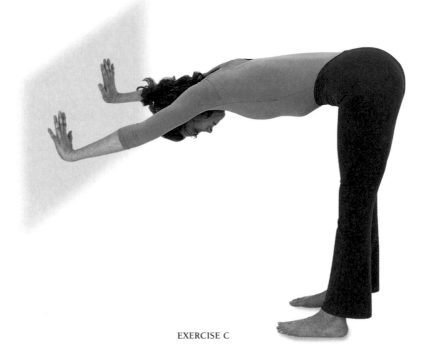

EXERCISE C

Yoga is good business

HAVE YOU EVER NOTICED how creativity flows when you have a chance to slow down and relax? As one experienced meditator, Joanne Steele, has expressed it, "Problems that were waiting, unresolved, seem to fall so beautifully into place as I meditate."

INTERNET

www.jps.net/dkgamow

More fascinating statistics can be found on David and Karen Gamow's web site. They run stress reduction and meditation seminars in the workplace for clients such as NASA and the San Francisco Police Academy.

When stress and pain are gone, productivity and creativity return. This is the logic of bringing yoga and meditation into the workplace. In short, what is good for the employees is good for the employer. Stress management programs that include yoga and meditation are popping up all over the corporate world, and no wonder. Just look at some of these stress statistics:

- $200 billion a year is lost to industry from stress-related illness.
- 75–90 percent of employee visits to hospitals are for ailments linked to stress.
- Chronic pain, hypertension, and headache alone – all stress-related ailments – account for 54 percent of all job absences.
- 30 percent of adults report high job stress nearly every day.

A REAL-LIFE STORY OF CORPORATE YOGA

Göran Boll is a Kundalini yoga teacher in Sweden. Since 1996 he has taught yoga in the workplace to more than 100 of Sweden's largest corporations and government agencies. It all started with the Swedish airline SAS, which hoped that yoga could alleviate stress among their flying personnel. The telephone company, two of the country's largest banks, Ericsson, Hewlett Packard and other computer companies, the Red Cross Hospital, and The Royal Swedish Parliament then followed. Boll is also involved in several major research projects on Kundalini yoga in Sweden.

Through his organization Lifeforce (www.lifeforce.nu), Boll aspired to bring yoga's benefits to that world. In his words:

I see the results every day – calm and serene faces, comments on how yoga practice makes them stronger, happier, and better equipped to handle a tough day at work. I am deeply grateful to be able to share this wonderful gift with so many people.

Yoga for your personal best

IT IS SAID THAT COMPETITION brings out the best in an athlete – and it brings out the stress, too. Yoga, as we know, is the great stress-reliever. For this one worthwhile reason, yoga would be valuable to athletes. But stress relief is only the starting point of yoga. There is so much more.

Yoga and meditation help the athlete "stretch" mentally, too. The more athletes are in touch with their inner strength and ability to be aware in the present moment, the more capable they are of reaching their personal best.

I am reminded of the well-known book by Phil Jackson, *Sacred Hoops*, in which Jackson reveals how he directs his world champions Chicago Bulls to be aggressive without anger and stay focused in the moment, based on the practice of Zen meditation.

Yoga, runners, and cyclists

You don't have to be a professional athlete to appreciate running and cycling. Being outdoors, hopefully in fresh air, or on an asphalt bike trail or a city street, you feel the freedom of the body's movement, almost as if you were in flight. But how you feel afterward, or a few years later, may depend on how consciously you maintained the health of your body before and after your "flight." Because yoga focuses on alignment, breath, and relaxation, it is the perfect complement to running and cycling. *Power Yoga* author Beryl Bender Birch teaches athletes Ashtanga yoga, which she says therapeutically aligns the body and protects and rehabilitates it from injury.

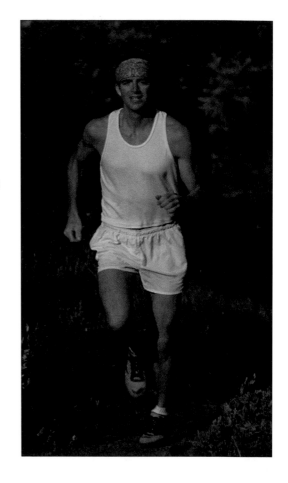

■ **One of the benefits of yoga** *is that it protects the body. If you enjoy vigorous physical activity, such as running, a regime of yoga will reduce the possibility of injury.*

A RUNNER'S UNEXPECTED BONUS

Buck Hales is a dedicated runner who discovered yoga through an injury. Now, when he's not running or teaching yoga, he's writing articles to help other runners on the web site www.yogacircle.com.

I had injured my iliopsoas muscle – a deep injury where the psoas inserts through the pelvis. [The psoas muscles attach to the lower spinal column and control certain movements of the thigh.] *I damaged it running full speed down a very steep hill. My track coach gave me some stretches to strengthen the abdominal muscles, but try as I might I was unable to access the tightness. I ran three marathons with this injury, and it kept getting worse. After a while any running aggravated it.*

My wife and I enrolled in a yoga class at the local community center. I didn't really know what to expect, but imagined yoga was a passive, meditative practice, good for relieving stress, with some modest stretches. My first impression of Hatha yoga was that it was hard! I had no idea just how tight I was. I couldn't sit comfortably with my back straight and my legs forward. Standing with legs straight, bent over at the waist and touching my hands to the floor? Not a chance. The tightness in my legs stopped me well short of the floor.

Within a few weeks, though, I noticed that I was already more limber. We learned a few positions that specifically targeted the tightness in my hip. I worked on my hips, and my sore iliopsoas improved with time. I avoided running down hills, and began to incorporate yoga into my pre- and post-run stretching routines.

The benefit of yoga to my running is inarguable. The benefit of yoga to my life is the unexpected bonus. Yoga is about balance. When I came to yoga, I just wanted to learn some good stretches. Not only did I learn those stretches, I have also experienced a tremendous period of personal, emotional, and spiritual growth. I have a way to seek balance in my busy life. The yoga way.

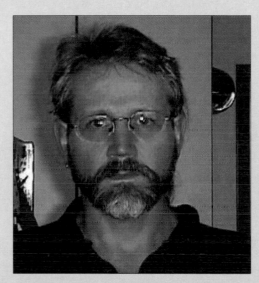

BUCK HALES

YOGA AND THE OLYMPICS

In 1974, a fellow Kundalini yoga teacher, Guruka Singh Khalsa, became the official yoga coach for the Ohio State University synchronized swim team. Under the farsighted coaching program of Mary Jo Ruggieri, which had at its core yoga, bodywork, healthy diet, and team counseling, the team practiced Kundalini yoga from 1974 to 1995. The team became the NCAA Collegiate National Champs for 17 years, won ten consecutive championships, and sent swimmers to the Pan Am Games and the Olympics in 1984, 1988, and 1992. In addition to the 44 young women in the A and B teams, Guruka Singh also worked with all the Olympic athletes. These elite athletes went on to be individual Olympic winners, two in 1988 (Silver), and one in 1992 (Gold). Mary Jo herself became known internationally as a world-class coach. This is her story:

Kundalini yoga saved my life as a coach. I would not have coached without it. The mainstream stretching techniques, which most sports coaches work with, are not going to give the edge in high-pressure competition. Nor do they affect the whole person. Kundalini yoga uses specific exercise sets that address very real needs. For example, the girls practiced yoga sets for the glandular system because often their hormones were off balance, and their adrenals were exhausted. They did breath of fire every day, which helped tremendously to expand their lung capacity for swimming. Anorexia and bulimia were fairly common among the girls, so Guruka Singh would give them yoga specifically for digestion and mental balance.

The pressure these young people faced was phenomenal. Yoga, meditation, and chanting drew them into their center and gave them focus in the face of challenge.

Sports are so physical, and yoga gave the girls the ability to integrate the physical with the mental and spiritual. People don't realize how disconnected these kids are with all the pressure they face, and the rigorous discipline they go through: 6 hours a day in the pool, ballet and weight lifting, high academic standards, no partying. Their lives belong to swimming.

In high-intensity sports, there is often a disconnection between what I think of as the internal "energy circuits." It's like this: You can build a great house. It looks good, but if the energy circuit breakers are not working, your house will not be able to function. Yoga integrates the neuromuscular energy system, which helped in every aspect of the team's performance.

When push came to shove, I could see it in their performance. There was something in their consciousness that gave them the edge. That something was yoga.

One of the most special gifts that yoga gave year after year was the team spirit. Before the girls went out, they always huddled in a circle with their arms around each other and chanted the traditional Kundalini yoga song: "May the long-time sun shine upon you, all love surround you, and the pure light within you guide your way on." They pulled their energy into the circle in this way for 20-something years. Last year I went to the 20-year OSU synchronized swimming reunion. Alumni and friends made a circle all the way around the pool, arms around each other, and chanted their song. With tears in their eyes, their hearts were united in a spirit that included, yet went beyond, those 20 years of teamwork.

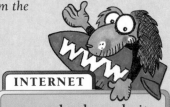

INTERNET

www.columbuspolarity .com

Mary Jo Ruggieri retired from coaching in 1995 and opened a polarity therapy center in Columbus. You can find information at this web site about how she practices Kundalini yoga and integrates it with her work.

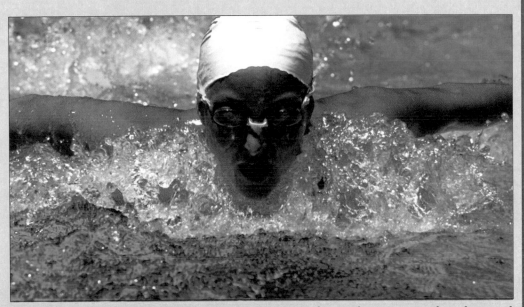

■ **The intensive training** that Ohio State University's synchronized swim team undertook ensured their physical fitness, but it was yoga that gave them the mental strength and emotional stability to win.

Golfer's yoga

Many PGA and LPGA professionals utilize yoga to sharpen their game. In the words of one such pro, Gary McCord, "Preparing for golf, from the viewpoint of a professional, is an exhaustive task. You have to tighten your swing, practice your short game, get in the right frame of mind, and get physically fit. Or you can practice yoga and accomplish all of the above."

INTERNET

www.yogaforgolfers .com

This is Katherine Roberts's web site, where she offers great yoga tips for golfers.

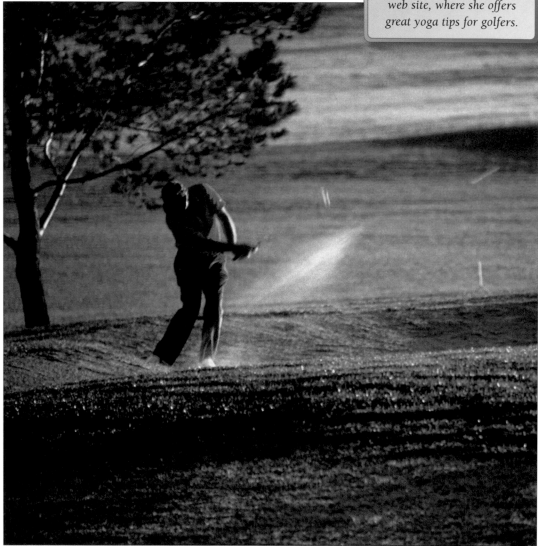

■ **Professional golfers have also turned to yoga**, *recognizing how beneficial it can be to their game. Yoga helps improve general fitness and flexibility, and helps achieve the right frame of mind for competition.*

Katherine Roberts is a nationally recognized speaker and writer on yoga and golf fitness, and the creator of the video "Yoga for Golfers . . . Because Your Body Doesn't Get a Mulligan." She says that once you make the commitment to enhance your golf game through yoga, you will see tremendous benefits in distance, focus, recovery time, and overall wellness.

A simple summary

✔ Most techniques for stress management that are used in the corporate world are based on the mind/body/spirit connection that is at the core of yoga.

✔ Yoga works to alleviate the number one work-related health problem: stress. By practicing yoga, you'll be more productive as you increase blood flow to the brain, which makes it easier to concentrate and think clearly.

✔ Repetitive stress injuries such as Carpal Tunnel Syndrome can be avoided by staying alert to what the body needs in order to stay healthy.

✔ When stress and pain are gone, productivity and creativity return. This is the logic of bringing yoga and meditation into the workplace, which many employers are doing by offering classes at lunchtime or after work.

✔ Competition brings out the best in the athlete, and it brings out the stress, too. Yoga is the great stress-reliever. But with yoga, stress-relief is only the starting point.

✔ Yoga and meditation help the athlete "stretch" mentally, too. The more you are in touch with your inner strength and your ability to be aware in the present moment, the more capable you are of reaching your personal best.

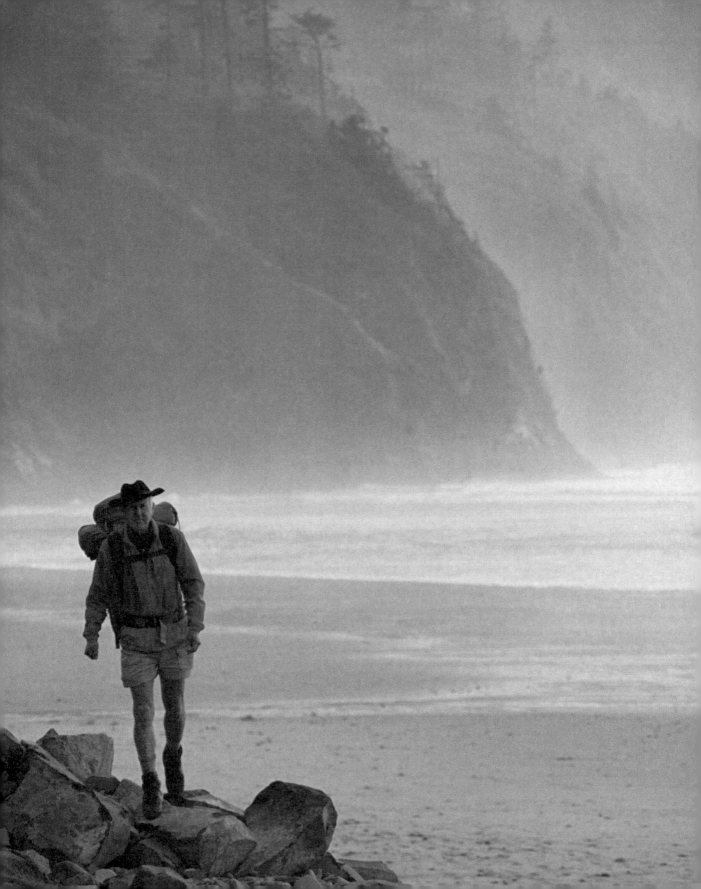

Chapter 19

Yoga, Meditation, and Medicine

HEALTH IS ON EVERYONE'S MIND these days. Healthcare issues concern individuals and families, whether it's health insurance, jobs with medical benefits, or simply staying healthy. My motto is to live to your best and prepare for the worst. Remember that you and the universe form a partnership, and focus on the positive steps you can take for your well-being. Yoga, meditation, and a holistic lifestyle will help take you there.

In this chapter...

✓ Patient, heal thyself!

✓ Yoga as therapy

✓ Healing in the "sacred space"

✓ Applying the medicine of meditation

✓ Projecting into the future of medicine

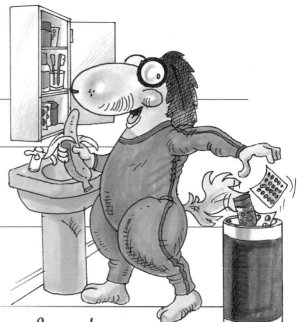

A HOLISTIC LIFESTYLE COMBINED WITH YOGA AND MEDITATION WILL HELP KEEP YOU FIT AND HEALTHY

Patient, heal thyself!

THOMAS EDISON ONCE SAID, *"The doctor of the future will give no medicine, but will interest his patients in the care of the human frame, in diet, and in the cause and prevention of disease." In many ways, we are still waiting for that future, but at the same time, we are creating it ourselves. One way you are creating your own healthy future is by reading this book and practicing the techniques you find here.*

The two systems of health care that are available today are conventional Western medicine and alternative medicine, which is the name given to holistic health care. Please keep in mind that the title "alternative medicine" was coined in response to the powerful medical establishment. In China, for example, where acupuncture, herbs, and Tai Chi are the norm, these practices are not called "alternative." They are respected practices and remedies that have been keeping people healthy for thousands of years.

The World Health Organization reports that many alternative, or complementary, treatments are the traditional medicine upon which two-thirds of the world relies as the main source of health care.

■ **Using herbs and spices** *to make medicines in China is a well-respected practice that goes back thousands of years.*

Rescue or prevention?

Conventional medicine is superb when it comes to surgery, emergency, and trauma. But, time and time again, alternative medicine has proven to be a more effective treatment over the long term, without disturbing side effects, and at a much lower cost. Increasingly, it is being found that chronic degenerative diseases such as cancer, heart disease, and arthritis, as well as common ailments like asthma, headaches, colds, and digestive disorders, can many times be cured or controlled with alternative medicine.

The more the established medical community and the alternative healthcare community can unite and respect each other, and the more we take responsibility for our own health by choosing healthy lifestyles, the sooner we will relieve ourselves of high-cost health care and pharmaceutical dependency, and experience a life of health and well-being.

Trivia...

According to a report from the American Association of Naturopathic Physicians, "We wait for illness to develop and then spend huge sums on heroic measures, even then ignoring the underlying lifestyle-related causes. This is the equivalent of waiting for a leaky roof to destroy the infrastructure of a house and then repairing the damage without fixing the leak."

There is no single approach that works for all people, or for all conditions. Using the best of both Eastern and Western medicine keeps all of our options open.

Many people feel that health care will not become prevention-oriented as long as physicians earn their living and gain renown primarily by delivering rescue medicine (interventions that repair immediate health crises or simply treat symptoms), since this is the way they can benefit most.

COST MANAGEMENT?

From Dr. Dean Ornish's Program for Reversing Heart Disease come these sobering facts: If a doctor performs bypass surgery on a patient, the insurance company will pay at least $30,000; for a balloon angioplasty, at least $7,500. If a doctor spends the same amount of time teaching a heart patient about nutrition and stress management techniques, the insurance company will pay no more than $150. And if the doctor spends the same amount of time teaching a well person how to stay healthy, they will not pay at all.

Drug drag

Doctors and patients alike are perplexed by a failure of drug-based therapies to bring relief. Patients often become trapped in a cycle of dependency on doctors to monitor and constantly adjust their medications rather than becoming empowered to change their lifestyle in ways that might help them regain health.

Of course, drugs, whether they be over-the-counter or prescription, have their place, but all too often there are alternatives that patients don't even know about. Often times, we would do well to "just say no to drugs" and say "yes" to the exploration of safe and effective alternatives.

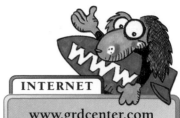

INTERNET

www.grdcenter.com

The GRD Center for Medicine and Humanology is a non-profit foundation that provides health education using yogic methods to people with chronic or life-threatening illness, such as HIV, cancer, and chronic pain.

TAKING DRUG ALTERNATIVES

In Burton Goldberg's excellent book *Alternative Medicine: The Definitive Guide*, 350 leading physicians address the treatment of over 200 health problems with alternative medicine. One physician, John R. Lee, M.D., had this to say about drugs:

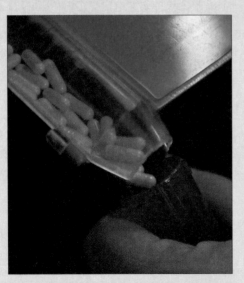

PRESCRIPTION DRUGS

Most over-the-counter, and almost all prescribed drug treatments, merely mask symptoms or control health problems, or in some way alter the way organs or systems . . . work. Drugs almost never deal with the reasons why these problems exist, while they frequently create new health problems as side effects . . . . [People] are seeking answers that address the root causes of their health problems, and aid in restoring normal, healthy body function. This is not to say that treatment of the symptoms of a condition is wrong. What would be wrong would be to think that by eliminating the symptom we have dealt with the problem itself.

Yoga as therapy

SOME PROGRESSIVE DOCTORS RECOMMEND *yoga to their patients, especially when their complaints have to do with nervous tension, weight gain, high blood pressure, or heart problems. When a doctor and patient catch and turn around a potentially dangerous illness through healthy life choices such as yoga, everyone benefits. The patient benefits, of course. But in addition, the doctor earns the patient's trust by honoring him or her with options that are holistic, rather than routinely prescribing drugs that often have undesirable side effects. Ultimately, the entire healthcare system of a country will benefit from preventive healthcare choices.*

Maintaining internal balance, throwing off stress, and boosting the body's self-healing powers are crucial to long-term health and well-being. This is what yoga does best. The belief that the body has a natural tendency toward homeostasis is at the heart of traditional health systems such as naturopathy, Chinese medicine, and Ayurvedic medicine, which includes yoga and meditation.

> **DEFINITION**
>
> Homeostasis *is the body's natural state of balance, in which all systems function smoothly.*

■ **Instead of prescribing drugs**, *an enlightened doctor may recommend yoga and a change in lifestyle to patients with high blood pressure.*

I find yoga to be one of the best healers I know. Yes, you have to apply yourself — you can't just take a pill. But once you get over the hump of procrastination and begin classes or practice on your own at home or with your partner, I think you will find yoga to be your best friend and therapist.

Integrative Yoga Therapy

Yoga can help bring the body into homeostasis and then help maintain it, especially for those who have physical challenges. Yoga therapy has spread across the land as a means of custom-tailoring yoga to individual needs through one-on-one sessions.

INTERNET

www.iytyogatherapy .com

Integrative Yoga Therapy offers training programs that include mind-body health sciences, as well as in-depth understanding of yoga postures. For more information, see their web site.

Integrative Yoga Therapy (IYT), founded by Joseph Le Page, M.A., is one of the most well-established yoga therapy programs today. The therapist designs a program of yoga practice to meet the needs and goals of the student, selecting, adapting, and modifying the practices of yoga appropriately for the individual, with respect to age, culture, religion, and specific physical challenges, in order to facilitate optimum health and healing. The therapist serves as a guide in the journey of self-healing and self-discovery, and some trained IYT instructors hold advanced degrees in physical therapy, psychology, or health education as well.

Trivia...

There is a new attitude among senior citizens these days; instead of degenerating as they age, many are regenerating themselves through yoga. Take a look at The New Yoga for People Over 50 *by Suza Francina, as well as books on gentle yoga, restorative yoga, and chair yoga.*

Phoenix Rising yoga therapy

Developed by Michael Lee in 1984, Phoenix Rising yoga is a combination of classical yoga poses (from the Kripalu style) and mind–body psychology. It incorporates 16 basic poses, done with a therapist who gently holds the student until emotional tension surfaces and is released. In a Phoenix Rising yoga session, feelings may arise, which are a natural part of the opening-up process of yoga. The feelings can range from sad to joyful and everything in between. Through the yoga poses, guided breathwork, and nondirective dialogue, Phoenix Rising helps to connect the physical and emotional parts of ourselves.

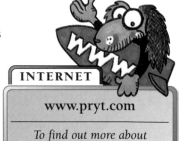

INTERNET

www.pryt.com

To find out more about teacher training and therapists in your area, go to Phoenix Rising yoga therapy's web site.

Healing in the "sacred space"

MIRACULOUS RECOVERIES. *We read about them, we may even know someone who is a walking miracle. Do they happen only by the grace of God? Do we have any part in them? These are tough questions that can digress into philosophical or intellectual discussions – but that is not our purpose in this section. Instead let us turn to our own consciousness for answers. Time for an experience.*

The yogic approach to healing

In the yogic approach to healing called *Sat Nam Rasayan*, the healer opens to a sensitive process of awareness, creating a space in which healing can occur naturally.

INTERNET

www.gurudevsnr.com

It is always best to have a trained Sat Nam Rasayan teacher guide you in person. At this web site, you will find locations of teachers and training sessions.

> **DEFINITION**
>
> Sat Nam Rasayan, *from Sanskrit, literally means "universal remedy of manifested truth."*

Rather than a technique, Sat Nam Rasayan is based on learning how to bring oneself into a state of heightened awareness and neutrality while holding an intention to heal. The healing branch of Kundalini yoga, this system was passed in secrecy through the centuries until taught by Yogi Bhajan to his student Guru Dev Singh. A systematic approach to the healing "sacred space" was then created by Guru Dev, a method that anyone can practice individually or in study groups.

Using this approach, time and space have no relevance. Whether it is called the "sacred space" or the "nonlocal mind" (coined by Dr. Larry Dossey, MD, in his book *Reinventing Medicine*), all healing can happen in this state of consciousness: Healing of yourself, someone you are with, someone at a distance, a particular situation that needs healing, and even the planet.

Borrowing from Subagh Singh Khalsa's exquisite book *Anatomy of Healing*, I will accompany you in touching the essence of this treasured healing system.

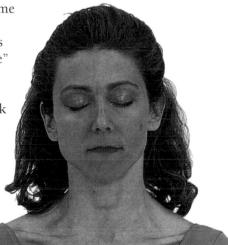

■ **To enter** *a state of heightened awareness in preparation for yogic healing, begin to feel all the various sensations that arise, such as the feel of your breath entering and exiting.*

THINGS TO KNOW ABOUT YOGIC HEALING

(a) Yogic healing, or Sat Nam Rasayan, is very simple. It is a specific and clearly defined state of awareness that happens in your neutral, meditative mind.

(b) All spiritual traditions teach how to reach sacred states. In order to learn Sat Nam Rasayan, all you need to do is to recognize when you are in this particular sacred space, and then become able to hold yourself stable in it.

(c) In Sat Nam Rasayan, you will find yourself enjoying deeper, more blissful meditations, feeling more loving, more aware, and more sensitive in all aspects of your life, and more able to deal with whatever challenge you face. But all of these are side effects and not Sat Nam Rasayan's primary purpose. Its purpose is to heal.

(d) If you decide to study Sat Nam Rasayan further than these few instructions, you will find that there is not as much to learn as there is to practice.

Practicing yogic healing

(1) Sit with a straight spine, and close your eyes. Tune in with the Kundalini yoga mantra from Chapter 11, Ong Namo, Guru Dev Namo.

(2) Gradually become aware of whatever sensations you are experiencing in your body at this moment. Feel the obvious sensations of your breath, the air on your skin. Also feel the more subtle, quiet sensations between the more obvious ones. Take your time and allow still more sensations into your awareness.

(3) Begin to include everything that appears in your awareness but concentrate on none of it. Take your time with this. Not concentrating on any one sensation will gradually lead you to an equal awareness of all sensations.

(4) Select from among the sensations a single one, the one that is most uncomfortable. Don't concentrate on this one sensation but remain aware of it along with everything else. Recognize the resistance that you may have to this sensation and allow the sensations of that resistance also to be there without any concentration. Continue this way until the discomfort is resolved.

(5) If you would like to go further, the next part involves a partner. It is called "healing with your presence." Have someone lie down beside you. First practice the first four instructions listed here. Then touch your partner lightly on the arm. Don't worry about technique. The simpler the better. Notice as you touch your partner that you feel new sensations, ones that arise in relation to him or her, but do not focus on these either. Just allow them. Resist your temptation to try to understand your partner.

This is the point at which practitioners, especially those with some healing experience, can fall into the trap of trying to "feel" or heal the other person. You are not doing any of that here because those ideas create a belief in separation between you and the other person. They create a "point of view."

(6) Allow all the new sensations, along with all the sensations that have already appeared, and equalize again to stabilize yourself in the sensitive space.

Working with the sensitive space is very subtle, and gets even more so with a partner. Learn it slowly, practicing over time. I have found it invaluable in opening me to an inner place of neutrality, where I am not holding a point of view.

(7) This process of entering the sensitive space is the beginning of healing with your presence. With practice, the internal state that you enter is a sacred space of unconditional love. And it is unconditional love that heals.

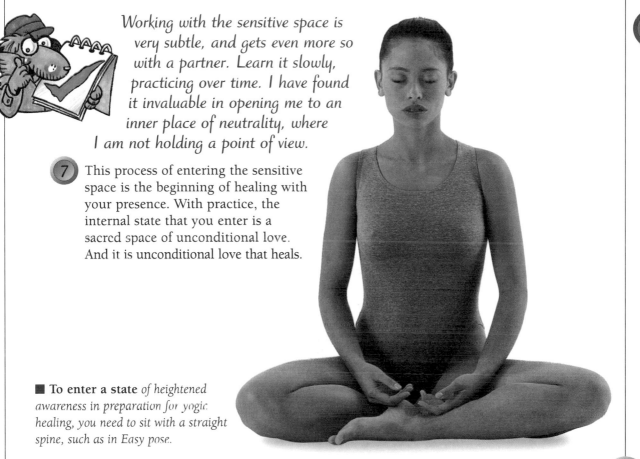

■ **To enter a state** *of heightened awareness in preparation for yogic healing, you need to sit with a straight spine, such as in Easy pose.*

311

Applying the medicine of meditation

WHEN WE THINK OF MEDICINE, what comes to mind? A pill or liquid that we ingest in the hope that it will cure us? Medicine has other meanings, too. In the old tribal traditions, the Medicine Man is the revered healer, and the shaman the transformational force of the community. Meditation as medicine is aligned with the image of this transformative power – the Medicine Man of earthly, yet mystical, might.

Dr. Dharma Singh Khalsa, MD, author of *Brain Longevity* and *The Pain Cure*, continues his groundbreaking work in his book *Meditation as Medicine*. This book is filled with documented medical success stories of patients who are using meditations that go beyond what he terms "passive" meditations into the realm of Medical Meditations. Medical Meditations utilize breath, posture and movement, mental focus, and mantras.

Sa Ta Na Ma, as you may remember from Chapter 14, is practiced by applying pressure to each consecutive finger. Dr. Dharma says that if you watch a PET scan of someone moving their fingers into different positions, you will see many areas of their brain light up. This demonstrates that various finger movements have a direct impact upon brain function.

When you chant Sa Ta Na Ma, the upper palate is struck and vibrational energy is relayed to the hypothalamus. The effect of the movement of the tongue, coupled with the sound waves resonating in the brain, stimulates the hypothalamus to secrete all of the necessary hormones, neurotransmitters, and peptides that can speak the brain's own language. Basically, your internal body systems have a dialogue with themselves, which causes them to spontaneously begin to "right" whatever is wrong within your internal makeup.

INTERNET

www.brain-longevity.com

For more information about Dr. Dharma Singh Khalsa's books and work, check out this web site.

TREATING HIV

Dr. Dharma relays the following story about the effects of sound currents on one of his HIV patients:

One patient who seemed to benefit from the vibratory effects of sound currents was a young woman who had contracted HIV from her boyfriend. Her Medical Meditation was intended to increase immunity, in part by stimulating the immune system's thymus gland (via the pituitary) by using sound vibrations. This naturalistic form of ultrasound seemed to have an almost immediate effect, judging from her white blood cell count. Using primarily just Medical Meditation and nutritional therapy, the woman has remained virtually symptom-free for more than 15 years. This result compares very favorably to even the best of the new pharmacologic approaches.

Projecting into the future of medicine

THERE ARE SO MANY EXCITING WAYS *that the best of Eastern and Western medicine are merging in our world today, but none more promising than the work being done by Dr. Dean Ornish with the Reversing Heart Disease Program. Studies done over a period of 19 years show that within a few weeks of using this program, patients reported a 91-percent average reduction in the frequency of chest pain due to heart disease. The progression of heart disease stopped or began to reverse in all but one of the study's participants who had cardiac PET scans after 4 to 5 years.*

Dr. Ornish's program is the only approach scientifically validated to begin reversing even severe coronary disease after only 1 year, without using cholesterol-lowering drugs or surgery. Instead, his self-help program utilizes yoga and meditation.

Dr. Ornish has spent many years studying the Integral yoga method, which is an essential component of his program. Other lifestyle changes that are part of the program are meditation and visualization, stress-management techniques, group support meetings, and following a low-fat vegetarian diet.

Medicare pays for selected patients who elect to follow this program at some participating sites. Health facilities from BroMenn Hospital in Bloomington, Illinois, to Highmark Blue Cross Blue Shield in Pittsburgh, Pennsylvania, now offer Dr. Ornish's program.

DWAYNE'S RECOVERY

One of the participants in Dr. Ornish's research was Dwayne, a man with severe coronary heart disease who, within a year after he started the program, experienced some overall reversal in his coronary artery blockages. In the book, *Dr. Dean Ornish's Program for Reversing Heart Disease*, Dwayne recounts a revealing and inspiring story of how illness can be a catalyst for transforming a person's life. This is an excerpt from his story:

Although he [Dr. Ornish] described the program to me, it didn't really sink in. If I had understood that I was going to have to do meditation and I was going to have to get in a group and talk about my life, I wouldn't have enrolled, because I thought it showed weakness . . . . I had been telling myself, "I can handle these problems myself. I don't need your help. If I need your help, you can operate on me and fix my heart physically, but don't touch me mentally or emotionally because I have it all together." That's the type of person I was . . . . [But] When I went to the research retreat, and some of these things were thrown at me, I said to myself, "You know, I think I'll try this. I'm going to try it on for size. If it helps me a little, then I'm going to take another step."

Before, I was all in a knot inside. I was tight all the time. My muscles were tight. I even learned that my blood vessels were tight and restricted. When you walk around that way for years and years and you're uptight all the time, then it takes its toll on your body.

I tell you, if I can do it, anybody can do it. And not only just the diet and exercise, but also the psychological part — getting rid of some of your animosities, hates, bigotry, all of that stuff that goes along with feeling bad about yourself. It's very helpful to have support of some kind . . . . When you ask for forgiveness, when you ask for understanding, when you ask for love, then you're able to give these too. That must be what the human body needs and what being human is all about. You know, it must be. Because it works.

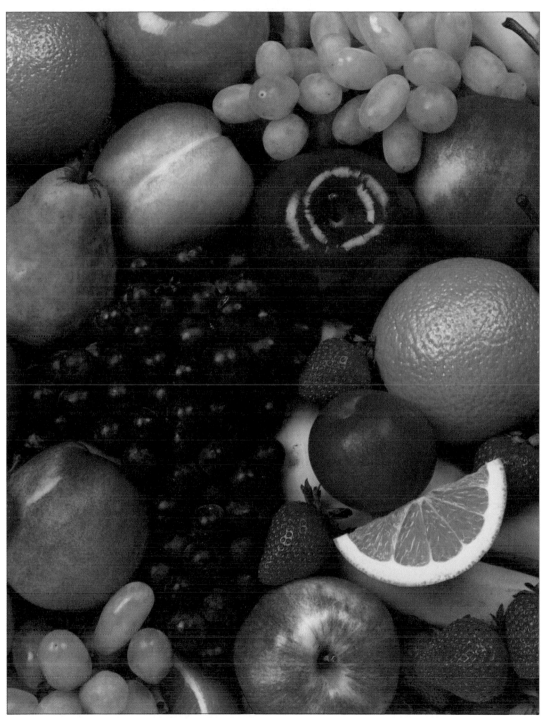

■ **A low-fat vegetarian diet**, *including plenty of fresh fruit, is an important part of Dr. Ornish's treatment program for reversing heart disease.*

Healing our lives and our hearts

Dr. Dean Ornish demonstrates that when we begin to heal our lives, our hearts begin to heal as well. It is a stirring proposition backed by examples of real people who in some cases had bypass surgery, sometimes more than once. Ultimately it was the lifestyle changes that reversed the blocked arteries.

Two completely different tests indicated the same findings: The major determinant of improvement in heart patients was not how old or how sick they were. The major factor was how much they changed their lifestyles by adding yoga, meditation, a vegetarian diet, and group support sessions.

According to Dr. Ornish, isolation can lead to stress and, ultimately, to illness, whereas intimacy can be healing. The forms that isolation come in are:

- Isolation from our feelings, our inner self, and inner peace
- Isolation from others
- Isolation from a higher force

Yoga includes breathing techniques, meditation, visualization, progressive relaxation practices, self-analysis, and altruism. All of these different methods have a common purpose, which is to heal our isolation.

INTERNET

www.my.webmd.com

Ths web site is a good choice for finding more information about Dr. Ornish's program, and for a list of participating licensed program sites. Click on Dr. Dean Ornish, MD, Lifestyle.

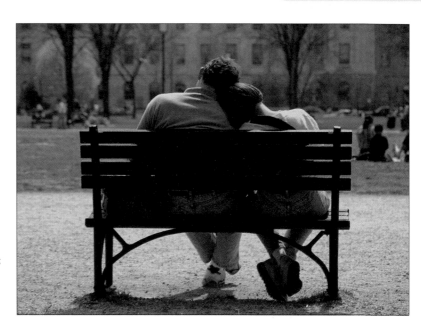

■ **Opening up** *to others and showing our affection prevents feelings of isolation, not only in ourselves but also in those we care about.*

A simple summary

✓ Conventional medicine is superb when it comes to surgery, emergency, and trauma, but alternative medicine can be more effective for many other medical situations without disturbing side effects and at a much lower cost.

✓ Patients often become dependent on doctors to monitor and adjust their medications rather than becoming empowered to change their lifestyle in ways that might help them regain health.

✓ Progressive doctors are beginning to recommend yoga to patients, especially when their complaints relate to nervous tension, weight gain, high blood pressure, or heart problems.

✓ Maintaining internal balance, throwing off stress, and boosting the body's self-healing powers are crucial to long term health. This is what yoga does best.

✓ Yoga therapy has sprung up as a means of custom-tailoring yoga to individual needs through one-on-one sessions. Two of the most well known are Integrative Yoga Therapy (IYT) and Phoenix Rising yoga therapy.

✓ In yogic healing, the healer opens to a sensitive process of awareness, creating a space in which healing can occur naturally.

✓ You can use meditation as medicine. Medical Meditations use breath, mantras, posture and movement, and mental focus.

✓ Yoga is an essential component of Dr. Dean Ornish's Reversing Heart Disease Program. Meditation and visualization, stress management techniques, group support meetings, and following a low-fat vegetarian diet are also part of the program.

✓ Our culture is starting to include alternative medicine, such as yoga, not only by offering healthy lifestyle choices to individuals, but also through Medicare and healthcare programs.

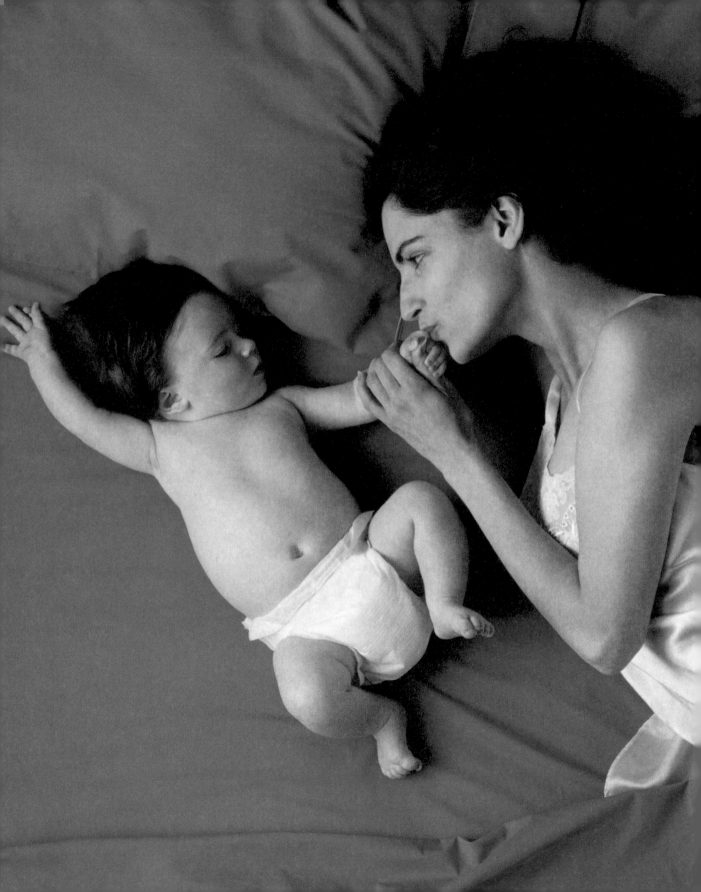

Chapter 20

Creating Peace Inside and Out

IN THIS LAST CHAPTER is the beginning – the beginning of our future. According to yogic teachings, the parts affect the whole, the whole affects the parts, and no action is wasted. In this chapter I will show you how to create peace through yoga – in our hearts, homes, and world.

In this chapter...

✓ The yoga of marriage

✓ Yoga for regular guys

✓ Ladies' choice

✓ Yoga for radiant children

✓ Peace through yoga

✓ Releasing fear through Dru yoga

✓ It all comes back to you

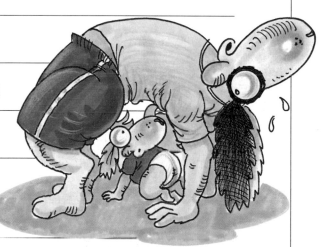

THE INNER PEACE THAT YOGA GIVES YOU WILL BE FELT BY OTHERS

The yoga of marriage

HEALTHY GENERATIONS *start with healthy marriages, which start with healthy couples. Ancient yogic wisdom says, "Don't call them married who sit together; they are married who are two bodies and one soul." Now, this doesn't mean you are supposed to lose your individuality. Instead, your unique gifts complement and merge together to create something that goes beyond what the two of you could be as individuals. That is the concept of two bodies and one soul.*

Marriage has been described as a "carriage unto infinity." Have you ever noticed what makes a really extraordinary marriage? In the best marriages, there is a commitment to the highest – in themselves, each other, and the entire world. The children who are born from this kind of marriage are exceptional.

"Okay now, so all of this sounds wonderful. How can these lofty concepts become reality?" you may think as you see your spouse hanging out in front of the TV set. There are no clear-cut answers, but I would say this: Start with yourself, and let the "cosmos" clear a path. Positive thinking, awareness of your breath, being truly empathetic and listening to points of view that are not shared by you, even simply smiling more, are some of the ways you can start. And, of course, begin a practice of yoga.

As you practice yoga, you will begin to feel different – more calm and happy. Your partner will begin to notice. Share something inspiring about your experience without the slightest hint of pressuring. If you sense an openness, invite him or her to join you.

A word of caution: Be conscious of allowing your partner to have his or her own experience. Rather than teaching your partner directly, try practicing together with a yoga video or going to a yoga class. In this way, you will both be students.

Trivia...

A yoga retreat is a wonderful way to regenerate and build your yoga practice at the same time. For many, both men and women, a retreat is a restful, uplifting getaway; for others, it's a life-changing experience. There are hundreds of yoga retreats offered nationally and internationally. A comprehensive resource is the book Yoga Vacations: A Guide to International Yoga Retreats *by Annalisa Cunningham.*

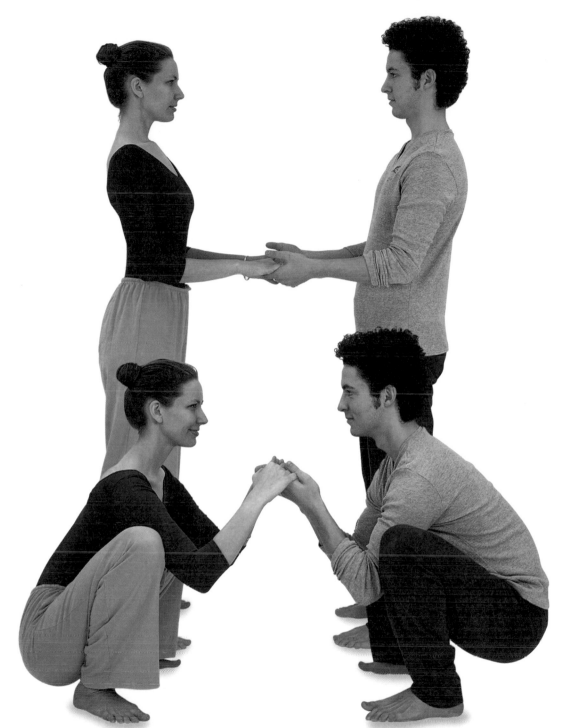

■ **Crow squats** *are ideal yoga poses for couples. Creating a physical link by holding hands and looking into your partner's eyes helps generate love and health.*

Yoga for regular guys

NOWADAYS YOGA IS FOR EVERYONE. Regular guys do it, too, and they are the better for it. If you look at all the yoga paths and their origins, almost all of them have been brought to the West by men. It is true that more women practice yoga than men, but that image is changing rapidly as men are discovering the treasures that yoga holds for them.

With the career and family responsibilities men have these days, they need all the stress relief they can get. As a result, more and more men are finding yoga to be the perfect way to let off steam and unwind.

Women have a natural affinity with yoga, as traditionally women have more flexibility and balance. Men have been more thoroughly trained in athletic endeavors, which require strength. Both are important in yoga, as we have seen. In yoga, you probably will not develop bigger muscles, but your muscles will be toned and hold your bones in place. Those who want a physical challenge may be drawn to styles of yoga like Ashtanga or Kundalini, or some of the more daring poses like handstands and Peacock pose, which require upper body strength and balance.

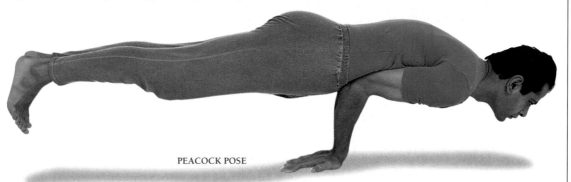

PEACOCK POSE

Yoga is not a sport, but it requires practice and perseverance like sports. As you now know, yoga is not about competition, unless you consider doing your best at each moment a contest with yourself. Done with awareness and care, this kind of inner competition can serve as a motivational tool.

Many of the ordinary activities that you do each day may not be exercising your body in a way that will bring health and flexibility. For example, sleeping is great for you, but does not reduce stress the way that yoga does. Lifting weights and bouncing the basketball in the driveway have their own value, but will not increase flexibility, or help you stay calm when things get tough. But yoga will. So, be brave, guys – *real* men do yoga!

Ladies' choice

IT IS NO WONDER THAT YOGA *is the practice of choice for women. Women resonate with the philosophy and practice of yoga effortlessly. And yoga helps women through all the many phases of their lives: From the beginning of menstruation through menopause, from prenatal to postpartum, and everything in between.*

A lovely book written with strength and grace, A Woman's Guide to Tantra Yoga by Vimala McClure, offers practical yogic guidance for women in every phase of life.

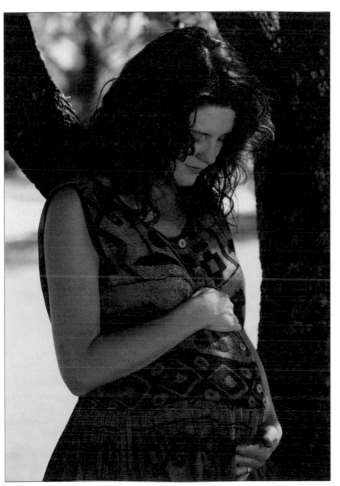

Yoga for pregnancy

Many women, especially those who want natural childbirth, discover yoga by seeking it out as a preparation for labor. As a result, many yoga centers have added prenatal and postpartum yoga classes to their schedules. Some HMOs and insurance carriers are now offering prenatal yoga care.

See the *K.I.S.S. Guide to Pregnancy* by Felicia Eisenberg Molnar for a comprehensive and easy-to-read guide on everything you need to know about pregnancy.

■ **Practicing yoga** *during pregnancy prepares both the mind and body for childbirth. It also helps you connect with the unborn child.*

PRENATAL YOGA

The following are some of the numerous benefits of prenatal yoga:

- Prepares the pelvic muscles, hips, and legs for childbirth
- Helps you process emotions from the increased hormonal activity
- Brings a greater awareness of the breath, how to use it during labor and to calm yourself
- Improves circulation, which is important because you are sharing your blood circulation with your baby
- Keeps the body supple and aligned while it changes to accommodate the life within
- Most importantly, helps you connect with your unborn child

When I learned the panting breath that is used to "ride out" contractions, I thought, "This is easy. It's really not very different from Breath of Fire which I've been doing for years." I was especially grateful for my yogic training when I was in the midst of full-scale labor and 40 miles from the hospital, using the panting breath to hold off the baby's birth!

Be wise and cautious

If you've never done yoga, it's best to consult your doctor or nurse practitioner before beginning during pregnancy. If you are considered high risk or have any health problems, make sure to seek medical advice first. Sometimes the recommendation will be to start yoga after the first trimester, as research shows that prenatal problems frequently occur within the first 3 months of pregnancy. And make sure to have a teacher who knows what kind of yoga is good for pregnancy. Among poses to avoid are those done lying on your stomach or flat on your back, strong spinal twists, and inverted poses such as headstands.

Be sure to consult your doctor before beginning prenatal yoga if you have hypertension, toxemia, diabetes, or are at risk for premature labor.

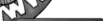

INTERNET

www.gurmukh.com

Connect with your baby heart-to-heart both inside and outside the womb with two great prenatal and postpartum yoga videos at this site.

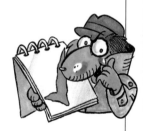

Women's phases of life

Most noteworthy among the many phases of a woman's life are the menopausal years, in which hormones can cause havoc. These years can be addressed quite beautifully with yoga, because hormones are controlled by the glandular system, and the glandular system is yoga's specialty. Women who have practiced yoga prior to menopause find both perimenopause (the stage right before menopause) and menopause to be easier and, in some cases, effortless. Yoga and meditation help release emotions and stress often associated with this phase of a woman's life. Yoga poses that balance glands, nerves, and muscular tension are good to do at this time.

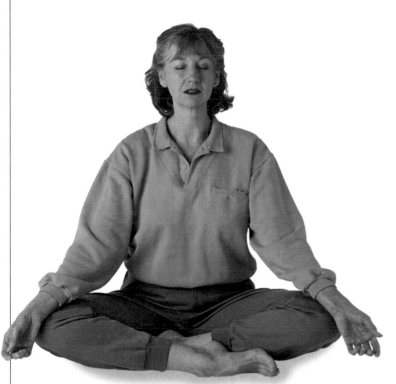

■ **Yoga practiced** *prior to and after the menopause will help make this time easier to bear, physically and psychologically.*

Trivia...

If you're experiencing hot flashes, find the nearest wall for some inverted poses, which help the endocrine glands regulate your hormone levels. Lie on the floor with your buttocks close to the wall, and put your legs up on the wall. Relax and breathe. Downward-facing dog is great also, or, if you are really adventurous, try a handstand against the wall. While in Downward-facing dog, bring your heels against the wall, then boost one foot at a time up onto the wall, balancing on your arms with your body straight for a few seconds.

When her children are grown, a woman's "empty nest" provides the perfect opportunity for her to grow in awareness and deepen her sense of purposeful work. Menopause can be a time of "pausing" in your tracks to open up to new possibilities of spiritual and personal fulfillment. Through yoga and meditation it is possible to develop a deep inner "knowing" and courageously move forward into exciting new areas.

Yoga for radiant children

A BRIGHT CHILD is bright not only in intellect but in spirit. Yoga, meditation, and a healthy diet help create children who are bright lights in this world. In my role of "Ms. Shakta," the traveling children's yoga teacher, I have taught up to 300 preschool and elementary children a week. I never fail to be awed by the way children naturally take to yoga, and the insights they come up with, like the 5-year-old girl who after class confided, "I feel happy in my heart when I do yoga."

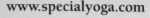

Although yoga has enjoyed popularity with adults for many years, it's only recently that we have understood how helpful it can be for children. Yoga not only increases their self-awareness, it builds their self-esteem and helps strengthen their growing bodies. It's truly a welcome oasis in a culture that offers little in the way of mindful, yet active, play. And, by the way, the key word is *play*. What children care about most is having fun. While adult yoga can be as serious as a person makes it, children's yoga has got to be a blast!

INTERNET

www.specialyoga.com

Go to this site for therapeutic yoga for children with cerebral palsy, Down's syndrome, and learning disabilities. Sonia Sumar's remarkable book, Yoga for the Special Child, *can be found here, too.*

The new generation of children is under tremendous pressure to achieve. Informational stimulation and media hype can be relentless. Yoga will help them relax and sort out what's important from what's not.

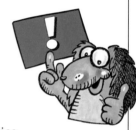

INTERNET

www.childrensyoga .com

Log onto this site to find my book, Fly Like A Butterfly: Yoga for Children, *and to try some children's yoga. You'll also find The Radiant Child yoga teacher-training program, and a comprehensive listing of children's yoga teachers.*

In addition to having a good time, children who practice yoga experience numerous benefits – increased learning capacity and mental alertness, better coordination, and improved self-discipline, to name a few. A child's yoga practice can also benefit the adult, since a happy child makes a happy parent.

In addition to books and videos for children's yoga, you might feel that having a teacher for your child is the way to go. Many yoga centers are beginning to offer classes for children. You will find the techniques and styles of yoga differ greatly from one center to the next, so explore and ask questions.

CHILDREN'S YOGA GUIDELINES

a The three main criteria of children's yoga: It has to be fun, moderately challenging, and create a positive internal change.

b Create a special time and place for yoga. Take some time in the morning or evening, and follow it with a deep relaxation.

c Begin by closing your eyes and taking a few deep breaths. Before beginning yoga, mentally or out loud recognize the inner guidance, and connect it to the universal guidance, however you perceive it to be. Share this centering technique with the children.

d With preschoolers, 15–20 minutes is a good start. Each exercise lasts 20 seconds, working up to 1 minute, as the children progress in their ability to stay focused. Make sure to have at least 2 minutes of relaxation at the end.

e Keep it short and imaginative with preschoolers (hissing in Cobra pose, leaping in Frog pose, for example).

f Elementary children can usually stay engaged for 20 minutes to a half-hour of yoga, preteens a half-hour or more. Include a few minutes of deep relaxation, and perhaps a 3–5-minute meditation.

g Challenge elementary and preteens with timers ("How long can you stay up in Bow pose?"). Tell them how the exercise or pose helps them ("Who wants to be calm for your exams? Try this deep breathing.").

FROG POSE

h Teens can do the same yoga that adults do. Keep it simple so they can be successful. Find out what their needs and goals are, and relate how yoga can help them with issues they face each day, such as feeling self-confident, being comfortable in their changing bodies, handling academic pressure, improving performance in team sports, etc.

i It is better to start simply and build gradually. Reach into children's inner selves using your intuition and lighthearted humor rather than your intellect.

Baby yoga

After I had practiced yoga for some time, it occurred to me how wonderful it would have been to have learned yoga as a child. I would have had so much less to "undo" – tight muscles, back strain, unhelpful habits, over-emotionality, insecurities, and on and on. So, being grateful that yoga found me at all, I knew that yoga would be a strong part of my child's life.

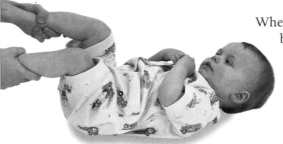

When our son was an infant, my husband and I bicycled his little legs and crisscrossed his arms while smiling and singing to him. In this way, the effects of yoga were imprinting on his unconscious mind. By the time he became old enough to practice on his own, doing yoga was as natural as brushing his teeth.

■ **You can introduce** *yoga very early on by "bicycling" your baby's legs, chanting and singing mantras, and smiling with them.*

When he was 3, my son began to close his eyes and meditate for a few minutes. He started to become aware of his breath. Sometimes he would say a little prayer, maybe for us or his dog and cat – those that made up his world, and brought out the love from his heart. Affirmations work well with young children. One that my son loved, as well as the children who came to my school, was "I am happy, I am good," chanted while moving his hands back and forth in rhythm with the mantra for energy and focus.

A child's best buddy

By the time he was 6 years old, my son could sit for 10 minutes or more and focus either internally or on his breath. One of his favorite meditations has been one for releasing negative thoughts and feelings. This is done by forming a cup with his hands, right hand inside the left, then bringing the cup up to the chest level. (Adults are welcome to try also.) With his eyes looking only into the cup, he inhaled deeply through his nose, then exhaled with a long, dry, spitting motion into the cup. Carried on that breath was one thought or feeling that he didn't want to have anymore.

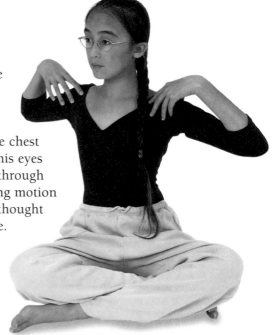

■ **Children between the ages of 9 and 12** *can perform many adult yoga exercises and meditation, although for shorter periods of time.*

I asked my son to tell me how he visualized this meditation working, and this is what he said: "You inhale and think of the thought you don't want. Then you exhale by blowing into your hands, and that bad thought or feeling will be destroyed by going down into your hands, which are like a pool of water, and the water sucks it in. That is the way I imagine it. You might imagine something else."

As he has gotten older, sometimes he doesn't want to slow down enough to let yoga work for him. But yoga, along with meditation, has given him the invaluable experience of knowing that his own best buddy is right inside, and that yoga will guide him there whenever he chooses.

Peace through yoga

CAN YOU IMAGINE A WORLD in which all humanity experiences the benefits of yoga? Where people are in touch with their inner centers, have healthy bodies and meditative minds, and make decisions based on their higher awareness? Is it just a pie in the sky dream? Or is it a very real possibility? Is it, perhaps, becoming a reality?

Karma yoga

There is a natural progression in your practice of yoga. The first phase you experience is opening up to new feelings and understandings. In the second phase, you root yourself in your newfound awareness. As you continue with your practice, you may reach a phase in which your needs are few and you have much to give to others, sometimes just with your presence. And, at some point during the second and third phases, there is a natural transition into the branch of yoga that is called Karma yoga.

DEFINITION

Karma is a Sanskrit word with several related meanings. Karma is a law of nature that is expressed by "as you reap, so shall you sow." It also refers to right action, selfless service, and taking action to uplift others.

Commonly the word *karma* brings forth the idea that "as you reap, so shall you sow" or "every action has an equal and opposite reaction." The experience of karma may be subtle, or it may not happen right away and you may not consciously experience the consequences of your actions, but karma still happens simply because it is a law of nature. So if we want to "reap" peace on our planet, we have to "sow" peace in our hearts – through forgiveness, through accepting ourselves and others, through remembering the good in everything that happens, and learning from our mistakes.

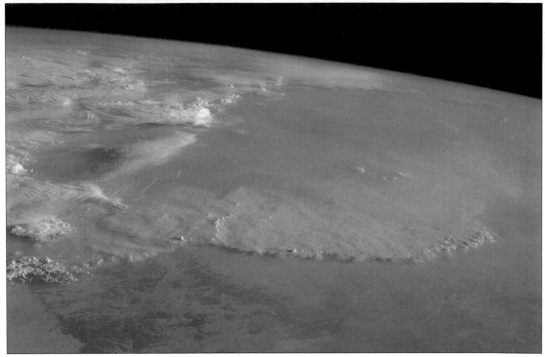

■ **Seen from a space shuttle**, *this awe-inspiring view of the Earth helps us realize that we all share in this beautiful "home," and by sowing peace in our hearts through yoga, we can reap peace on our planet.*

THE AGE OF AQUARIUS

According to yogic teachings, and confirmed by astrological understanding, our planet is moving through an auspicious time of great change that happens only every 2,000 years. We are transitioning from one astrological sign (Pisces) to another (Aquarius). In the age of Pisces, God was thought to be outside ourselves, and the theme was "I believe." In the age of Aquarius, God will be known to be within us, as a living, breathing God, and the theme will be "I know."

The cusp, or transition period, that we are currently experiencing will end in 2013, and is a time of great upheaval on every level of human existence. As a yoga practitioner, you are easing this transition by developing a clear, meditative mind and a caring heart. As your yoga practice evolves, you come to realize that we are all of the same identity, and that identity is infinite. This realization is the foundation of the new age.

One way to understand Karma yoga is from the point of view of energy moving through the chakras. Gradually, with a steady and sincere yoga practice, the lower chakras (root, sex organs, navel) get activated and energy is transformed to the higher centers (heart, throat, third eye, crown and energy field). Universal love and higher awareness become your guiding force. You may realize there is nothing left to do but to ask the question, "How can I help?"

Practicing selfless service

Every humanitarian and spiritual organization has an aspect of not-for-profit service. Yoga paths are no exception. One of the most common ways that yoga organizations serve is through donations of food, clothing, and shelter for the destitute and homeless. An example of this is the 3HO Foundation (Healthy, Happy, Holy Organization) of Los Angeles, whose members have consistently prepared and served a free healthy meal each day for over 15 years.

Yoga is filling a gap for natural self-help treatment in clinical settings, such as for mental health, chemical dependencies, and other addictions. Many community service organizations are adapting yoga, breathing exercises, and meditation in the form of stress-reduction exercises (yoga) and mind-focusing techniques (meditation).

Peace begins at home

One such successful organization based on the understanding that "peace begins at home" is the Institute for the Advancement of Service (IAS). IAS creates a bridge between personal growth and serving others by teaching students, parents, and healthcare and social workers (among others) mind/body/spirit concepts that can be applied in any work, group, family, or community setting.

Yoga, meditation, and affirmations play an important part in IAS. Members of the organization sustain a community of peace through the practice of inner peace, knowing that peace is not about changing or adjusting outer behavior. Rather, it is about changing our inner thoughts and motivations.

The Executive Director of IAS, Susan S. Trout, Ph.D., has written an enlightening book, *Born to Serve*, forwarded by His Holiness the Dalai Lama. Every facet of service to others is portrayed with insight and clarity by Susan Trout, who says, "In the process of my journey, I have learned a very important lesson: Being of service means doing whatever needs to be done with no attachment to the form of the task and with no investment in its outcome. I have also learned there is an integral relationship between service and my own personal healing process."

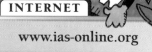

INTERNET

www.ias-online.org

For more information about the Institute for the Advancement of Service, go to its web site.

Yoga Inside

No one can take yoga away from you, as you carry its wisdom and experience with you wherever you go. For these reasons, yoga is the logical and enlightened response to incarcerated youth and children in protective shelters. Yoga Inside was created by Mark Stephens, a respected yoga teacher and part of the Los Angeles County Office of Education. The organization is built around a vision of freedom on the inside. As Stephens puts it, "They are always free – they're never really prisoners of anything. They are free to choose their thoughts, free to choose their reactions, free to be their true selves."

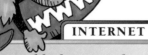

INTERNET

www.sivananda.org

Sivananda Yoga Center sponsors a Prisoner Outreach program.

INTERNET

www.yogainside.org

Yoga Inside gives the gift of yoga and meditations to prisoners, inner-city youth, children in protective shelters, and more.

In a dramatic and bold experiment, Stephens brought six Tibetan monks to visit the Kirby Center, a juvenile correctional facility, in a project called "Healing the Causes of Violence." The Kirby Center is surrounded by tall block walls topped with razor wire. Inside are about 100 of the county's most serious and violent juvenile offenders, all of whom have serious mental-health issues. The six Tibetan monks taught the boys how to meditate and create sand mandalas to peace. The profound change in the boys' attitudes following this event inspired the birth of Yoga Inside.

Yoga Inside is expanding its services to include inner-city public schools, mental-health treatment facilities, shelters for the battered and abused, and other similar facilities.

Into the war zones

INTERNET

www.blackyogateachers .com

Members of the International Association of Black Yoga Teachers teach yoga to inner city children. For more information, see their site.

Serving those who aid those in war and disaster zones is the brilliant contribution of the Life Foundation International. LFI goes into areas such as Bosnia, Northern Ireland, and East Africa and helps aid workers, field staff, therapists, and counselors overcome burnout and manage the stress and painful emotions of their intense work through self-help approaches – movement, breath, visualization, and humor.

The techniques LFI uses are based on a type of yoga called Dru yoga, which teaches how to balance body, heart, and mind by using the heart as the pivotal point around which all else revolves. It is characterized by beautiful flowing movements that channel the body's

YOGA FOR THE CITY

Sat Kartar Kaur Khalsa founded Kundalini Yoga for Youth, a yoga program for inner-city youth in Boston and Providence, in 1993.

Some of the stories she has told me are heart wrenching – such as children who feel safe when relaxing on their backs only if they have a shawl covering them because they are scarred by abuse.

Some are just as heartwarming – such as the boy in his mid-teens, a former hard-core gang member, who told Sat Kartar, "You saved my life."

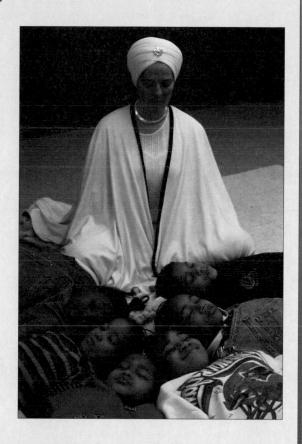

■ **With her yoga youth program**, *Sat Kartar Kaur Khalsa has brought peace and hope to many inner-city children.*

subtle energy through the heart to create healing. Over the past 5 years, this system has formed the basis for their de-traumatization work in the war zones of the world.

Dru yoga is proving particularly effective in war-torn areas because it allows a person to transform emotional pain without having to relive the experience of trauma.

There is a sequence of movements for every painful state we humans experience. For example, if you are experiencing grief, there is a specific sequence to transform the feeling into freedom and renewal. For anxiety, there is a sequence to transform this into the courage to move forward, and so on.

Releasing fear through Dru yoga

A LITTLE GEM CALLED The Dance Between Joy and Pain by Dr. Mansukh Patel and Rita Goswami, RGN, is filled with uplifting anecdotes and easy exercises for releasing emotions and cultivating inner strength. The following two sequences of Dru yoga can be done together or separately.

Releasing stretch

1. Interlock your hands behind your back. Breathe in and pull your hands up behind you.

2. As you breathe out, start to bend forward from your hips, raising your arms up straight as high as you can without straining. Soften your knees so they are not locked or strained. Breathe naturally for 30 seconds.

3. Slowly breathe in, uncurling from the base of your spine. Release your hands and exhale.

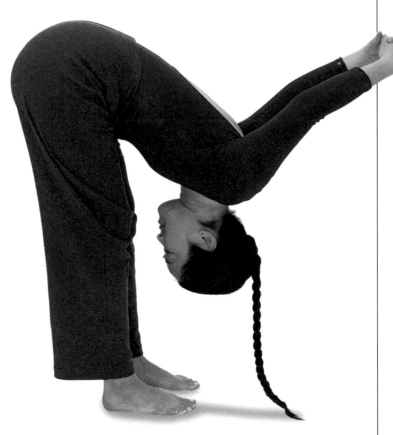

RELEASING STRETCH

Fearless flight

1 Raise your arms out to your sides to shoulder height. Bend forward, keeping your knees soft, as you breathe out. At the same time, gently swoop your arms down so that they meet in front of your feet. Your palms are facing upward with the right palm on top of the left. Breathe naturally.

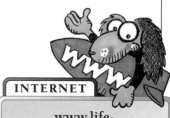

INTERNET

www.life-foundation.com

To find out more about the work of the Life Foundation, go to their web site.

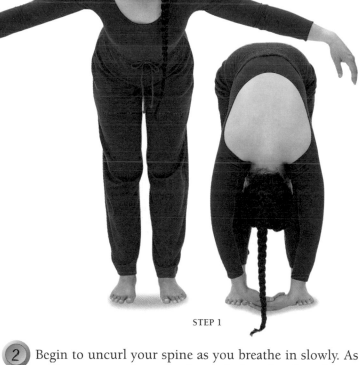

STEP 1

2 Begin to uncurl your spine as you breathe in slowly. As you do so, keep your palms together as before, but face them toward your body as you draw your hands slowly up the front of you 5 6 inches (12–15 cm) away from your body.

3 Continue inhaling slowly as you move your hands upward until your arms are raised above your head with your palms facing downward. Look up slightly.

4 Breathing out, bring your arms down to shoulder height in the starting position and begin the sequence again.

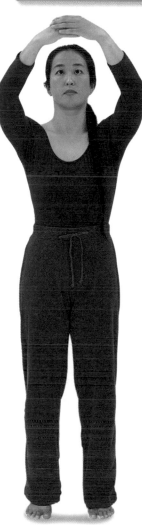

STEP 3

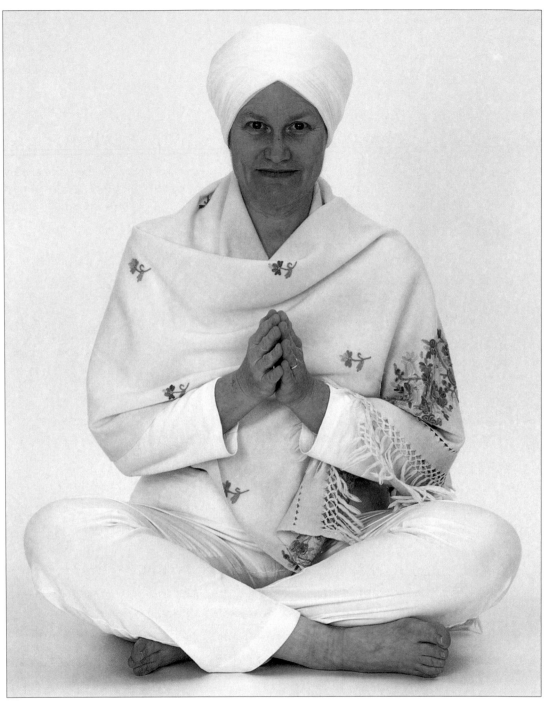

■ **In yoga, there is a beautiful tradition** *of placing the hands in Prayer pose and bowing slightly, as demonstrated by author Shakta Kaur Khalsa. This gesture says, "I honor the universal spirit in you," and is used both as a greeting and a farewell.*

It all comes back to you

WHEN YOU GET RIGHT DOWN TO IT, peace in our world is not the issue. Peace comes piece by piece, person by person, and moment by moment. Every time you feel peaceful and grateful, lovingly care for others, or live to your highest, you are strengthening the energy of peace in our world.

The chain of peace is made up of individual human links who know they are unbreakably clasped to every other human being in the world. To be this kind of human takes a body that is vital and strong, a mind that is grounded in awareness, a heart that is giving, and a spirit that is filled with the energy of the universe, of the One.

Yoga is your ticket to transformation. Simply begin and it is begun!

A simple summary

✔ Healthy generations start with healthy marriages, which start with healthy couples. In the best marriages, there is a commitment to the highest – in themselves, each other, and the entire world.

✔ Men and women who practice yoga together experience transformation in their own lives and in their family life.

✔ Yoga creates children who are bright lights in this world, increasing their self-awareness, building self-esteem, and strengthening their bodies.

✔ Karma yoga is selfless service. The word "karma" means "action." It means living your yoga, walking your talk, and taking action to uplift others.

✔ In order to "reap" peace on our planet, we have to "sow" peace in our hearts. Whenever you feel peaceful or give selflessly to others, you help to strengthen the energy of peace in our world. A practice of yoga can take you there.

Other resources

Books

Acu-Yoga
Michael Reed Gach,
Japan Book Publishers, Tokyo, 1999

Alternative Medicine: The Definitive Guide
Burton Goldberg,
Future Medicine Publishing,
Payallup WA, 1999

Ananda Yoga for Higher Awareness
Swami Kriyananda (J. Donald Walters),
Crystal Clarity Publications,
Nevada City CA, 1967

Anatomy of Miracles
Subagh Singh Khalsa,
Tuttle Publications, Boston, 1999

Asana Pranayama Mudra Bandha
Swami Satyananda Saraswati,
Bihar School of Yoga, Bihar, India, 1997

Autobiography of a Yogi
Paramahansa Yogananda,
Crystal Clarity Publications,
Nevada City CA, 1995

Ayurveda: The Ancient Indian Healing
Scott Gearson Ayurveda, MD,
Element Books, Rockport MA, 1993

Baby and Mom (video)
Gurmukh Khalsa,
Parade Videos, Peter Pan Ind., Newark NJ

Be Here Now
Ram Dass,
Crown, New York, 1971

Born to Serve
Susan S. Trout, Ph.D,
Three Rivers Press, Alexandria VA, 1997

Brain Longevity
Dharma Singh Khalsa, MD,
Warner Books, New York, 1999

Breathwalk
Yogi Bhajan, Ph.D, and
Gurucharan Singh Khalsa, Ph.D,
Broadway Books, New York, 2000

A Call to Women: The Healthy Breast Program and Workbook
Sat Dharam Kaur, MD,
Quarry Press, Kingston ON, 2000

Chanting: Discovering Spirit in Sound
Robert Gass,
Bantam Doubleday Dell, New York, 2000

Complete Guide to Integrative Medicine
Dr. David Peters and Anne Woodham,
DK Publishing, New York, 2000

The Dance Between Joy and Pain
Dr. Mansukh Patel and Rita Goswami, RGN,
Life Foundation Publications, 1995

Diet for a New America
John Robbins,
H.J. Kramer, Tiburon CA, 1987

Dr. Dean Ornish's Program for Reversing Heart Disease
Dean Ornish, MD,
Ballantine Books, New York, 1990

The Dynamic Laws of Healing
Catherine Ponder,
Devorss & Co., New York, 1966

The Five Fingered Family
Shakta Kaur Khalsa,
The Brookfield Reader, Sterling VA, 2000

Fly Like a Butterfly: Yoga for Children
Shakta Kaur Khalsa,
Sterling Publishers, New York, 1998

Foods for Health and Healing
Yogi Bhajan, Ph.D,
KRI Pub., Espanola NM, 1983

From Vegetables With Love
Siri Ved Kaur Khalsa,
Arcline Publications, San Francisco, 1989

Hands of Light
Barbara Ann Brennan,
Bantam Books, New York, 1987

The Heart of Yoga
T.K.V. Desikachar,
Inner Traditions International,
Rochester VT, 1999

How to Know God
Swami Prabhavananda and
Christopher Isherwood,
Vedanta Press, Hollywood CA, 1981

The Illustrated Encyclopedia of Well Being
Dr. Julian Jessel-Kenyon,
Sterling Publishers, New York, 1999

Integral Yoga Hatha
Swami Satchidananda,
Integral Yoga Distribution,
Buckingham VA, 1998

K.I.S.S. Guide to Pregnancy
Felicia Eisenberg Molnar,
DK Publishing, New York, 2001

Kundalini Yoga
Shakta Kaur Khalsa,
DK Publishing, New York, 2001

Kundalini Yoga: The Flow of Eternal Power
Shakti Parwha Kaur Khalsa,
Perigree, New York, 1998

The Light of Asia
Edwin Arnold,
Kessinger Publications, Kila MT, 1997

Light Emerging
Barbara Ann Brennan,
Bantam Books, New York, 1993

Light on Yoga
B.K.S. Iyengar,
Schocken Books, New York, 1979

Living Yoga
Georg Feuerstein and Stephan Bodian,
Putnam, New York, 1990

Meditation for Absolutely Everyone
Subagh Singh Khalsa,
Tuttle Publications, Boston, 1994

Meditation as Medicine
Dharma Singh Khalsa, MD,
Pocket Books, New York, 2001

The Moosewood Cookbook
Mollie Katzen,
Running Press, Philadelphia, 1996

The New Laurel's Kitchen
Laurel Robertson, Carol Flinders, and
Brian Ruppenthal,
Ten Speed Press, Berkeley CA, 1986

The New Yoga for People Over 50
Suza Francina,
Health Communications,
Deerfield Beach FL, 1997

The Pain Cure
Dharma Singh Khalsa, MD,
Warner Books, New York, 2000

The Power of Prayer
Larry Dossey, MD,
Harper Mass Market Paperbacks,
New York, 1997

Power Yoga
Beryl Bender Birch,
Fireside Books, New York, 1995

Prenatal and Post Natal Yoga (video)
Gurmukh Khalsa,
Parade Videos, Peter Pan Ind., Newark NJ

Radionics and the Subtle Bodies of Man
Dr. David Tansley,
Beekman Publishing, 1972

Reinventing Medicine
Larry Dossey, MD,
HarperCollins, New York, 1999

Relax and Renew: Restful Yoga for Stressful Times
Judith Lasater,
Rodmell Press, Berkeley CA, 1995

Sacred Hoops
Phil Jackson, Hyperion, New York, 1995

Shambhala Encyclopedia of Yoga
Georg Feuerstein,
Shambhala Publications, Boston, 1997

The Sivananda Companion to Yoga
The Sivananda Yoga Center,
Simon and Schuster Inc., New York, l983

Timeless Healing
Herbert Benson, MD,
Fireside Books, New York, 1996

Tofu Cookery
Louise Hagler,
Book Publishing Company,
Summertown TN, 1991

The Whole Soy Cookbook
Patricia Greenberg,
Three Rivers Press, New York, 1998

A Woman's Guide to Tantra Yoga
Vimala McClure,
New World Library, Novato CA, 1997

Yoga Breathing and Relaxation (video)
Richard Freeman,
Delphi Prod., Boulder CO, 1997

Yoga the Iyengar Way
Silva, Mira, and Shyam Mehta,
DK Publishing, New York, 1990

Yoga: Mastering the Basics
Sandra Anderson and Rolf Sovik,
Himalayan Institute Press,
Honesdale PA, 2000

Yoga: Mind and Body
Sivananda Yoga Vedanta Center,
DK Publishing, New York, 1998

Yoga: The Path to Holistic Health
B.K.S. Iyengar,
DK Publishing, New York, 2001

Yoga for the Special Child
Sonia Sumar,
Special Yoga Publications,
Buckingham VA, 1996

Yoga Vacations
Annalisa Cunningham,
Avalon Travel Publishing,
Emeryville CA, 1999

Yoga for Your Life
Margaret Pierce and Martin Pierce,
Sterling Publishers, New York, 1996

Yoga on the Web

CHECK OUT THE GROWING NUMBER OF SITES on the Internet dedicated to yoga. The following list contains some of the most useful. Please note, however, that due to the fast-changing nature of the Net, some of those listed may be defunct by the time you read this.

www.anusara.com
Contact this site for information about Anusara yoga, teachers, and teacher-training sessions.

www.ascentmagazine.com
Check this Canadian site to read mind-expanding articles on yoga and related topics, or subscribe to their quarterly magazine.

www.ashtanga.com
This site offers information about Ashtanga yoga. Click on "classes" to find a local trained Ashtanga teacher.

www.barbarabrennan.com
Barbara Brennan, a healer and former NASA scientist, works with the human energy field and chakras. Find out about the Barbara Brennan School of Healing here.

www.beyondanada.com

Swami Beyondanada is the cosmic clown who's been around as long as the yoga movement. Check his web site for some wise and witty plays on words.

www.bheka.com

This is a site specializing in yoga props.

www.bikramyoga.com

Check out this site for Bikram yoga, developed by Bikram Choudhury. It includes an international list of teachers.

www.blackyogateachers.com

The International Association of Black Yoga Teachers teaches yoga to inner city children and offers support for Black yoga teachers internationally.

www.brain-longevity.com

Gives information about Dr. Dharma Singh Khalsa's books and his work with yoga in the medical world, including natural ways to prevent Alzheimer's disease.

www.breathwalk.com.

Learn about the walking meditation program called Breathwalk. Instructor training programs are also offered.

www.childrensyoga.com

This site contains a wealth of children's yoga. Click here to find a sampling of children's yoga to try at home, a list of trained teachers (in the US) and holistic parenting tips.

www.columbuspolarity.com

The site for the Polarity Therapy Center of Columbus, Ohio, where Kundalini yoga is offered and integrated with Polarity Therapy work.

www.comnet.org/iynaus

Among other valuable information, you'll find an international listing of Iyengar teachers here.

www.crystalclarity.com

Find out about Ananda yoga books, audios, and videos.

www.dosseydossey.com

This is the site for Larry Dossey, MD, author of several books linking medicine, healing, and prayer.

www.downwarddog.com

The Downward Dog is an Ashtanga yoga center in Toronto, offering classes and teacher training.

www.earthsave.org

EarthSave International leads a global movement to promote healthy food choices for the well-being of all life on Earth. The Pulitzer Prize nominated book *Diet for a New America* by John Robbins prompted the formation of EarthSave International.

www.expandinglight.org

Visit this site to discover more about Ananda yoga, teachers (in the US), and how to enroll on teacher-training courses at the Expanding Light's beautiful Nevada City center in California.

www.extensionyoga.com

This site is a vital resource for every yoga practitioner who wants to learn how to minimize risk and maximize the benefits of yoga. Sam Dworkis is the host, a well-known author of two books, *Ex Tension* and *Recovery Yoga*.

www.fishcrane.com

A site that specializes in yoga props.

www.grdcenter.com

The GRD Center for Medicine and Humanology is a nonprofit foundation that provides health education using yogic methods to people with chronic or life-threatening illness, such as HIV, cancer, and chronic pain.

www.gurmukh.com

Connect with your baby both inside and outside the womb with two prenatal and postpartum yoga videos.

www.gurudevsnr.com

Provides information on the yogic healing art, Sat Nam Rasayan, and locations of teachers and training sessions in the US.

www.himalayaninstitute.org

Contact the Himalayan Institute to find out more about their programs, or to find a trained teacher. They are the source for the well-known magazine *Yoga International*, as well as the Himalayan Institute Press.

www.huggermugger.com

Offers specialist advice on yoga props.

www.ias-online.org

This is the site for more information about the Institute for the Advancement of Service, which uses yoga, meditation, and other self-help processes to help those in service organizations, such as social workers, healthcare providers and educators.

www.iyengar-yoga.com
Contact this site for a world of Iyengar yoga resources.

www.iytyogatherapy.com
Integrative Yoga Therapy offers training programs in the US that include mind-body health sciences, as well as in-depth understanding of yoga postures.

www.jps.net/dkgamow
David and Karen Gamow conduct stress reduction and meditation seminars in the workplace. Among their clients are NASA and the San Francisco Police Academy.

www.kashi.org
Ma Jaya Sati Bhagavati, who is known simply as "Ma," helps those who are dying of cancer and AIDS and raises the children of AIDS victims at her center in Florida.

www.kfa.org
This is the site for the Krishnamurti Foundation of America, founded by J. Krishnamurti in 1969.

www.kinfonet.org
This site features volumes of books and articles by J. Krishnamurti.

www.kripalu.com
Find out about year-round yoga workshops and programs offered at the Kripalu Center. Also contains a directory of US teachers and information about teacher-training.

www.kundaliniyoga.com
Provides a wealth of information about Kundalini yoga as taught by Yogi Bhajan. Click on IKYTA (International Kundalini Yoga Teachers Association) for local teachers.

www.lifeforce.nu
A Swedish-based web site (also offered in English) that has taken yoga into the corporate world and workplace. Provides a sampling of yoga for the office.

www.life-foundation.com
Find out more about the work of The Life Foundation, which brings self-help resources, such as Dru yoga, to those in war and disaster zones around the world.

www.moreyoga.com
Offers yoga and relaxation tools and yoga T-shirts.

www.morinu.com
Log onto this site for tasty tofu recipes and tips.

www.mydailyyoga.com
With clear animation that's easy to follow, Ellen Serber demonstrates over a dozen yoga exercises that anyone can do while sitting or standing at a desk.

www.my.webmd.com
Log onto this site for more about Dr. Ornish's Reversing Heart Disease program, and a list of licensed program sites.

www.ottawayoga.com
A Rama Lotus Yoga Centre in Ottawa offering classes in Kundalini, Hatha, and Bikram yoga.

www.pierceprogram.com.
Viniyoga teachers Martin and Margaret Pierce give information on books, teachers, and training.

www.power-yoga.com
This is Beryl Bender Birch's web site, which has lots of great information, especially for athletes.

www.pryt.com
Go to this site to find Phoenix Rising Yoga Therapy's teacher-training and therapists in the US.

www.sivananda.org
This is the official site for everything about Sivananda yoga, including their retreat centers, classes, teacher training, and their Prisoner OutReach program.

www.specialyoga.com
Details on Therapeutic yoga for infants and children with special needs, such as cerebral palsy, Down's syndrome, ADD, and other disorders, can be found at this site.

www.SpiritVoyage.com
Listen to and order music of mantras and uplifting songs to go with your yoga practice. Order books, too.

www.springhillmedia.com
Visit this site to find out more about the music of Robert Gass and his chanting workshops.

www.stressaway.com
Check out this site for software you can purchase that will help you exercise away your stress in the workplace.

www.taoskundalini.com
Provides information on the Kundalini yoga center in Taos, New Mexico, and how to order potassium alum, used in cleaning the mouth and throat.

www.thecleanse.com

Another good source of potassium alum. The Cleanse is also a comprehensive internal cleansing program using diet, Chinese herbs, yoga, and meditation.

www.3ho.org

Contains services and inspiration for a healthy lifestyle, courtesy of the 3HO (Healthy, Happy, Holy Organization).

www.truefoodnow.org

Greenpeace's site is one of the best for information about GMOs (genetically modified organisms). Check their Truefood Shopping List, where you can find out which products have GMOs.

www.unitywoods.com

Check this site for the Unity Wood Yoga Center in Bethesda, MD, founded by John Schumacher. It is one of the most well-established yoga centers for Iygengar yoga.

www.viniyoga.com

Gary Kraftsow's American Viniyoga Institute, teacher training, and books on Viniyoga are located at this site.

www.yogaalliance.com

As well as working to design a unified minimum standard of training for yoga teachers, Yoga Alliance is a voluntary group dedicated to providing support and upholding the rights of yoga teachers. Go to this site to find out more information, and how to register.

www.yogacircle.com

Contains articles for athletes about the benefits of yoga.

www.yogafinder.com

This site is designed to help you find classes and teachers of all types of yoga, wherever you are in the world.

www.yogaforgolfers.com

Katherine Roberts is an expert on yoga and golf fitness. Her site will inspire you to improve your golf game and your life through yoga.

www.yogainside.org

Yoga Inside gives the gift of yoga and meditation to prisoners, inner-city youth, children in protective shelters, and many more.

www.yogainternational.com

The Himalayan Institute's *Yoga International* magazine contains thought-provoking articles and book reviews, and includes an annual directory of yoga teachers.

www.yogajournal.com

The *Yoga Journal* web site contains articles about yoga, book reviews, information about yoga retreats, and much more, including an annual directory of yoga teachers.

www.yogalines.com

Canadian yoga props provider.

www.yogamovement.com

Created for both beginners and experienced yoga practitioners, this site is a great source of everything yoga related.

www.yogapro.com

This site specializes in yoga props.

www.yogaprops.net

This is another site specializing in yoga props.

www.yogasite.com

This is an Internet-based resource center for anything yoga related. Lots of great yoga information, answers to questions, and links provided.

www.yogastudio.ns.ca

The Yoga Studio is a yoga center offering classes and teaching training in Halifax, NS.

www.yogaville.org

See photos of the beautiful LOTUS Temple and find out more about Integral yoga at this site.

www.yogawest.ca

Yoga West is a 3HO Kundalini yoga center situated in Vancouver, BC.

www.yogatoronto.com

Yoga Centre Toronto offers Iyengar yoga classes and special needs programs.

www.yogaworkshop.com

Visit the web site of Richard Freeman, one of the foremost teachers of Ashtanga yoga, for videos and information.

www.yogitea.com

The Yogi Tea web site is where you will find healthy and tasty herbal teas, such as the Original Spice Yogi Tea latte.

www.yrec.org

Check this site for an in-depth understanding of the who, what, and where of yoga. Its founder, Georg Feuerstein, is one of the top yoga scholars, and has authored numerous books on yoga.

Yoga organizations

Ananda Yoga/The Expanding Light
1618 Tyle Foote Rd., Nevada City,
CA 95959
1-800 346-5350

Anusara Yoga
722 Shenandoah Drive, Spring, TX 77381
1-888-398-9642

Ashtanga Yoga
325 E. 41st St., #203
New York, NY 10017
(212) 661-2895

B.K.S. Iyengar Yoga
National Assoc. of the U.S.
PO Box 941, Lemont, PA 16851
1-800 889-9642

Federation of Ontario Yoga Teachers
107 High Street, South Hampton, ON
Canada N0H 2L0
(519) 797-1818

Himalayan Institute of Canada
4083 Fieldgate Drive, Mississauga, ON
Canada L4W 2C6
(905) 238-7168

Integral Yoga
Satchidananda Ashram-Yogaville
Buckingham, VA 23921
(804) 969-3121

International Association of Black Yoga Teachers
PO Box 360922
Los Angeles, CA 90036
(213) 833-6371

International Kundalini Yoga Teachers Assoc.
Route 2, Box 4, Shady Lane
Espanola, NM 87532
(505) 753-0423

Kripalu Center for Yoga and Health
PO Box 793, West St.
Lenox, MA 01240

Kundalini Yoga for Youth
368 Village Street
Millis, MA 02054

Life Foundation School of Therapeutics (Dru Yoga)
Maristowe House, Dover St.,
Bilston, W. Mids WV146AL, UK
(+44) 01902 409164

Montreal Yoga Teachers Association
1361 Greene Avenue
Westmount, Quebec
Canada H3Z 2A8
(514) 574-0948

Phoenix Rising Yoga Therapy
PO Box 819
Housatonic, MA 01236

Sivananda Yoga Vendanta Center
243 W. 24th St., New York, NY 10011

Viniyoga/T.K.V. Desikachar
The Pierce Program,
1164 N. Highland Ave., N.E.
Atlanta, GA 30306

Yoga Alliance
120 South Third Ave.
West Reading, PA 19611
1-877 964-2255

Yoga Association of Alberta
Percy Page Centre
11759 Groat Road
Edmonton, AB
Canada T5M 3K6
(780) 427-8876

Yoga College of India/Bikram Yoga
8800 Wilshire Blvd., 2nd floor
Beverly Hills, CA 90211

The Yoga Workshop
2020 21st St.
Boulder, CO 80302
(303) 449-6102

A simple glossary

Acupressure An ancient Oriental method of healing that directly presses and manipulates the body through systems of points and meridians.

Acupressure points The key places in the body's energetic system where the life force energy can be tapped.

Affirmation A method of creating change based on the belief that the body is pliable to human thought and feeling in both negative and positive ways. Therefore, to affirm, a person "makes firm" a positive concept.

Ahimsa (Ah HIM sa) The quality of being non-violent. Harmlessness.

Ajna See Third-eye point.

Alternative medicine The name given to holistic healthcare.

Ananda (Ah NUN dah) Bliss, divine happiness.

Anusara (An ah SAHR ah) A Sanskrit word meaning "flowing with grace" or "following the heart."

Apana (Ah PAHN ah) The process of releasing waste or toxins on the outbreath. Can also refer to the eliminative energy of the body.

Asana (AH sun ah) The term used to describe the physical postures of yoga, literally meaning "steady pose." The asanas are practiced to develop control over the mind and body.

Ashram (AH shrum) A spiritual community. It may consist of one house or many in close proximity, and exists to support mind/body/spirit health and growth.

Ashtanga (Ahsh TUN gah) From the Sanskrit, "ast" (eight) and "anga" (limbs), referring to the eight limbs or principles of the Yoga sutras.

Atman, or Atma (AHT Mun) The soul, or transcendental self.

Aura The energy field that surrounds and interpenetrates the body. It is considered by yogis and many healers to be the energetic framework upon which the physical body rests.

Ayurveda (Ah Yur VED ah) A holistic system of medicine from the Sanskrit words meaning "life" and "knowledge," or the knowledge of life.

Bandha (BUN dah) Literally "lock," "bond," or "tie" in Sanskrit, an internal contraction of the body's muscles used to create "locks" in order to focus concentration, stimulate internal heat, and, ultimately, control the flow of prana.

Bean curd See Tofu.

Bhakti yoga (BHAHK tee) The branch of yoga that focuses on devotion and selfless love.

Biofeedback Feedback applied to biological functions. A biofeedback machine is any device that makes a person more aware of an internal bodily function.

Breath of fire One of the most well-known breathing exercises of Kundalini yoga, used to energize and purify.

Brow point See Third-eye point.

Chakras (CHAH krahs) Literally "circles" or "wheels" in Sanskrit, these are the energy centers, or vortices, that flow through and around the human body.

Corpse pose The relaxation yoga pose that is done by lying on your back with your hands at the sides of your body, palms up. No energy need be expended to hold the body in this position.

Dharana (Dha RAH nah) The process that focuses on one-pointed concentration.

Dhyana (Dha YAHN ah) The process that instills a deep inner space of awareness and meditation without focus on an object.

Diaphragm lock (Uddiyana bandha) Uddiyana means "to fly up," and this body lock refers to the action of the navel, which is pulled inward and upward, usually on the held exhale.

Endorphins Natural chemicals released by the brain that relieve pain and induce a feeling of euphoria after physical exertion.

Epinephrine A fast-acting hormone produced by the adrenal glands that prepares the body for dealing with stress or danger by increasing heart and breathing rates.

Ghee (hard "g" as in "go") Clarified butter, which is butter cooked on a low flame until the impurities separate and are strained out, yielding a clear golden liquid.

Guru (gu ROO) Literally one who takes you from the darkness to the light. Often used casually to denote a teacher or master.

Gyan mudra (hard "g," as in "go": Gi YAHN) Gyan means "wisdom." Mudra means "lock" or "seal." A hand position in yoga, Gyan mudra corresponds to the area of the brain that activates wisdom and knowledge.

Gyan yoga See Jnana.

Hara (HAH rah) According to Eastern teachings, this is the internal center of power, and is located just below the navel.

Hatha yoga (HAH tah) Ha means" sun," and tha is" moon." This is often interpreted to mean the balance of opposites (male and female) within the person. Another meaning of hatha is "forceful" or "effort," signifying transformation through the effort or force of the physical body.

Holistic An approach to health that considers the whole of a person's being (body, mind, and spirit), rather than the separate parts.

Homeostasis The body's natural state of balance in which all systems function smoothly, even in a dynamic state.

Ida (EE da) The left nerve channel residing in the spine, which carries the cooling, lunar, receptive energy.

Intuition Immediate insight or understanding without conscious reasoning.

Jalandhara bandha *See* Neck lock.

Japa (JUP ah) Repeating a mantra as meditation.

Jnana, or Gyan yoga (JAH nah) The branch of yoga that focuses on contemplation and wisdom.

Kapalabhati (Kup ah la BAH ti) An important yogic breathing practice, also called the "skull-shining breath," so named because it increases the amount of oxygen to the brain, clearing the mind and improving concentration.

Karma (KAR mah) A Sanskrit word with several related meanings. Karma is a law of nature that is expressed by "as you reap, so shall you sow." It also refers to right action, selfless service, and taking action to uplift others.

Karma yoga The branch of yoga that focuses on right action.

Kicheree (KICH er ee) An Indian word for a highly digestible, well-balanced food made with rice and mung beans.

Kirlian photography A means of taking pictures of the patterns of energy and force fields usually unseen by the human eye.

Kripalu (Kri PAH lu) Comes from the Sanskrit "kripal," which means compassion or mercy.

Kriya (KREE ya) Sanskrit for "action," this is a yoga posture or sequence of postures that improves the well-being of specific areas of the body, mind, and spirit.

Kundalini (Kun dah LI nee) Comes from the root word "kundal" in Sanskrit, which means "the lock of the hair from the beloved." The uncoiling of this energy is the awakening of the kundalini – the unlimited potential that already exists in every human.

Loincloth A very small body covering traditionally worn by Indian yogis, made from a piece of cotton that wraps through the groin and around the pelvis.

Maha bhanda (MAH hah) Maha means "great" in Sanskrit. The great lock is all three locks (neck, diaphragm, and root) applied together.

Mala (MAH lah) Yogic prayer beads used in the repetition of mantra to keep focused and for counting repetitions.

Mantra (MUN trah) Literally means "mind projection," and is a yogic technique of focusing on an external or internal sound to create a personal transformation. Concentrated repetition (internal or out loud) produces vibrations within the individual's entire system hat are in tune with the universal vibration or energy.

Masala (Mah SAHL ah) Literally meaning "blend" in Sanskrit, masala is a combination of spices and root vegetables cooked together.

Meridians The acupressure pathways through which the life force flows.

Mula bandha *See* Root lock.

Naad (Nahd) The essence of all sound. Naad yoga is the experience of how sound currents, which are usually chanted and linked with the breath, affect the body, mind, and spirit.

Nadis (NAH dees) The subtle channels within the body that supply energy (prana) to every organ and cell of the body.

Nauli (NAU lee) Abdominal churning that massages and invigorates all the internal organs.

Neck lock (Jalandhara bandha) A body lock that is applied by drawing the chin slightly in toward the throat, making sure the spine and neck are straight. It is usually applied at the end of an exhalation, and often done with the diaphragm lock.

Neti (NEH tee) A yogic technique for cleansing the nasal passages.

Niyamas (Nih YAH mahs) The "do's" of yoga: purity, contentment, chastity, self study, and awareness of the spirit.

Organic produce Food that is grown without the use of harmful pesticides and artificial fertilizers. Instead, crops are grown using natural fertilizers, biological pest control, and crop rotation.

Pingala (Pin GAH la) The right nerve channel residing in the spine, which carries the warming, solar, projective energy.

Prana (PRAH na) The vital life force in all things. Prana also refers to the vital energy that is drawn in to the body on the inhalation.

Pranayama (Prah na YAH ma) From two Sanskrit words, prana, meaning "life force," and yama, which means "discipline." Pranayama practice is the discipline or technology of breathing.

Pratyahara (Praht ya HA rah) The process that focuses on becoming aware of and controlling the thought waves of the mind.

Props Yoga tools that assist and support the practitioner in stretching in ways that he or she would not be able to do otherwise.

Pure water Water that has been filtered to remove nitrates, pesticides, and metal traces.

Raja yoga (RAH ja) Literally means "royal," and often refers to the path of yoga that focuses on meditation.

Rajas (RAH jas) The quality of being overstimulating or overactive.

Repetitive stress Refers to the stress that is placed on localized areas of the body by repetitive movements over a period of time.

Restorative yoga Yoga that uses restful poses with props to stimulate and relax the body as it moves toward balance.

Root lock (Mula bandha) The contracting and lifting of the perineum and the perineal muscle, which is located between the genital and the anus.

Samadhi (Sah MAH di) The ecstatic state of being in which the meditator becomes one with the object of meditation.

Sat Nam Rasayan (SUT Nahm Rah SAH yun) From Sanskrit, literally means "universal remedy of manifested truth," a meditative yogic healing modality.

Sattva (SUT vah) The quality of being pure, calm, and clear.

Shushmana (SHUSH mun ah) The master nerve channel in the central column of the spine.

Sitali (Si TA lee) A cooling breath that relaxes the body while keeping the mind alert.

Spirituality A state of being, beyond dogma, that transcends physical existence, and creates a sense of wholeness, peace, and higher purposefulness in a person.

Spring water Water that is naturally pure, as it comes directly from a mountain spring.

Sthira (STEER ah) A Sanskrit word that means "steadiness" and "alertness."

Sukha (SUK ha) "Ease" or "comfort" in Sanskrit.

Sun salutation (Surya namaskar) One of the most well-practiced series of postures known to yoga, consists of a sequence of 12 positions that move the spine in various ways and promote flexibility in the limbs.

Surya namaskar See Sun salutation.

Swami (SWAH mee) Title for a spiritual master.

Tamas (TUM as) The quality of being inert or lethargic.

Tantra (TUN trah) Literally means "the place where opposites meet and become one."

Third-eye point Refers to the sixth chakra, or the intuitive center, located between the eyebrows and about 1 in (3 cm) below the surface. Also called the Ajna, or the brow point.

Tofu Also called bean curd, this high-protein food is made by curdling the mild white "milk" of the soybean.

Toning The utterance of an elongated vowel sound. The practice of toning uses the vowel sounds for healing and spiritual development.

Turmeric An Indian root, which is ground into a bright yellow powder and is healing to the joints of the body.

Uddiyana bandha See Diaphragm lock.

Ujjayi (Oo JAH yee) Literally "victorious" in Sanskrit. This breathing exercise is for energy and purification.

Vini (VI nee) From the Sanskrit, "special" and "individual." It can also mean step-by-step and gradual.

Vinyasa (Vin YAH sah) A sequence of breath-synchronized yoga movements.

Vishnu mudra (VISH noo) A hand position used for alternate nostril breathing.

Yamas (YA mahs) The "don'ts" of yoga: no violence, stealing, lying, possessiveness, or excess.

Yoga (YO gah) From Sanskrit, meaning "to yoke," "to unite," "to join together." Yoga's aim is to unite the body, mind, and spirit.

Yoga sutras (SU trahs) The codification of yoga's principles into a written system, which was developed thousands of years ago by the physician sage Patanjali.

Yogi (YO gi) An accomplished male student of yoga.

Yogini (Yo GI ni) An accomplished female student of yoga.

Index

Acknowledgments

Author's acknowledgments

This has been such an expansive and exciting project! Foremost, my thanks go to Lavonne Carlson, my project publisher, whose conviction in my capabilities initiated this book; to Jennifer Williams, the best editor in the world (at least I think so!); and to Lisa Lenard and Gretchen Fruchey who expertly edited the book with a perceptive touch. I would also like to thank Caroline Hunt, Mary Thompson, Mandy Lebentz, Helen Ridge, Mandy Earey, Dave King (Dave King Studio), Simran Kaur Khalsa, and Maki Yamamoto.

Many thanks go to all of the yoga teachers and students who added their voices and inspiration to these pages. I am ever grateful to my teacher, Yogi Bhajan, my husband, Kartar Singh Khalsa, and my son, Ram Das Singh Khalsa, who have been my biggest supporters and inspiration.

Publisher's acknowledgments

Dorling Kindersley would like to thank Neal Cobourne for designing the jacket; Melanie Simmonds, Marcus Scott, and Hayley Smith for picture research; and Jessica Clark for legal advice.

Packager's acknowledgments

Cooling Brown would like to thank Alison Bolus, Fiona Wild, Margaret Doyle, Kate Bresler, and Patricia Coward for editorial assistance; Barry Robson for illustrating the dogs and bringing them so vividly to life; and Mira Mehta for permission to use photographs from the book *Yoga the Iyengar Way* by Silva, Mira, and Shyam Mehta.